Implementing A Reproductive Health Agenda In India: The Beginning

Editor

Saroj Pachauri

Technical Editor

Sangeeta Subramanian

Assisted by

Stina Almroth

Publication Coordinator

Anjali Nayyar

Population Council
South & East Asia—Regional office

The Population Council is an international, non-profit, non-governmental institution that seeks to improve the well being and reproductive health of current and future generations around the world and to help achieve a humane, equitable, and sustainable balance between people and resources. The Council conducts biomedical, social science, and public health research and helps build research capacities in developing countries. Established in 1952, the Council is governed by an international board of trustees. Its New York headquarters supports a global network of regional and country offices.

Population Council
Regional Office
South & East Asia Region
Zone 5A, Ground Floor
India Habitat Centre
Lodi Road, New Delhi 110 003
India

Design and Production: Spectra VisualWord

Contents

FOREWORD

This book performs the much needed role of tracing the revolutionary change that has taken place in India since the International Conference on Population and Development (ICPD) in 1994. The reader will be given a roadmap in time and space of the major issues involved in providing quality reproductive health care. But questions will come to the minds of some – "How do these new developments affect the outcomes of programmes earlier targetted at reducing population growth? Does the ICPD mean that we don't care about demographic projections?" The good news is that there is common cause – a great common cause – between those whose primary concern is reproductive health, and those vitally concerned about demographic change.

The concerns about programmes inspired by demographic goals are well known:

- The existence of targets is seen as disrespectful of women (whose use of family planning far exceeds that of men); it treats them as numbers.
- Targets drive family planning workers to emphasise quantity. The world is watching India's search for new management models.
- Coercion has too often accompanied family planning programmes – from the days of India's emergency programme, to the ill-fated Pakistani programmes, to China, to some of the early NORPLANT campaigns in Indonesia.

• Some contest that there is too much medical dependency; that contraceptives have been so developed that they keep women dependent on service providers.

• There are concerns that inadequate service capacity, particularly in government programmes which are too often underfunded and undertrained, means that the level of service will not be appropriate for high technology contraceptives or for contraceptives requiring extensive follow up. This is certainly a concern in India, despite the admirable outreach of India's health services.

These concerns, drawn from a reproductive health focus, make us reflect on the impact of programmes on individual women. They also draw our attention to the fact that lack of reproductive choice for women will be helped by the search for better technology. There are some real unmet needs that we at the Population Council will try to meet during the next decade. Science is not predictable, but we hope to develop contraceptives for men, post-coital contraceptives, menses inducers and medical abortificients, and perhaps most important, for the health of the women and men of the world, contraceptives under the control of women that would also offer protection against sexually transmitted infections, particularly HIV.

But technology is far from the totality of the solution and family planning alone will never be enough to meet demographic targets. At the Population Council, we will strive with our partners around the world to demonstrate, in ever more compelling ways, that we must go beyond family planning to find those sources of population growth which centre on the role of women in society. Many of these relate directly to reproductive health concerns.

As societies, we would rather ignore the socially inconvenient aspects of reproductive health and population. We would prefer to see it as a passing phase or a cultural imperative that girls are too often treated very differently from boys. We would prefer not to know that violence plays a role in reproductive health and that all reproductive health problems are grounded in the roles and status of women in our societies. It would be nice to solve population issues without tackling these eclipsed issues, but we cannot.

We must work toward eliminating gender inequalities in schooling and the marketplace; we must strive for a reduction in unproductive domestic labour; and, for a far more equitable distribution of responsibilities in the family, especially with regard to the care of children.

From a population and human welfare perspective, there is no compelling reason why the father-child link is any less important than the mother-child link. At the level of programme, policy, and social debate, there must be discussion on the value of the father's role, and the expectations of fathers. There should be incentives for "good" fathering and sanctions for "poor" fathering.

We must create conditions – through selective, creative and ethically sound social investment – for women and couples to seek a lower number of surviving children. And these investments, if they are to find political constituents and acceptance by people in the highest fertility societies, must be affirming of women, men and children of this generation, not simply laying the foundation for a better life for the next generation. The demand to limit families is growing in ways we do not yet understand. The economic imperative of smaller families is more and more the reality for the world's families.

There is well documented and researched data which demonstrates that a desirable demographic outcome can be reached only when women are treated differently than they are now in most countries. Preferences for high fertility and the underlying social and economic insecurity are fundamental causes of high birth rates and rapid population growth. There are differing incentives for men and women with regard to child numbers. Men and women have markedly different time and financial obligations to children in many cultures, hence women hold a clear self-interest in limiting their fertility, which men may not share.

This means that countries, which are concerned about reaching demographic goals, have to take seriously the elimination of gender inequality. This cannot just be a philosophy. It must be underpinned by a systematic set of policies and norms. Legal frameworks which seem abstract to people's lives do, nonetheless, set norms.

Late marriages in many societies could have as significant a demographic effect as the introduction of new contraceptives. Teenage pregnancy has a demographic effect, as well as an often-devastating human effect. There have been many calls to increase the age of marriage for girls. There need to be more, and the political and social leaderships need to be involved. Many countries have laws mandating ages of 17 and 18 for marriage, that are regularly violated. But if we look at the local level, we will find some solutions to the complex task of giving reality to these laws. It is the local community, which is likely to provide guidance for the kind of social reforms that will empower girls to resist early marriage pressures from their families and society as a whole.

Less conflict exists between demographic imperatives and humanitarian actions, than may seem to be the case. We want girls and women in school. It will enhance their lives in immeasurable ways and will dramatically bring down population growth rates by reducing both the numbers of children wanted and increasing the age at first childbirth. We want babies later, babies who are healthier and do not die, and we want to give girls a chance to be educated and to find values that we know will also lead to smaller families. We want infant mortality to decline because it is wrong that babies and young children should die, that families should suffer, and because there is no country on earth where fertility has declined before infant mortality has fallen. We want better quality of care because people should be well treated and given choices. This promotes contraceptive prevalence and therefore a different demographic outcome. We want to meet the unmet demand for family planning because it is wrong that women should have fertility outcomes which they do not want. We want good reproductive health because it counts to people – and people are what count.

Margaret Catley-Carlson
President
Population Council, New York

ACKNOWLEDGEMENTS

I thank the many people whose contributions have made this book possible. This book is the culmination of the dedication and hard work of the authors who responded to my requests in record time. They critically examined key policy and programme issues to discuss the current state-of-the-art in their chapters.

I greatly appreciate the painstaking efforts of Vijaya Ranganathan and Nomita Jain in copy editing the manuscript. Sagri Singh deserves credit for her help in reviewing and editing, and Sneh Rewal for her assistance with many other tasks.

Monica Bhalla and H.C. Nangia deserve special appreciation for their untiring efforts and hard work in typing numerous drafts of the manuscript. Vatsala Kalyanaraman, Atul Khurana, Asha Matta and Anita Srivastava also assisted with secretarial work.

I would also like to convey my appreciation to the dedicated Population Council team without whose support this work could not possibly have been accomplished.

Special credit goes to Bindu Badshah and Sudhir Pillai for their amazing responsiveness in designing and publishing a high quality volume within a very tight time frame.

Finally, I am indebted to the MacArthur Foundation for providing the financial support for this publication.

Saroj Pachauri

INTRODUCTORY ESSAY

Saroj Pachauri

Moving Towards Reproductive Health: Issues and Evidence

Introduction

At the International Conference on Population and Development (ICPD) at Cairo in 1994, consensus was reached on a new agenda for population and development. The ICPD was a triumph for those seeking an end to the great debate that had plagued the population field since the first World Population Conference at Bucharest in 1974; a debate between advocates of development who believed that development is the best contraceptive and, therefore, a necessary precondition to sustained fertility decline and those who asserted that family planning services must be implemented to meet the high demand for fertility control which they believed existed. A notably wide gulf remained between these two essentially academic positions. The practical result was ambivalence and ambiguity in many countries about which approach to take. The ICPD took giant strides toward resolving this conflict by placing the population problem squarely in the development context and focussing attention on individual needs instead of demographic targets.

At the ICPD, the nations of the world agreed that governments should give special attention to the education of girls, the health of women, the survival of infants and young children, and in general, the empowerment of women. At the same time, comprehensive reproductive health services should be provided to enable couples to achieve their reproductive goals, and determine freely and responsibly the number and spacing of their children (United Nations, 1994). The ICPD consensus implied that if governments ensure that this basic package of social policies and reproductive health services is in place, they will simultaneously make strides toward greater social equity and reduce high rates of population growth (Sinding and Fathallah, 1995). Using groundbreaking language, the ICPD Programme of Action, strongly endorsed the concepts of reproductive and sexual health and rights, and the need for services to achieve those ends.

Translating the ICPD Agenda: The Policy Process in India

Well before the Cairo conference – at least a decade earlier – several NGOs, researchers, women's groups, and donors in India, had sought to change programme direction by moving away from demographic targets and numbers and focussing on how to address the needs of clients, especially women. NGOs and feminists who had formed pressure groups were in the forefront of advancing this agenda. These grassroots voices were heard along with similar echoes from around the world at the ICPD which provided a platform where consensus, on what had been very widely debated issues, was finally reached.

Soon after the Cairo conference, the Government of India set in motion a process to translate the ICPD Programme of Action within the national context. In November 1994, a joint mission of the Government of India and the World Bank was set up to undertake a sectoral review. In 1995, the World Bank submitted a report entitled 'India's Family Welfare Program: Toward a Reproductive and Child Health Approach' to the Government of India (World Bank, 1995). The government decided to adopt the policy and as a first step, in April 1996, removed method-specific contraceptive targets nationwide. This was an essential prerequisite for translating the ICPD agenda in India. On October 15, 1997, the reproductive and child health programme was launched (Ministry of Health and Family Welfare, undated).

Shifting paradigms: from demographic goals to individual needs

In India, shifting to the reproductive health approach implies sending new implementation signals to 250,000 family welfare staff, that now client satisfaction is the programme's primary goal, with demographic impact a secondary, though important concern. Consequently, broadening the existing package of services is necessary and improving the quality of services top priority. To achieve these goals two major challenges must be addressed. First, it is necessary to create an understanding of the paradigm shift i.e. a reconceptualisation of the population problem by all stakeholders. And second, service delivery programmes must be redesigned to effectively address the reproductive health needs of people (Pachauri, 1995).

The new reproductive and child health programme requires an ideological change in the culture of the programme, from a focus in the past on achieving method-specific contraceptive targets, often using coercive means, to providing client-centred, quality services. For achieving the demographic goal of reducing the rate of population growth at the macro-level, broader social and economic policies – especially those designed to improve education and enhance employment opportunities for women – must be promoted.

Addressing clients' needs: essential package of services

Addressing reproductive health needs means reducing unwanted fertility as well as the burden of reproductive morbidity and mortality. An essential package of reproductive and child health services to address clients' needs is beginning to be operationalised in India. The rationale for suggesting a package of services is to enable programme planners to: (1) assess the feasibility and management implications for implementing various combinations of health services at different levels of the health service system in diverse settings; and, (2) examine the cost, financing and sustainability implications for implementing these health services (Pachauri, 1995).

Designing a cost-effective package of good quality services that can be made available and accessible to all, especially to the poor, is a real challenge. Although providing comprehensive reproductive health services is a desirable goal, the extent to which the programme can expand without compromising the quality and effectiveness of existing services has to be seriously considered. There is clearly a need to prioritise and to develop a phased approach with an incremental addition of health interventions that require greater skills and resources. Since it is not possible to prepare a blueprint for the entire country, a framework has been proposed for implementing the package of services. The criteria used for prioritising services to be included in the essential package are: (1) levels of fertility and mortality; (2) disease burden; (3) cost-effectiveness of available health interventions; and, (4) the capacity of the health system to deliver health services (Pachauri, 1995).

A fear which has been articulated by policy planners, programme managers and others concerned about population numbers is that family planning efforts will be 'diluted' if broader reproductive health services are provided. The reality is that family planning forms the centrepiece of the proposed package and good quality contraceptive services cannot be provided without addressing related reproductive health needs. Long years of experience have shown that contraceptive acceptance and continuation depend on ensuring the safety and quality of services. For example, reproductive tract infections are widely prevalent among women and their management is important, not only to relieve the suffering and pain they cause, but to ensure that contraceptive methods can be provided safely and effectively. Sterility, pelvic inflammatory disease, stillbirth and abortions are some of the serious complications that arise if these conditions are left untreated. The fear of sterility and delayed child bearing have been major barriers to contraceptive acceptance. Therefore, the stress on integrated services.

To be implemented nationwide over a five to ten year period, the package of essential reproductive and child health services includes services for the prevention and management of unwanted pregnancy; the promotion of safe motherhood and child survival; nutritional services for vulnerable groups; services for the prevention and management of reproductive tract infections and sexually transmitted infections as well as reproductive health services for adolescents.

Three points deserve emphasis with respect to the package of essential services:

- First, most of the services in the essential package are already included in the family welfare programme but have often not been provided for want of resources, adequate training, and other reasons.

- Second, improvements in health depend on making the whole set of services available because their effectiveness depends on ensuring that they are integrated. Therefore, no priorities are set for services included in the essential package. If sufficient resources are not available, the whole package should be introduced in phases rather than attempting to strengthen individual services on a piecemeal basis. The services included in the essential package are among the most cost-effective.

- Third, although adding new services and improving quality are major challenges, they do not require a quantum increase in resources. It is increasing coverage by filling current gaps in staff and infrastructure that requires substantial additional resources (Measham and Heaver, 1995).

Operationalising the package of essential services

To operationalise the package of essential services, it must be integrated within the existing primary health care system. However, the capacity of the health delivery system is not uniform in the country and there is tremendous diversity among regions, states and even within states. Therefore, the design of programme strategies must be context-specific.

Since men and women have multiple reproductive health needs, the challenge is to provide integrated services to address these needs. However, most health services have so far been provided through vertical programmes. There is a growing understanding that horizontal integration of services must be achieved if reproductive and sexual health and rights are to be universally realised. There must be a convergence of services at the users' level. If services are administered through vertical programmes that originate from different government departments and are funded by various donors, with their own agendas, the result is multiplicity and fragmentation which is wasteful and inefficient. It would be counterproductive to have reproductive health as yet another vertical programme. In fact, the reproductive health approach provides an opportunity for integrating services. The challenge is to strengthen services that are in place by expanding their reach and improving their quality and by effectively integrating reproductive health services within ongoing programmes (Pachauri, 1996).

India has initiated the process to implement the reproductive health agenda – to make a paradigm shift and to address the needs of the people. This volume provides a glimpse of the processes that are underway.

Rationale and Scope of the Book

The significant policy shift by India was an outcome of a process of experiential learning that had been underway in the country for several years. Many constituencies in India had opposed coercive, top-down population control policies. Strong arguments had been made to improve the quality of services; to address the reproductive health needs of people, especially women; and, to decentralise programme planning and monitoring. This thinking was in consonance with the larger efforts at democratic decentralisation in the country. The 72nd and 73rd Amendments to the Indian Constitution mandated one-third reservations for women in elected bodies at the village level to give a voice to women in decentralised planning processes. Similar views were voiced at the ICPD. The global endorsement of these concepts provided the legitimacy and the additional spark that was needed to catalyse the process of policy change at the national level.

The questions now being asked are: What has been the process of implementing this new policy? What progress has been made since India proposed the paradigm shift? Although it is much too soon to measure impact or draw conclusions, this volume makes a modest attempt to understand the processes underway in the country. The contributors to this volume are scholars and practitioners who have been engaged with these issues in their respective fields of work. They have made an effort to critically examine key policy and programme issues by using empirical data and drawing lessons from the field.

Although by no means exhaustive, this volume brings together a number of important initiatives that are at different stages of development in the country. It provides an analysis of the fertility transition in India; the outcome of removing method-specific targets that had driven the family planning programme for several decades; the design of new methodologies, indicators and processes for monitoring and evaluating decentralised programmes; and, the financial and human resource needs for implementing the reproductive and child health programme. In addition, efforts to forge new partnerships for effectively operationalising the programme, as well as to promote advocacy for making the paradigm shift a reality for India, are discussed.

Services to address reproductive health problems, such as HIV/AIDS, maternal mortality, unsafe abortion, and reproductive tract infections that are being implemented in the country, are assessed. Neglected population groups, particularly adolescents and men, have been brought into the framework of discussion. Gender and sexuality are cross-cutting themes. Conspicuous by its absence, is a discussion on reproductive rights which reflects a gap in the current discourse.

The chapters in this volume are organised within three broad themes: (1) implementing reproductive health policy; (2) reaching neglected population groups; and, (3) addressing reproductive health problems.

Implementing Reproductive Health Policy

This section includes a discussion on: the fertility transition in India; the causes and consequences of withdrawing method-specific targets; monitoring and evaluating decentralised programmes; advocacy initiatives; management of financial and human resources; and, promoting partnerships.

The fertility transition

Jain's chapter on fertility transition in India provides a backdrop for subsequent discussions. The author examines the huge disparities in gender equity, levels of fertility, and education. His question is: Can fertility transition, which has been underway in India over the past 20 years, contribute to just social policies for reducing gender and regional disparities in health and education? The rationale for reducing population growth through fertility reduction is to improve social and economic conditions. It is, therefore, important to ascertain the extent to which ongoing fertility transition has contributed to the reduction of disparities and socially valued outcomes. The author examines the positive relationship between women's education and fertility decline and shows that fertility declines sharply with education where female education is low, but this gap narrows where fertility levels are low. He argues for a redistribution of resources to promote women's education in states that have low female literacy and high fertility.

Although fertility decline is underway in India, there is continued concern about 'controlling the population'. This debate continues at different levels even after the government has changed policy. It is clearly premature to measure the impact of a programme that was launched only 15 months ago. However, a question that could be legitimately asked is: What are the processes underway in different parts of the country and what is the direction of change? Analyses by Khan and Townsend, Visaria and Visaria and Murthy address this question.

Removal of method-specific targets: A debate

Method-specific targets were removed nationwide in April 1996. Their sudden and abrupt removal was a dramatic change, a change that shook the system. Its reverberations were felt nationwide. The removal of targets was a necessary first step for making the paradigm shift i.e., changing from an emphasis on population numbers to a focus on quality of services. But because targets had driven the programme for many decades and all policy and programme efforts had been focussed on the achievement of targets, their sudden withdrawal without preparation and without putting in place any alternative monitoring system caused considerable confusion at the field level, especially since the performance of all programme staff had been measured by how effectively they achieved their targets.

Consequently many professionals critiqued the policy change. Some were vociferous in their articulations and predicted chaotic outcomes for India (Ross, 1998). Several people questioned why targets were removed? What was the impact of removing targets on programme performance? What was the effect on birth rates? Would the programme lose momentum under the target-free approach? In their chapter, Khan and Townsend analyse seven case studies to examine state level experiences. Their analysis shows that: (1) 18 months after targets were removed, implementation of the target-free approach varied considerably across the country. In some states the target approach, in a variant form, was still functional. (2) Most of the states would have preferred a gradual approach to the withdrawal of targets. (3) The consensus of senior state officials was that the target-free approach should be continued and problems in implementing the new policy should be addressed on a priority basis.

The analysis by Khan and Townsend also showed that there was a decline in programme performance in the first year because of the abrupt introduction of the target-free approach. This trend has since been reversed. In the first year, more than three-fourths of the decline in acceptors of sterilisation and IUDs was contributed by three of the four least developed states (Bihar, Madhya Pradesh and Uttar Pradesh). Rajasthan, the fourth such state, actually registered an increase in the use of all methods.

Khan and Townsend reviewed data over a 10-year period to examine the trend in the crude birth rate (CBR). The CBR continued to decline during 1995-1996 (from 28.3 in 1995 to 27.5 in 1996 and 27.2 in 1997); the greatest decline was recorded during 1996-97 (0.9 per 1,000). A continued decline was reported even in states with persistent high fertility such as Uttar Pradesh where the CBR decreased from 34.8 per 1,000 in 1995 to 34.0 in 1996 and to 33.5 in 1997. In addition, operations research in two districts of Uttar Pradesh showed a decline in the total fertility rate during this period. There was no evidence of reduction in contraceptive prevalence under the target-free approach.

Evidence from the field

Visaria and Visaria undertook research to assess the impact of removing targets at the field level. Qualitative research was undertaken in two contrasting states, Tamil Nadu in the south and Rajasthan in north. These researchers enquired into issues such as the work load of health staff, whether or not the programme had become more responsive to the needs of the people, and whether the functioning of the programme had changed at the field level. Their analysis showed that in Tamil Nadu, immunisation services, antenatal visits by health workers, and mothers' meetings at the village level had increased significantly over the past 7-8 years, even prior to the ICPD. Workers in Tamil Nadu enjoyed a better status as health care providers than they did when they provided family planning services only. While improvements had begun in Rajasthan, progress was much slower. Services for safe abortion and management of reproductive tract infections were yet to be implemented in both states. Some efforts had begun in Tamil Nadu where there was a higher demand for the government's health services but in Rajasthan these services were yet to be organised.

The results of operations research by Khan and Townsend in Uttar Pradesh showed an improvement, although modest, in the quality of services. For example, field workers had begun to provide a range of services and a broader choice of contraceptive methods. Clients were informed about more methods and some women reported less pressure to accept sterilisation which had been the dominant method for years. These results indicated that while the quality of services was still well below the desired standards, the changes that had occurred since 1995 were in the right direction.

Monitoring and evaluating decentralised programmes

For decades, the impact of the family planning programme had been measured in terms of its contribution toward the increase of contraceptive prevalence and decrease in fertility. Since these indicators neither reflected the impact of service quality, nor assessed morbidity and mortality, they were not adequate for measuring the impact of reproductive health services. New monitoring systems to assess the quality of health services from the perspective of the client were needed (Pachauri, 1995).

In her chapter, Murthy examines the issue of decentralised planning and monitoring. The specific questions that she addresses are: How are quality and client satisfaction ensured? Has there been an increase in the range of services? Do locally determined targets reflect local needs? Have planning and management responsibilities been decentralised? Is community involvement encouraged, and if so how? The author concludes that decentralised participative planning which replaced the target system has brought about several qualitative changes. The new *mantra* (chant) of concern for quality and client satisfaction is beginning to be sanctified. Health workers are becoming increasingly aware of the range of services to be provided; as a result, their self-esteem has improved.

Murthy describes the conceptual framework for planning and monitoring the reproductive and child health programme. The new system uses three tools: (1) activity reports by the workers; (2) technical assessment reports on service quality; and, (3) clients' reports of access, quality and attitudes of service providers. Another new feature is regular household and facility surveys which provide managerially useful information and also give clients a 'voice' to express their views.

Has this policy change had any impact on field operations? Murthy's analysis shows that as there is now no pressure to meet contraceptive targets, almost all states have begun to report an improvement in prenatal care and to focus their attention on providing safe delivery services. The acceptance of reversible methods by younger couples has increased and health workers get credit for identifying contraceptive side effects. Some states have even begun to provide safe delivery services. However, services for emergency obstetric care, safe abortion and treatment of reproductive tract infections and infertility are still not in place. In addition, there are unaddressed issues that relate to the involvement of women and decentralising decision making to the grassroots.

Murthy recommends that research should be undertaken to seek answers to key questions such as: What are the barriers that clients' face in accessing services? What criteria do clients use to judge service quality? How do clients' judgements differ from those of health staff and professionals? Is the policy change improving the effectiveness of the programme? Who provides services at the community level and how do people choose among different providers?

Pathak, Ram and Verma complement Murthy's analysis. They describe the system of monitoring and evaluation that was used in the past and discuss the new indicators for assessing access to services and the quality of care. Rapid household surveys to assess service coverage and quality, and clients' health seeking behaviours and satisfaction, have been designed to monitor the programme at the district level. These household surveys are complemented by surveys of the health facilities. All these surveys are conducted by independent agencies. The authors conclude that the new monitoring system is a marked departure from the earlier top-down system. They discuss the challenges ahead as they foresee that various states in India may eventually emphasise different indicators because their needs and priorities differ significantly.

The role of advocacy

Even though reproductive health rhetoric is now used by many, there are major information gaps at all levels ranging from a lack of understanding of the reproductive health and rights concepts to questions about what short-term and long-term strategies are needed to operationalise the programme. This presents a major deterrent to implementing the new policy. Therefore, strong advocacy efforts are needed to translate the rhetoric into reality. A range of different constituencies, including the government, donors, NGOs, activists, feminists, and researchers must be informed and empowered to catalyse a process of networking with a growing number of stakeholders so that the ideology and the ethos embodied in the paradigm shift is effectively internalised and programmes responsive to clients' needs are designed and implemented (Pachauri, 1995; 1997b).

India implemented a population control policy for about four decades when the programme was wedded to a top-down, bureaucratic, target-driven system. In her chapter, Nayyar argues that advocacy is urgently needed to change the mindset of all concerned constituencies. Decision-makers at the national level must send signals to the state level to facilitate the process of policy implementation.

Different stakeholders must understand the need for change and get engaged in the advocacy process. Although it is difficult and time-consuming to engage in discussion with diverse groups holding different points of view, it is essential to build coalitions and alliances to prepare common ground. After the ICPD, many donors have decided to fund reproductive health programmes. However, there are serious gaps in their understanding of the concepts and the issues which must be addressed so that donors can be more effective. Therefore, advocacy with donors is needed. To implement reproductive health services, technical issues need to be understood. It is, therefore, important to involve those that have the expertise such as obstetricians and gynaecologists, physicians, paramedical staff as well as researchers and trainers. Demographers who have led the population field for decades are natural allies for promoting the reproductive health and rights agenda.

Nayyar underscores how media, a powerful tool for disseminating information and sensitising large numbers of people, can be used for advocacy. However, it is necessary to complement media initiatives with advocacy efforts with the government, NGOs, *panchayats*, and the people. She discusses advocacy programmes that are being implemented and draws lessons from these experiences. She asserts that while past efforts were focussed on advocating against an insensitive population policy, now advocacy tools should be used to support government and NGO efforts to facilitate programme implementation.

Financial and human resource management

There is widespread concern that the cost of providing reproductive and child health services to a predominantly rural population will be substantial. Visaria and Visaria review the actual expenditure on the family welfare programme since 1985-86 (both in current and real terms). They show that over the Eighth Plan period 1992-97, the per capita expenditure on family welfare in India increased in two of the five years, fast enough to lead to a modest rise in real terms over the five-year period. Their detailed analysis of activity-specific expenditure over the five years also showed faster expenditure increases in the delivery of services. While consistent with the goals of the ICPD, these changes cannot really be attributed to it. The recent success of the Government of India in mobilising external assistance augurs well for expanding resource flows to improve the range and quality of services. In the long run, however, the country will have to rely primarily on domestic resources, both public and private, for ensuring the health and welfare of its people.

Human resources and their management are key to implementing the programme. Mavalankar focusses on this important issue in his chapter. He reviews the current situation of training, supervision, accountability and performance appraisal of programme functionaries and argues for making systemic changes to improve programme management.

Reproductive health is qualitatively and conceptually different from the previous vertical programmes. Therefore, it not only needs strong technical inputs, but also requires a different philosophy of work. To radically change the system's perspective towards client-oriented ways of providing services, training, supervision, performance appraisal and reward systems need to change so that there is an incentive and support for staff to change their work behaviours, styles of management and patterns of planning. The author proposes a comprehensive approach for human resource management. There is clearly an urgent need to improve the work ethic if client-centred, gender-sensitive services are to be implemented.

Partnerships to advance the agenda

Since India's independence 51 years ago, the government has been the major actor in promoting population, health and development programmes, especially for the poor. Several public sector programmes have been designed and implemented. In recent years, however, there has been increasing involvement of the non-government sector. Although progress has been slow, there is a clear move towards developing partnerships between the government, the NGOs and the rapidly growing private sector.

The paradigm shift requires that the top-down approach be replaced with planning by the people. The importance of community involvement, both in defining and articulating needs as well as in monitoring service quality is underscored. The assumption is that if people are involved in planning, they will have an ownership in the programme which will be reflected in better utilisation of services and improved health outcomes. NGOs have been particularly effective in bringing into the public domain, the needs and problems of the people, especially of the poor. NGOs have also pioneered innovative ways of providing quality services that are responsive to people's needs (Pachauri, 1994a).

In recent years, the *panchayat* is beginning to be seen as an important partner to involve the community; to provide a voice for the community; and to make programmes accountable to the people. The challenge is how to involve *panchayats*, which are as yet nascent institutions. With 33 percent reservations for women, there are now some 800,000 women in *panchayats*. Potentially, they represent a strong political force in decision-making at the grassroots. If their capacity for local governance is strengthened, they could have a significant impact on the process of democratic decentralisation and on enhancing women's roles in this process. Several NGOs and researchers are beginning to work with *panchayats* and some are involving *panchayats* in the efforts to address the reproductive health needs of the people.

Mukhopadhyay and Sivaramayya examine these issues by drawing upon the experience of an action research project that they are undertaking in three states. They explore the possibility of utilising NGOs as catalysts within the constitutionally mandated structure of local governance through *panchayats*. Their project is designed to use reproductive health services as an entry point to empower women and to enhance their political participation at the grassroots. The authors assert that while reproductive health is a natural focal point for women's empowerment, the reproductive and child health programme does not adequately address women's needs. There is little in the design of the programme that envisages genuine participation by women at the grassroots. The problem is further compounded by the fact that health is not a priority for *panchayats* and that the latter have yet to develop strong systems of governance.

The researchers urge that participatory approaches be used to involve women in action and research. More importantly, support structures are necessary to catalyse a process of empowerment for the powerless. It is here that NGO involvement is needed. By locating such initiatives within a collaborative structure involving the *panchayats*, it would be possible to ensure long-term sustainability. Therefore, more NGOs should be encouraged to work with *panchayats* to facilitate these processes.

Client expenditure on health

What costs do women incur in seeking health care? What are women's health seeking behaviours? Bhatia and Cleland seek answers to these important questions in their chapter. They review studies undertaken in India and report on their own research in Karnataka. Their study focussed on adult women to assess the utilisation of government and private sources of health care as well as self-medication. The researchers examined illnesses for different socio-economic groups of women, by their perceived severity, duration and diagnostic category.

For some illnesses, especially genito-urinary problems and anaemia, that are seen as 'a part of life', women frequently resorted to self-medication. A practitioner was, however, consulted for all illnesses perceived to be severe. The results of their study reinforce the findings of others about the dominance of the private sector, that includes qualified and unqualified practitioners, in the provision of health care. The average cost women incurred was Rs 75 ($2.41) to visit a private practitioner and Rs 66 ($1.9[1]) to visit a government practitioner. The average annual cost incurred by a woman on health care was Rs 172 ($5.5).

Although government services are theoretically free, in 75 percent of the cases women incurred costs when they consulted a government practitioner. Because government practitioners were often involved in private practice, the distinction between the private and the public sectors tended to get blurred. The authors suggest that while there is a need to improve the quality of care at government facilities and make them more affordable for the

---

1 Average exchange rate in 1993-94 was Rs 31.40 per $1.
(Source: Economic Survey 1997-98. Ministry of Finance, New Delhi, India.)

weaker sections of society, there is also a need for regulatory and supporting policy interventions to promote a viable and efficient private sector.

Reaching Neglected Population Groups

The contributors draw attention to population subgroups including adolescents and men whose needs have not been addressed by past programmes. There is a growing realisation that their involvement is critical for the achievement of reproductive health goals.

Adolescents: growing numbers, growing needs

Adolescents have been by-passed in past programmes and consequently their needs have neither been assessed nor addressed. Health services for adolescent girls have special significance in India where there is strong son preference and where adolescent pregnancy is the norm. These services would not only impact on the adolescent girls' own health but would also have long-term intergenerational effects by reducing the risk of low birth weight and minimising subsequent child mortality risks (Gopalan, 1989). Malnutrition is an underlying problem that seriously affects the health of adolescent girls and adult women and has its roots in early childhood. About 85 percent of women in India are anaemic. The association between anaemia and low birth weight, prematurity, perinatal mortality and maternal mortality has been extensively documented in India (Pachauri and Marwah, 1971; Ramachandran, 1992) but the problem has yet to be successfully addressed.

As India witnesses the entry of the largest ever generation of adolescents, compelling arguments are being made for examining the special needs of this neglected and vulnerable population subgroup (adolescents, 10-19 years of age, represent about a fifth of India's population). Early discussions are beginning to focus on how adolescent programmes should be designed and implemented.

Should special programmes be targetted at adolescents or should sexual and reproductive health services be mainstreamed within existing primary health care programmes? What strategies should be designed to reach adolescents in school and out of school? How should programmes target boys and girls? What strategies can most effectively involve parents, teachers, and communities? How can the multiple needs of adolescents be addressed holistically and sensitively? These are among the many challenges facing stakeholders attempting to address the social and biological needs of adolescents in India (Pachauri, 1998a).

Singh examines the policy environment in the country and discusses recent policies and programmes that aim to address the multiple needs of adolescents and youth. She asserts that the ICPD provided a platform, a space and a vocabulary for a discourse on the needs of adolescents, but that there remains a paucity of information on how to address these needs. She argues that while policy makers in India have long recognised the potential of youth, their approach to harness this potential has remained paternalistic. The ICPD redefined adolescents and youth within the framework of rights and choices. The author underscores the need to further the understanding of the government and the civil society so that effective strategies can be designed to translate rights into the reality of adolescents' lives.

Singh discusses the many cutting edge policies that have been recently formulated for youth, and more particularly for girls, and draws on innovative government initiatives. Her key messages are: (1) the government and NGOs must form true partnerships to move this agenda forward; and, (2) youth must be brought in as equal partners in the process of designing policies and programmes to address their needs.

By examining the nascent but valiant efforts of pioneering NGOs implementing community-based programmes, Mamdani draws attention to the problems faced by married and unmarried adolescents and provides insights into strategic approaches that NGOs employ to address them. Through her analysis, she integrates national data with information gleaned through NGO experiences in different parts of the country. She explores the special risks to adolescents of early marriage, unwanted pregnancy, abortion, malnutrition, HIV/AIDS and sexually transmitted infections.

The author weaves within her discourse, an analysis of the social, cultural, and political contexts within which these problems arise and are perpetuated. As she discusses the work of NGOs with adolescents in rural, urban, and tribal communities, she focusses on the adolescent girl who, because of gender differentials, is particularly disadvantaged. She discusses the prevailing gender norms that impede access to health and education and underscores the importance of designing appropriate services for adolescents. Mamdani assesses early efforts made to address the needs of adolescents in resource poor settings, within culturally hostile environments. This documentation of NGO experiences should provide useful lessons for government and non-government organisations that are currently grappling with these urgent and challenging problems.

Men as responsible partners in reproductive health

Since gender inequalities favour men in patriarchal societies and sexual and reproductive health decisions are made by them, there is a growing realisation that unless men are reached, programme efforts will have limited impact. While focussing on women and addressing their reproductive health needs, special efforts should be made to encourage men to take responsibility for reproductive health as responsible sexual partners, husbands and fathers (Pachauri, 1997a).

Research on HIV/AIDs and sexuality has highlighted the inadequacy of strategies that target only women. Because of unequal gender-power relations, women are especially vulnerable as they are unable to negotiate changes in sexual behaviour to prevent unwanted pregnancy and to practice safer sex. Research on sexual negotiation strategies has dramatically underscored the need for involving men in programmes that aim at bringing about changes in sexual behaviour for the prevention of infection. However, such behaviour change is as relevant for addressing other reproductive health problems. Therefore, men's involvement as responsible partners is essential. Besides, men, too, have reproductive and sexual health needs that should be addressed (Pachauri, 1997a).

In her chapter, Raju analyses men's roles in reproductive and sexual health matters by drawing upon the experience of NGOs working with men to address reproductive health problems in poor rural, tribal and urban slum communities. In most cases, men have been included in programmes that aim to improve women's health within the existing paradigm of gender relations in which men's roles continue to be defined in traditional ways. Obviously, the NGOs themselves operate within the same contexts and face the same dilemma as the people. While NGOs have not engineered major social change, their very efforts to include men have meant questioning the prevailing gender construct, but within limits. The author exemplifies how these issues are addressed at the grassroots. A related concern is whether involving men might jeopardise women's right to privacy and control over their bodies. The experience of some NGOs shows that this fear is unfounded when women themselves demand men's involvement.

NGOs are undertaking a variety of innovative and creative programmes that can provide important lessons. But is there an enabling policy environment within which these experiences can be upscaled? Raju's examination of government policy shows scarce recognition of these concerns even as India makes a paradigm shift. Men's roles do not find a place in the design of reproductive health programmes. Although there is some discussion on increasing the use of male methods such as vasectomy and condoms, there has not been a discourse around issues of male responsibility and there is little mention of these issues in government documents. On the other hand, there is growing momentum at the policy and programme levels within government departments that are concerned with improving women's status and reducing gender disparities. The women's movement has propelled this agenda.

Raju argues that unless efforts are mainstreamed within public sector programmes, men's involvement in reproductive health will remain a marginalised issue. In a country where gender differentials are so rigidly defined, this is a real challenge. Rapidly changing societal norms, values and aspirations; an unprecedented spread of messages through the media; and, a strong women's movement that is now beginning to take roots at the village level, provide new opportunities and challenges. Joint efforts by the government, NGOs and the civil society can make a difference.

Addressing Reproductive Health Problems

Several reproductive health problems including HIV/AIDS, reproductive tract infections, safe motherhood and abortion are discussed by the contributors to this volume. Sexual health and sexuality are cross-cutting issues.

HIV/AIDS: A problem denied

India is now thought to have more HIV positive persons than any other country in the world but denial of the problem has impeded action. After the first AIDS case was reported in India in May 1986, some 6,600 AIDS cases were reported by September 1998 (NACO, 1998). These figures are believed to be a gross underestimate. Over the years, there has been a steep rise in the reported seropositivity rate – from 2.5 per 1,000 in 1986 to 22.0 per 1,000 in 1998 (NACO, 1998). The prevalence of HIV infection has been on the rise in practically all states and all population groups in India. The increase is observed irrespective of when the infection reached any particular state. The dominant mode of HIV transmission is heterosexual which accounts for about two-thirds of the infections in India. Therefore, promoting safer sexual behaviours lies at the heart of strategies for preventing HIV/AIDS (Pachauri, 1994b; 1997c).

In her chapter, Ramasubban traces the development of efforts to address the HIV/AIDS problem and draws attention to the serious gulf between rhetoric and reality. The author examines the problem within the country's political and socio-cultural context and analyses the impeding and fostering factors. She argues that:

> *"AIDS, as no other disease before it, holds up a mirror to Indian society, compelling both policy makers and members of the civil society to bring on centre-stage policies, social processes, social groups and behaviours that had hitherto been relegated to the margins."*

Ramasubban weaves into her discussion of the national programme, two best practices, one of which is state-led in Tamil Nadu and the other is an NGO-led effort in West Bengal. The strategic approaches employed in these two examples differ widely, underscoring the importance of designing programmes to respond to local contexts, needs and opportunities. These case studies provide insights into how challenges to confront politically and culturally sensitive issues related to gender and sexuality can be creatively addressed. To advance the HIV/AIDS agenda, a wider public discourse and frank discussion on these issues, that have been carefully skirted in the past, will be necessary. The author concludes that HIV/AIDS prevention and care is not as yet a part of the mainstream social process. She make a case for bridging the gap between women's powerlessness and the uncharted terrain of men's sexual behaviours; between AIDS control measures and primary health care strategies; and, between health policy formulation and its implementation.

Sethi's chapter complements Ramasubban's by providing an overview of the government's programme. In 1992, the government launched a national response through a well conceptualised programme that was designed to promote partnerships within government bureaucracies, as well as with NGOs, the corporate sector and other players. A comprehensive plan was formulated to decentralise authority to the states; establish sentinel surveillance systems; promote condom use; rationalise blood safety; and, initiate hospital infection control procedures. In addition, pioneering behavioural research was conducted to help design appropriate intervention strategies. Efforts were also initiated to address social, ethical and legal issues. Although well conceived, the denial of the problem and the near absence of political will resulted in poor implementation of the programme. Thus, the country lost precious time because of a faltering programme that never took roots.

Over the last couple of years, there has been a 're-awakening'. National programme efforts are being revived once more. The new agenda that has been framed is based on lessons learned from past experiences, nationally and globally. And although many of the challenges underscored in Ramasubban's chapter still remain to be addressed, advocacy efforts are underway at all levels of the bureaucracy to generate the political will. In addition, carefully carved designs to decentralise programmes are being creatively prepared. Sethi discusses the new agenda.

The author also draws attention to the shared concerns between the reproductive health and AIDS control programmes. The ideological underpinnings of a commitment to uphold human rights, provide informed choice, promote gender equity, and implement people-centred, need-based services as well as to encourage non-judgmental, inclusive attitudes to sexuality, are virtually the same. Programmatically, too, there are several areas of convergence related to sexually transmitted infections, safe motherhood, child survival, and safe sex. Thus, there is a strong, mutually supportive relationship between the processes and philosophy globally endorsed at the ICPD and the direction in which the national response to HIV/AIDS is developing.

In their chapter, Verma, Bhende and Mane discuss the NGO response to HIV/AIDS and focus on NGOs that are addressing women's needs. The authors study programmes that focus particularly on empowering women as well as those focussing on controlling HIV/AIDS. The experience of NGOs that are integrating these services within broader reproductive health programmes is also discussed. Their research shows that NGOs are employing diverse strategies to combat the problem.

The authors examine a variety of innovative strategies employed by NGOs to involve and mobilise communities and provide health services. Interventions targetted at adolescent girls and boys at the community level and within schools and colleges are discussed. Deriving lessons from these experiences, the authors

In his chapter, Mavalankar reviews the status of the safe motherhood programme, which he states was a major departure from the maternal and child health (MCH) programme of the past. He finds that the safe motherhood programme received low priority at the policy and implementation levels. There was little political commitment. Most strategies that were designed were not implemented. There was a lack of co-ordination between inputs, processes and outputs. And because monitoring systems were not put in place, it was difficult to assess impact. However, it was evident from available information that the objective of the programme, which was to save mothers' lives, was not met.

One might ask why is it that maternal mortality rates have continued to stagnate in India? A maternal and child health programme made no dent in 40 years and even after a special safe motherhood programme was implemented, no impact was perceptible. Do mothers' lives not matter? Or are the forces that perpetuate gender discrimination so strong in society, of which the health service system is but a part, that no programme can make a difference?

The reproductive health approach represents an effort to redress this neglect. Although critiqued by some as a 'feminist agenda', the need for this shift in paradigm can hardly be minimised. However, there is clearly a need to learn from past experience and to ensure that the reproductive and child health programme does not suffer the same pitfalls. The reproductive health approach aims to involve the community and to make the programme accountable to the people. It is necessary to ensure that accountability mechanisms are put in place so that the programme is indeed responsive to clients' needs and is implemented in the spirit in which it has been conceptualised.

Unsafe abortion: A pervasive problem

Unsafe induced abortion is the single greatest cause of maternal mortality, and at the same time, the most preventable. Of all the major causes of maternal death, those that lead to abortion deaths are the best understood. Women need not die or suffer medical consequences from abortions because abortions do not kill women; it is unsafely performed abortions which kill (Maine, 1991). Although abortion was legalised in India over 27 years ago, it is still a neglected problem. Access to safe abortion services remains problematic for poor women, especially in rural areas.

The conceptual link between family planning and abortion is fundamental. Effective contraception is an important means of preventing unwanted pregnancy thus preempting the need for abortion. In the absence of safe contraceptive backup, however, women will continue to be forced to employ unsafe means for terminating unwanted pregnancies with attendant high maternal mortality and morbidity. However, even with the best family planning programmes, there will always be a need for safe abortion services.

Khan and co-authors review the literature on abortion in India and show widely differing annual estimates ranging between 5 to 6 million and more. A situational analysis of services for the medical termination of pregnancy in the public sector in four states of India shows that there are many systemic problems in delivering services. There are serious issues of access, quality and cost, especially for the poor. There is a wide gulf between the demand and availability of safe abortion services. Consequently, women resort to unsafe abortions, risking their lives. Abortion contributes to 12 percent of maternal deaths in India (Registrar General of India, 1990).

The researchers conclude that while there is a need to equip more facilities to provide safe abortion services, merely increasing the number of facilities will not solve the problem. A proportion of government approved facilities that could provide safe abortion are not doing so because of the lack of trained staff. Also, many women do not know that abortion is legal. The social distance between service providers and users presents a major barrier. Can menstrual regulation services by paramedical staff be considered for India? Would the medical establishment allow for such a possibility? The authors recommend that the Medical Termination of Pregnancy (MTP) Act be modified and demedicalised so that it is more responsive to women's needs. The momentum generated post-ICPD should be harnessed to promote a wider public debate. The challenge is to achieve these objectives without creating a controversy around this sensitive issue.

Sexuality: A cross cutting theme

Reproductive health is related to sexual health in particular and to sexuality in general. In past programmes, these issues were carefully skirted. A discussion of sex and sexuality was taboo because of its political and cultural sensitivity. Ignoring the linkages between family planning, reproductive health and sexuality resulted in several programmatic distortions. Many reproductive and sexual health needs were not addressed and many client groups neglected (Pachauri, 1994; Germaine, et al 1994). For example, the needs of adolescents and young people who constitute a large proportion of the population and who are sexually active both within and outside marriage, were ignored.

The problem of HIV/AIDS has opened up a discussion on sex and sexuality because persuading people to have safe sex is at the core of programmes for AIDS prevention. Women's special vulnerability because of gender disparities has become evident. Women's sexuality represents the interface between two of the most potent and insidious forms of oppression that prevail in Indian society, gender and sexuality (Ramasubban, 1995). The reluctance to address these issues has limited the effectiveness of programmes designed to improve women's health, promote family planning, and prevent HIV and other sexually transmitted infections (Pachauri, 1994c).

As issues related to sexuality are inextricably linked to reproductive health, they are discussed in several chapters in this book. Pelto, however, addresses these issues explicitly in his chapter. The author traces the tenor of the discourse from the 1980s to the present by drawing on research on sexuality undertaken in India. His articulation provides insights into an area where there has been little documentation. In his state-of-the-art paper, the author discusses the experiences of several sub-categories of men and women in rural, tribal and urban slum areas of India. These include sexual experiences of married women as well as women with multiple sexual partners; experiences of unmarried men and men's first sexual experiences; sexual behaviours of adolescents and sex with relatives. The author illustrates the complexity of the problems by providing quotes from the field. These voices bring to life and humanise the problems that people face in the real world.

Pelto identifies the challenges ahead and argues that if effective interventions are to be designed, more sophisticated research will be needed to understand sexual negotiation strategies between spouses; issues related to domestic violence and sexual coercion; and, sexual practices of men who have sex with men who are a hidden risk category. A major challenge is to develop and refine methodological and conceptual research tools to undertake evaluative research so that interventions relevant to people's lives can be designed.

Addressing Challenges Into the Next Century

The contributors to this volume have analysed India's first steps in making a paradigm shift. The challenges ahead are many, some more formidable than others, but the first challenge of changing policy in the largest democracy in the world, has been overcome. India is now on the threshold of change as it operationalises the new agenda. There is now no turning back.

The inevitability of moving this agenda forward is established despite concerns articulated by many, especially those who still support policies to control population numbers, even when these have been coercive and violated reproductive rights. The proponents of this ideology have continued to critique India's policy change. For example, when targets were removed, the initial problems at the field level were presented as evidence that the decision to change policy was ill conceived (Ross, 1998; Narayana, 1998).

Such a conclusion is premature, as it is based on very early evidence, focussing narrowly on the immediate aftermath of the removal of method-specific targets alone. Although the authors of this volume also document problems, they extend their assessment well beyond targets and examine the broader reproductive and child health programme as it is being planned and operationalised in the country.

Considering that this programme was officially launched only 15 months ago, the momentum achieved in implementing policy is significant. Several essential first steps have been taken. For example, decentralised planning processes are now underway; new monitoring and evaluation systems are being operationalised; human resource development strategies are being re-examined; innovative ways to provide information are being tried; a discourse on how to address the needs of adolescents is on the national agenda; there is a growing momentum for enhancing women's empowerment; and, efforts have been initiated to address sexual and reproductive health problems of women and men.

While important first steps have been taken, many unaddressed problems still remain. Reproductive health is inextricably linked to the issue of rights. The removal of method-specific targets implies that people can now make informed contraceptive choices. Contraceptive choice is linked to larger reproductive choice issues and to reproductive rights. Poor women in India have few life choices. Is reproductive choice a reality in this context? Reproductive rights have not as yet been brought into the national discourse.

Reproductive rights cannot be realised if gender disparities prevail. If policies that promote social justice, women's empowerment and reproductive health can converge; if NGOs, governments, activists and researchers can together promote advocacy initiatives; and, if these growing networks can raise the resources and influence macro-level policy, only then can reproductive rights become a reality for India.

Advocacy efforts should be enhanced to promote an understanding of the paradigm change. The shift in paradigm has mind-boggling implications because it calls for a change from a top-down, male-dominated, bureaucratic, target-driven programme, to client-friendly, gender-sensitive services that respond to people's needs.

The government alone cannot achieve these ambitious goals. It must, therefore, actively seek partnerships with NGOs, the private sector, *panchayats* and the people. Such partnerships are necessary not only to complement the government's own programme but also to ensure its accountability to the people. Efforts by the government, NGOs, and the private sector must be supported by those of the people, the civil society at large, to sustain the momentum to operationalise reproductive health and rights, and to bring about social change.

The analyses presented in this volume validate that the programme is moving on the right path. A strong political will and concerted efforts of all stakeholders will be needed to create the synergy to move the new agenda forward.

References

Ascadi, G.T.F., and Johnson-Ascadi, G. 1990. Safe Motherhood in South Asia: Socio-cultural and Demographic Aspects of Maternal Health. Background Paper for the Safe Motherhood South Asia Conference, Lahore.

Fortney, J.A., and Jason, B.S. (eds.). 1996. The Base of the Iceberg: Prevalence and Perceptions of Maternal Morbidity in Four Developing Countries: The Maternal Morbidity Network. Family Health International, Research Triangle Park, USA.

Germaine, A., Nowrojee, S., and Pyne, H.H. 1994. Setting a New Agenda: Sexual and Reproductive Health and Rights. In: G. Sen, A. Germaine, and L.C. Chen, (eds.). Population Policies Reconsidered: Health, Empowerment and Rights. Harvard Series on Population and International Health. Boston: Harvard University Press.

Gopalan, C. 1989. Women and Nutrition in India - General Considerations. In: C. Gopalan and S. Kaur (eds.). Women and Nutrition in India. 1-16. Nutrition Foundation of India Special Publication Series 5.

Government of India. 1997. Reproductive and Child Health Programme. Ministry of Health and Family Welfare. New Delhi, India.

International Institute of Population Sciences. 1994. National Family Health Survey, 1992-93, India Introductory Report. Mumbai, India.

Jain, A.K. 1992. Conclusions: Recommended Next Steps. In: A.K. Jain (ed.). Managing Quality of Care in Population Programs, USA: Kumarian Press.

Jain, A., and Bruce, J. 1994. A Reproductive Health Approach to the Objectives and Assessment of Family Planning Programs. In: G. Lin, A. Germaine, and L.C. Chen (eds.). Population Policies Reconsidered: Health Empowerment and Rights, 192-211. Boston: Harvard School of Public Health.

Maine, D. 1991. Safe Motherhood Programs: Options and Issues. Columbia University Center for Population and Family Health, New York, USA.

Measham, A., and M. Heaver. 1995. India's Family Welfare Program: Moving to a Reproductive and Child Health Approach. Directions in Development. World Bank, Washington D.C., USA.

National AIDS Control Organisation. 1998. *Nexus*. Population Services International, New Delhi, India.

Narayana, G. 1998. Summary. The Policy Project. Targets for Family Planning in India. An Analysis of Policy Change, Consequences, and Alternative Choices. The Policy Project, the Futures Group, New Delhi, India.

Pachauri, S. 1998a. Adolescents in Asia: Issues and Challenges. *Demography India,* Vol. 27, No. 1.

Pachauri, S. 1998b. Unmet Reproductive and Sexual Health Needs in South Asia. *Journal of Health and Population in Developing Countries,* 1(2):29-30.

Pachauri, S. 1997a. Point of View. In: Toward a New Partnership: Encouraging the Positive Involvement of Men as Supportive Partners in Reproductive Health. Population Council Newsletter No.3, November 1997.

Pachauri, S. 1997b. Advocacy for Reproductive Health. Lecture at Maharaja Sayajirao University and Society for Operations Research and Training, Baroda, India, July 16, 1997.

Pachauri, S. 1997c. Breaking the Silence. In: S. Solomon, and R.P. Rajan, (eds.). Whispers from Within: Unheard Voices of People with HIV/AIDS. Chennai: Navshakti.

Pachauri, S. 1996a. A Shift from Family Planning to Reproductive Health: New Challenges. In: K. Srinivasan, (ed.). Population Policy and Reproductive Health. Population Foundation of India. New Delhi: Hindustan Publishing Corporation.

Pachauri, S. 1995. Defining an Essential Package of Reproductive and Child Health Services. In: India's Family Welfare Program: Towards a Reproductive and Child Health Approach. Population and Human Resources, Operations Division, South Asia Country Department (India, Nepal and Bhutan). World Bank, Washington D.C., USA.

Pachauri, S. (ed.). 1994a. Reaching India's Poor: Non-governmental Approaches to Community Health. Sage Publications, New Delhi, and Thousand Oaks, London.

Pachauri, S. 1994b. Women's Reproductive Health in India: Research Needs and Priorities. In: J. Gittlesohn, M.E. Bentley, P.J. Pelto, M. Nag, S. Pachauri, A.D. Harrison, and L.T. Landman, (eds.). Listening to Women Talk about their Health Issues and Evidence from India. The Ford Foundation and Har-Anand Publications, New Delhi, India.

Pachauri, S. 1994c. Relationship between AIDS and Family Planning Programmes: A Rationale for Developing Integrated Reproductive Health Services. *Health Transitions Review*, Supplement to Volume 4: 321-347.

Pachauri, S., and Marwah, S.M. 1971. A Correlation Study of Birth Weight and Some Maternal Factors. *Indian Journal of Medical Research*, 25(9): 604-612.

Ramachandran, P. 1992. Anaemia in Pregnancy. In: S.S. Ratnam, B.K. Rao, and S. Arulkumaran (eds.). Obstetrics and Gynecology for Postgraduates, Volume I. Madras: Orient Longman Ltd.

Ramasubban, R. 1995. Patriarchy and the Risks of HIV Transmission. In: M. Dasgupta, T.N. Krishnan and Lincoln Chen (eds.). Women, Health and Development in India. Mumbai: Oxford University Press.

Ross, J.A. 1998. The Policy Project. Targets for Family Planning in India. An Analysis of Policy Change, Consequences, and Alternative Choices. The Policy Project, the Futures Group, New Delhi, India.

Registrar General of India. 1990. Survey of Census of Death, (Rural) Annual Report, 1990. Office of the Registrar General, New Delhi, India.

Sinding, W.S. and Fathalla, M. 1995. From Demographic Targets to Individual Needs: The Great Transition. *The UNFPA Magazine Populi*, 22(8):18-21.

United Nations. 1994. Report of the International Conference on Population and Development, Cairo, September 5-13. A/CONF.171/13.

World Bank 1995. India's Family Welfare Program: Toward a Reproductive and Child Health Approach. World Bank Population and Human Resources Division, South Asia Country Department II, Report No. 14644-IN. World Bank, Washington D.C., USA.

PART ONE

Implementing Reproductive Health Policy

1

Fertility Transition in India: Implications for Social Policies

Anrudh Jain

Paper published in: *Reproductive Change in Brazil and India.*
Editors: George Martine, Monica Das Gupta and Lincoln Chen.
Oxford University Press.
Grateful thanks to United Nations Development Programme (UNDP) for giving us permission to use this paper.

Introduction

Rapid population growth, at times, is blamed for all social ills facing the human race, including global warming, environmental degradation, tribal and racial conflicts, widespread hunger and poverty. Furthermore, rapid population growth in a country has been assumed to impede its economic development and, therefore, its ability to provide basic services and to improve the conditions of its people. One of the main rationales[1] behind the investment of public resources in family planning programmes is the belief that a decline in population growth rate would lead to a faster rate of economic development and, thus, would also enhance a country's ability to improve the condition of its people. This belief is based on the reasoning that a growing base of the population pyramid (size of the cohort aged 0 to 4 years) requires increasing resources for such basic services as education and health. Governments are unable to allocate these resources because of slow economic growth. Poor health and education of the labour force in turn slows the pace of economic development even further.

A reduction in the population growth rate through a reduction in fertility decreases the size and the proportion of the population base and, therefore, lowers the demand made by education and health sectors for government resources. Thus, per capita availability of resources for health and education increase even in the absence of any increase in the total allocation of government resources for

[1] Other rationales for investing public resources in family planning programmes include the improvements in maternal and child health and the basic human right to have access to the means of regulating ones own fertility.

these services. This improves the health and education of the labour force and, thus, accelerates the pace of economic development.

Now that fertility transition in India has been ongoing for the past 20 years, can it provide a substitute for just social policies, for example, those oriented to remove gender and regional disparities in health or education? The analysis presented in this paper suggests that while the recent change in age distribution would enhance the government's ability to improve the wellbeing of the Indian people, it cannot depend upon these changes alone to achieve the overall objective of improving health and education conditions of its people throughout India.

Our conclusion is based on various observations. Social justice and fertility decline are closely interlinked, but the degree varies from state to state. Reduction in infant mortality, an improvement in female education and a decrease in gender disparity are among the conditions that contribute to fertility decline. We find changes in age structure much more pronounced in states which have already achieved higher education, lower infant and child mortality and gender equality. In other states, however, we find both social justice and fertility decline relatively less advanced.

The policy and budgeting framework of India today means, however, that potential savings due to changes in the age distribution and in the resources required for education and health in one state cannot be transferred to another state. Policies must be developed that allow those transfers and determine priorities within each state for more investment.

Within the Indian context, education and health – the levels and distribution of which are key indicators of social justice – are under the domain of the state government. The progress made in closing the gaps of regional disparities in infant mortality is to some extent, the result of centrally sponsored and financed activities like the universal immunisation programme (UIP). Given the variable degree of background gender equality, levels of resources going to education and commitment to girls' access to schooling, improvements in female education across the various states would require a similar centrally sponsored and financed programme. Such a programme could mitigate the effects of social and cultural factors that impede female education and undercut universalising primary education, especially in rural areas.

These observations are based on the analysis presented in the subsequent three sections. The first section analyses the state-level data from National Family Health Survey (NFHS) to identify some of the key determinants of fertility. The second analyses the data from censuses, Sample Registration System (SRS) and NFHS to show the extent of the progress made in terms of improving equality in education and health in selected states. The last section brings together these data to identify implications of India's fertility decline for future social policy.

Determinants of Fertility

Conditions that promote high fertility include disparities within and among households. Parents are believed to have large families in order to enhance their own welfare, for reasons such as old age security, to provide extra help in domestic and field work, and to support other siblings. Thus, a shift in parents' thinking toward an improvement in the welfare of children and a more equitable sharing of the cost and benefits of children between men and women would create conditions conducive to fertility decline.

There is no unique set of prerequisites necessary for fertility decline to occur and fertility has declined under a variety of conditions. While socio-economic development would ultimately lead to fertility decline and family planning programmes have been shown to decrease fertility even under poor conditions, the best results are obtained by a good programme under good social settings. Conditions conducive to fertility decline include:

a. a family planning programme that offers services and information of good quality;
b. low infant and child mortality; and
c. high female literacy and education, at least upto the primary level.

The role of social development (female education and health) in fertility transition in Kerala is well established (Krishnan, 1998). How social development has influenced the course of fertility decline in other states is less well documented. This section briefly outlines the roles of infant mortality and female education in fertility transition in India.

The NFHS conducted in 1992-93 confirmed that fertility in India has declined. Not only has it declined in Southern states like Kerala and Tamil Nadu, but also in Northern states like Uttar Pradesh. In fact, fertility has declined throughout the country during the 1980s. The total fertility rate (TFR) in India, according to the SRS, has declined from 5.7 births per woman in 1970-72 to 4.5 in 1980-82 and to 3.7 in 1990-92. The TFR estimated by NFHS for the 1990-92 period, however, was 3.4 births per woman. Notwithstanding the difference in the TFR estimates of SRS and NFHS, it is certain that fertility in India has declined during the last 20 years by at least two births per woman[2].

Table 1 shows the classification of 16 major states by the level of infant mortality and female education (% of married women aged 15-49 years who have at least primary level education). The TFR for each state is shown within parentheses. The TFR is less than 3.1 births per woman in states where both the infant mortality rate (IMR) is low to medium (i.e., less than 75) and female education is medium to high (i.e., more than 27 percent). There are two exceptions to this rule – Orissa and Haryana. The TFR in Orissa is lower than what would be expected on the basis of levels of infant mortality and female education. The situation is reversed for Haryana. The level of IMR in Rajasthan is medium but the level of

---

[2] The National Family Health Survey (NFHS), carried out between April 1992 and September 1993, included a nationally representative sample of 89,777 ever-married women in the age group 13-49 years from 24 states and Delhi. It collected information on fertility, family planning, mortality, and maternal and child health. The Sample Registration System (SRS) was initiated in 1964-65 on a pilot basis and on a full-scale in 1969-70 to provide dependable estimates of vital rates at the national and state levels. Initially, the SRS underestimated the "true" level of birth and death rates. The accuracy of SRS estimates is believed to have improved over time (Bhat, forthcoming).

TABLE 1. Classification of 16 Major States by Level of Female Education and Infant Mortality Rate, 1992-93.

Female Education (% of married women in reproductive age with at least primary level education)	Infant Mortality Rate per 1000 Live Births		
	HIGH (85-110)	MEDIUM (65-75)	LOW (24-55)
LOW (19-23%)	Bihar (4.0) M. P. (4.0) Orissa* (2.9) U. P. (4.8)	Rajasthan (3.6)	
MEDIUM (27-36%)	Assam (3.5)	A. P. (2.6) Gujarat (3.0) Haryana* (4.0) Karnataka (2.9) W. B. (2.9)	
HIGH (39-45%)		Tamil Nadu (2.5)	Jammu (3.1) Maharashtra (2.9) Punjab (2.9) Kerala (2.0)

Total fertility rate for each state is shown in parentheses.

** The levels of TFR in Orissa and Haryana are different than what would be expected on the basis of the levels of infant mortality and female education in these states.*

Source: NFHS, 1992-93

female education is low, whereas the level of female education is medium in Assam and the level of IMR is high. The TFR in these two states is lower than the level in the remaining three states – Bihar, Madhya Pradesh and Uttar Pradesh – where both female education is low and infant mortality is high. A reduction in infant mortality and an increase in the level of female education in these three states will help them to move rapidly toward the replacement level fertility.

The role of infant & child mortality

Fertility decline observed during the last twenty years has been accompanied by a substantial decline in infant and child mortality. The overall IMR in India, according to SRS estimates, has declined from 132 to 80 deaths per 1000 births between 1970-72 and 1990-92, while TFR declined from 5.7 to 3.7 births per woman. The overall relationship between state-level IMR and TFR is reflected by the correlation coefficient of 0.619 between the two, which suggests that states with high infant mortality also have high fertility. There is a two-way connection between infant mortality and fertility.

The implication of high infant and child mortality for fertility behaviour is reflected by a gap between the average number of surviving children and the average number of live births per woman. For example, the average number of children born and surviving among women aged 40 to 44 years, according to NFHS, were 4.8 births and 4.0 children, respectively. The difference between the two in Uttar Pradesh with high infant mortality, however, was much higher than that in Kerala with low infant mortality (1.2 vs. 0.2 births). The number of births a woman has is included in the numerator for estimating indices of fertility such as TFR and crude birth rate (CBR). However, when a woman says that she wants a certain number of children she refers to surviving children and not to live births. This means that a reduction in infant and child mortality would reduce the number of births she must have to reach her desired number of surviving children, which in turn would reduce TFR without reducing the desired family size.

This connection between IMR and TFR reflects both the biological and behavioural effects of high infant mortality on fertility. For example, the duration of breast feeding for a child who dies in infancy is considerably shorter than for the child who survives for a longer period. Thus, the birth interval in the absence of contraceptive use following an infant death is usually shorter than that following the child who survives for more than one year. Moreover, a desire to replace a lost child in the subsequent birth interval may be implemented by adjusting the timing and frequency of coitus.

The relationship between IMR and TFR also reflects the fact that high fertility in a community means a higher proportion of high parity births and the fact that IMR is also high among births of high parity. Hence, a reduction in TFR achieved through a reduction of high parity births would also reduce infant mortality. However, direct interventions to reduce infant mortality at all parities, and especially at the first parity, are most likely to reduce TFR. Such policies need special attention in Assam, Bihar, Madhya Pradesh, Orissa, and Uttar Pradesh where the level of IMR is estimated to be as high as 85 deaths or more per 1000 births.

The role of female education

Female education in many societies has been found to be associated with a decrease in indicators of fertility and mortality. India is no exception. The assumption about the fertility reduction effect of education is based on the observation that the advancement in female education leads to: (i) a decrease in the demand (ideal or desired) for children; (ii) an increase in age at marriage; (iii) an increase in the use of contraception; and (iv) a decrease in the incidence and duration of breast feeding and postpartum abstinence (see Table 2).

TABLE 2. Total Fertility Rate and its Proximate Determinants by Level of Female Education in India, 1992-93.

Female Education	Fertility Rate			Contra-ceptive Prevalence Rate	Median Age at Marriage Among Women 25-29 Yrs.	Median Number of Months of Postpartum Non-susceptibility
	Total	Wanted	Un-wanted			
Illiterate	4.03	3.15	0.88	33.9	15.3	11.4
Literate	3.01	2.31	0.70	50.4	17.1	9.2
Middle school	2.49	1.95	0.54	50.8	18.7	7.9
High school & above	2.15	1.78	0.37	54.7	21.7	6.2
TOTAL	3.39	2.64	0.75	40.6	16.6	10.2

Source: NFHS, 1992-93

FIG 1: Total Fertility Rate by Female Education for Major States in India: 1990-1992

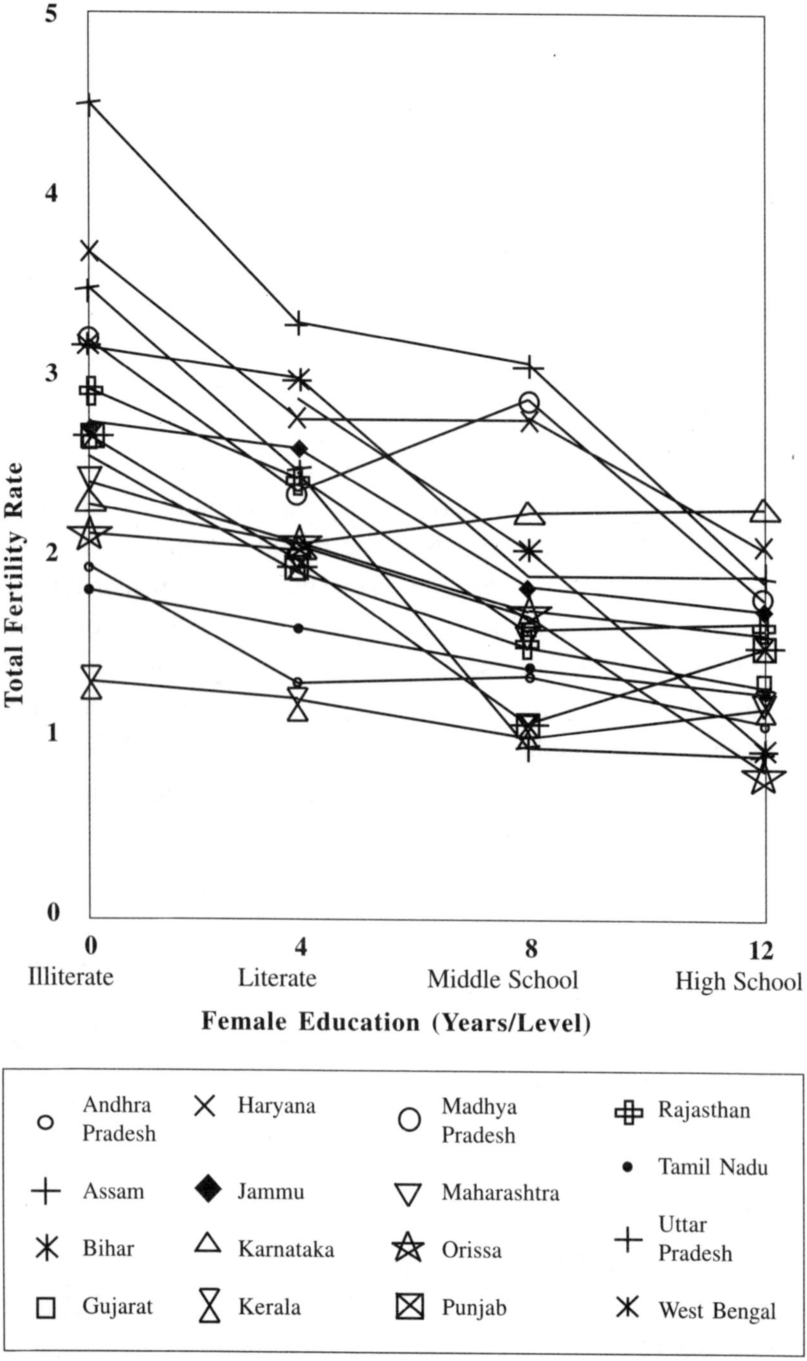

According to NFHS there is no state in which TFR among females with little education is higher than that among women with no education. Even if there was such a state, its resources are wasted and social justice goals failed if girls' dropout rates from grades one to four are not minimised. Thus, even without the amply demonstrated fertility decline rationale, policies must work to increase the proportion of girls completing primary level of schooling (Jain, 1981).

The effect of education on fertility is measured by the slope in a regression equation, which was found to vary from place to place and state to state in India (see Figure 1). For example, TFR in Uttar Pradesh decreases from 5.4 births among women with no education to 2.6 births among women with at least high school education, which implies a regression coefficient of - 0.220. In Kerala, in comparison, TFR decreases from 2.3 to 2.0 births per woman with a regression coefficient of - 0.029. The effect of female education measured by the slope of the regression equation in Kerala is lower than in Uttar Pradesh (-.029 vs. -.220). This is what one would expect at different stages of demographic transition. At the beginning of demographic transition, TFR is likely to be uniformly high in all education groups. As women with better education start to regulate their fertility, the relationship between TFR and education becomes pronounced as depicted by the pattern in Uttar Pradesh. Toward the end of the demographic transition, the fertility becomes uniformly low in all education groups as depicted by the pattern in Kerala.

If the relationship between female education and fertility simply reflects the stage of demographic transition, will improvement in female education in, for example, Uttar Pradesh reduce fertility? The answer would depend upon a better understanding of why the effect of education on fertility varies from state to state. Two distinct situations under which the individual-level effect of education on fertility could vary among countries or communities within a country are schematically shown in Figures 2(a) and 2(b).

In the pattern shown in Figure 2(a), the average fertility of women with little or no education is similar across countries whereas fertility of educated women differs markedly across countries. In

FIG 2: Hypothetical Relationship Between Female Education & Fertility for Five Countries

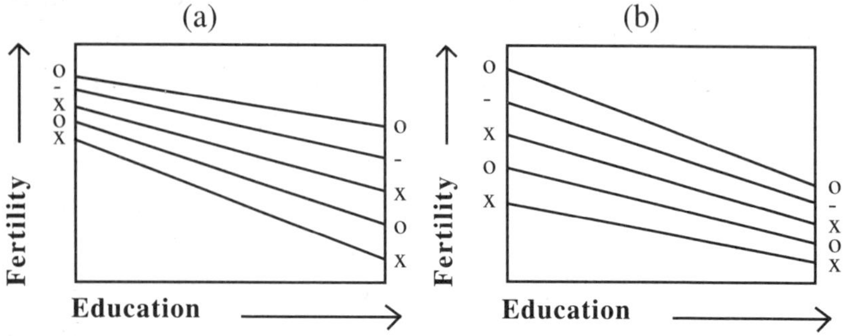

this pattern, the variation in the effect of education on fertility is due to the variation in the fertility of educated women. The variation in the fertility of educated women across communities could reflect differences among communities in such factors as levels of economic development, opportunities for, and actual participation by, educated women in the paid labour force and, therefore, to differences in the economic value of education. If so, an increase in female education is unlikely to reduce fertility without simultaneous improvements in economic opportunities. This is the most prevalent interpretation about the differential effect of female education on fertility.

In the pattern shown in Figure 2(b), the average fertility of educated women is similar across communities whereas fertility of women with little or no education differs markedly across communities. In this pattern, the variation in the effect of education on fertility is due to the variation in the fertility of women with no education. The fact that fertility of educated women is similar across communities with different opportunities would imply that fertility behaviour of women in part depends upon their education. In this case, attention must be given to understand causes of differences among communities in the fertility behaviour of women with no education, which could reflect the impact of differences in post-partum amenorrhea and abstinence, differences in infant mortality, and the differential impact of family planning programme, i.e., differential use of contraception among women with no education.

The pattern in India (Figure 1) is similar to the one shown in Figure 2(b). While TFR among women with no education varies from a low of 2.3 in Kerala to a high of 5.4 in Uttar Pradesh, TFR among women with at least high school level education is quite close to 2 except in Bihar, Haryana, Karnataka, Madhya Pradesh and Uttar Pradesh. In these states, TFR varies between 2.6 in Bihar and Uttar Pradesh and 3.0 in Karnataka. Thus, the difference between regression coefficients for Kerala and Uttar Pradesh (-.029 vs. -.220) is primarily due to the difference in fertility among women with no education (5.4 vs. 2.3) rather than due to the difference in fertility among educated women (2.6 vs. 2.0). Women with high school education appear to be more similar across state boundaries than women with no education (the standard deviation of TFRs among women with no education is 0.79 in comparison to 0.42 among those with high school education). This means that there might be something more to female education (that holds across state boundaries) than an increase in their potential to participate in economic activities (which varies among states). Improvements in female education, therefore, can be expected to influence fertility behaviour even without simultaneous changes in other factors such as increased opportunities for them to participate in the paid labour force[3]. A similar conclusion was drawn by an analysis conducted with data from 11 countries (Jain, 1981).

[3] Improvements in girls' education will reduce fertility as they move through their reproductive period. Will children's education reduce parental fertility in the short run? This is unlikely to be the case in high fertility societies especially if laws about compulsory education and prohibition against child labour cannot be enforced. There are two reasons for not expecting a feedback loop of children's education to parental fertility. The first reason is based on demographic realities and the second on the belief that parents in high fertility societies tend to maximize their own welfare rather than their children's.

In high fertility societies, by the time the eldest child is likely to complete primary education, the mother would be about 30 years of age and, on an average, would have completed about 70 percent of her marital fertility. If the effect of a child's education on parent's fertility is postponed until she/he completes secondary school, the mother will be close to completing her childbearing process.

If benefits to parents from their children's education are higher than the corresponding costs, they are unlikely to reduce their fertility because more children would mean higher benefits. On the other hand, if benefits from their children's education are lower than the corresponding costs, the outcome is likely to be no education for children rather than high education for children and low fertility for parents. In brief, children's education is unlikely to have a negative feedback effect on parent's fertility unless parents are assumed to maximize the welfare of their children at an early stage of childbearing. But if that were the case, parents would already have small families (Jain, 1982).

Potential effect of improvement in female education

What can be achieved by focusing upon female education? To address this question we compare two states, Kerala and Uttar Pradesh, in regards to the effect of female education on total and wanted fertility rates and infant mortality rates. The results, from NFHS, are shown in Table 3; panel A for total fertility rate, panel B for wanted fertility rate, and panel C for infant mortality rate.

Seventy-six percent of women of the reproductive age in Uttar Pradesh have no education in comparison to 16 percent in Kerala. If the education of women in Uttar Pradesh was the same as the education of women in Kerala, the overall TFR in Uttar Pradesh would have been 3.9 instead of 4.8 births per woman. This means that out of a difference of 2.8 births in TFR between Uttar Pradesh and Kerala, 0.9 births are accounted for by the fact that women in Uttar Pradesh have lower education than those in Kerala. The remaining difference of 1.9 births reflects the effect of differences between Kerala and Uttar Pradesh in education specific fertility rates. Women in Uttar Pradesh have higher fertility than women with similar education in Kerala. The differences between the two states, however, decreases from 3.1 births for women with no education to 0.6 births for women with high school education. The narrowing of fertility differences with improvement in education suggests that the differential effect of macro-level factors on TFR between the two states is more pronounced among women with no education than among the educated women. The lower fertility of women with no education in Kerala, perhaps, reflects the fact that the services for health and family planning in Kerala are better than in Uttar Pradesh. Women with high school education in Uttar Pradesh, on the other hand perhaps, have similar access to these services as women with comparable education in Kerala. Thus, simultaneous improvements made in Uttar Pradesh in the quality and availability of education, health, and family planning services would contribute to the reduction of overall TFR in the state.

The wanted fertility in Uttar Pradesh decreases from 4.3 among women with no education to 2.1 among those with at least high

TABLE 3. Total and Wanted Fertility Rates and Infant Mortality Rates by Female Education in Kerala and Uttar Pradesh, 1992-93.

	Education	Kerala	Uttar Pradesh	Ratio (Kerala/U.P.)
A. TOTAL FERTILITY RATE	Illiterate	2.27	5.36	0.424
	Literate	2.16	4.16	0.519
	Middle School	1.95	3.81	0.512
	High School	1.95	2.55	.0765
	TOTAL OBSERVED	2.00	4.82	0.415
	TOTAL ESTIMATED*	2.00	3.92	0.510
	Constant	2.26	5.29	
	Regression Coefficient	-.029	-.220	
B. WANTED FERTILITY RATE	Illiterate	1.98	4.30	.0460
	Literate	1.92	3.30	0.582
	Middle School	1.81	3.00	0.603
	High School	1.86	2.10	0.886
	TOTAL OBSERVED	1.82	3.80	0.479
	TOTAL ESTIMATED*	1.82	3.13	
	Constant	1.96	4.21	
	Regression Coefficient	-.012	-.173	
C. INFANT MORTALITY RATE	Illiterate	60.4	127.4	0.474
	Literate	33.6	72.7	0.462
	Middle School	22.7	83.0	0.273
	High School	14.5	54.6	0.266
	TOTAL	23.8	99.9	0.238
	Constant	55.1	115.6	
	Regression Coefficient	-3.72	-5.20	

Source: NFHS, 1992-93.

**Assumes that the education composition of women in Uttar Pradesh was the same as that in Kerala.*

school level of education[4]. It is of interest to note that the level of wanted fertility among women with high school education in Uttar Pradesh is quite close to the corresponding level among women with no education in Kerala. In both groups the level of infant mortality is approximately the same. Thus, decline in wanted fertility would require a substantial decrease in infant mortality or a substantial increase in female education. However, improvements in both female education and health would perhaps decrease wanted fertility faster than the improvements in any one of the two factors.

As far as the reduction in infant and child mortality is concerned, the effect of female education is complementary to that of health services. In fact, under certain circumstances, the effect of the two factors may even be synergistic, because both facilitate changes in health seeking behaviour. This point can be illustrated by comparing education-specific infant mortality rates between Kerala and Uttar Pradesh. The infant mortality rate in Kerala declines from a level of 60 among women with no education to 14 among those with at least high school education. In comparison, IMR in Uttar Pradesh decreases from 127 among women with no education to 55 among those with at least high school education. The effect of education on infant mortality measured by the slope of the regression equation is -3.72 in Kerala and -5.20 in Uttar Pradesh. This means that improving female education in Uttar Pradesh will reduce the overall IMR. However, even if all women in Uttar Pradesh receive a high school level education and nothing else changes in terms of health services, the overall IMR is likely to be reduced to 55 - the current level among high school graduates. In order for the IMR to decline

[4] Unwanted births are excluded from the numerator in calculating wanted fertility rate. According to NFHS: "a birth is considered unwanted if the number of living children at the time of conception was greater than or equal to the current ideal number of children, as reported by the respondent. Women who gave a non-numeric response to the question on the ideal number of children were assumed to want all their births". This procedure estimated that 24 percent of TFR was unwanted. Distribution of births during the four years preceding the survey and current pregnancies by fertile planning status indicated that only 9 percent of births were unwanted and an additional 14 percent were mistimed. The difference in unwanted fertility between the two procedures may reflect the effect of post-facto rationalisation, i.e., women are unwilling to call a child already born as "unwanted".

further, there have to be improvements in other factors including health services.

The gross effect of health services can be measured by differences in the education-specific ratios of IMR (shown in Column 4 of Table 3 in panel C). The effect of health services on IMR decreases with an increase in education, which simply means that the effect of health services on IMR among women with no educafion is much more pronounced than that among educated women. In other words, an increase in the spread of health services would reduce the effect of female education on infant mortality because women with no education would also be able to use these services. These comparisons make it clear that simultaneous improvements in both education and health services would reduce infant mortality faster than concentrating on any one of the two.

As far as the reduction in total fertility is concerned, the effect of female education is complementary to that of contraceptive and health services: improvements in female education reduces the desired family size (see panel B in Table 3) and improves women's ability to regulate their fertility, and improvements in contraceptive services provide women with the means to transform their desires into practice. Similarly, reductions in infant and child mortality and in fertility are mutually supportive. In sum, a faster decline in IMR and a faster increase in female education along with a good quality family planning programme is likely to accelerate the ongoing fertility transition in India.

Maximising the Social Benefits of Fertility Decline

When we think of the consequences/benefits of fertility decline, we need to consider them at different levels: the macro (all-India) level, the regional (or state) level, the family level and the individual level. We also need to consider whether the cost of fertility reduction and potential benefits are proportionately distributed among people of different segments. For example, the cost of fertility reduction and the benefits derived from low fertility may not be shared equally between rich and poor households, or between the man and the woman in the same household. This could happen when poor households (or women) are asked to reduce their fertility while other government policies tend to favour the middle class and the rich (or men).

While some of the assumptions about adverse economic consequences of rapid population growth, mentioned earlier, have recently been questioned, the adverse consequences of rapid population growth were recognised by the Indian economic planners as early as the 1950s. Even the Eighth Five-Year Plan document considered the implications of the rapid population growth of the past:

> *"The (population) growth started increasing rather fast after 1951 and reached a peak of 2.22 percent during the decade 1971-81. It is tempting to think that if only India had succeeded in containing her population growth rate after 1951 to around one percent per annum i.e. the rate China has achieved, how much difference this factor alone would have meant in terms of per capita income, consumption, and levels of living."* (Planning Commission, 1992).

A recent study (Dreze and Sen, 1995), however, suggests that if India could cut its population growth to China's level, its annual per capita gross domestic product (GDP) growth would go up slightly from 3.1 percent to 3.8 percent, i.e., a reduction in the rate of population growth would have little effect on the pace of economic development. The authors, however, support policies to reduce the rate of population growth on other grounds.

The effect of fertility decline on a government's ability to invest in human development is mitigated through changes in age distribution of the population. While India still has a young population, the age composition of her population has begun to change. The age composition has been quite stable until 1971 because of high fertility: about 41 percent between 0 to 14 years of age; about 5 to 6 percent over the age of 60 years; and the remaining about 53 to 54 percent in the working ages (15 to 59 years). The effect of the recent decline in fertility on the age composition has started to show in terms of a slight decrease in the percent of population aged 0-14 years (from 41 percent in 1971 to 36 percent in 1991) and a corresponding increase in the working age population from 54 percent in 1971 to 58 percent in 1991 (see Table 4). Consequently, the dependency ratio has decreased from 0.85 in 1971

Table 4. Age Distribution of Population in India and Selected States for 1961-1991.

Age (Years) (1)	1961 Census (2)	1971 Census (3)	1981 Census (4)	1991 SRS (5)	1992/93 NFHS (6)
		INDIA			
0-14	41	41	38	36	38
15-59	53	54	56	58	54
60+	6	5	6	6	8
Total	100	100	100	100	100
		KERALA			
0-14	42	40	35	30	30
15-59	52	54	57	62	62
60+	6	6	8	8	8
Total	100	100	100	100	100
		UTTAR PRADESH			
0-14	41	42	42	39	42
15-59	53	51	51	55	50
60+	6	7	7	6	8
Total	100	100	100	100	100
		TAMIL NADU			
0-14	37	38	35	31	32
15-59	57	54	59	62	60
60+	6	6	6	7	8
Total	100	100	100	100	100

to 0.72 in 1991. The overall dependency ratio is made up of two components: dependency burden of the young (0 to 14 years) population and the dependency burden of the old (over 60 years) population. The first component has decreased from 0.76 to 0.62 during the last 20 years, whereas the second component has increased slightly from 0.09 to 0.10.

There are two important implications of the young population in India. The first, is the phenomenon of momentum, which means that even if fertility is instantaneously reduced to the replacement level, the population will continue to grow until children already born pass through their reproductive period. This effect can be minimised by increasing the length of the generation which can be done by delaying the age at first birth, and by increasing the interval between subsequent births. The second issue has to do with the provision of health and education services. While the size of the cohort becoming eligible for education has started to decline in terms of the proportion of the total population, the absolute number of children becoming eligible for primary education is likely to grow for some time. On the other hand, while the proportion of elderly (60 or more years of age) has remained constant, the absolute number of elderly has increased substantially because of the growth in the total population size. Health and other needs of this elderly population will increasingly become an important and growing source of public expenditure. An important policy issue that must be addressed by Indian policy makers is how to meet the demands made by the growing elderly population on public expenditures without reducing the resources required to meet the needs of children.

These effects would be felt differently in each state, because of differences in the changes in age distribution. It is important to consider state level differences because both education and health are state domains, i.e., the state government invests the majority of resources required to improve the education and health conditions of its people. Under the current scheme, the savings realised in one state from education of young children as a consequence of the fertility reduction are not transferable to another state.

The age distributions of three states are compared in Table 4 to illustrate the point: Kerala and Tamil Nadu with low fertility, and Uttar Pradesh with high fertility. The age distributions in all three states were quite similar until 1971. The age distribution in Uttar Pradesh shows a very slight change since then, whereas the proportion of the population in the young age group, 0 to 14 years, in both Kerala and Tamil Nadu has declined substantially. The dependency burden of the young population in Kerala has declined markedly from 0.74 to 0.48 and in Tamil Nadu, it has declined from 0.70 in 1971 to 0.50 in 1991. The dependency burden of the young population in Uttar Pradesh, on the other hand, has declined slightly from 0.82 to 0.71. The dependency burden of the young population in Uttar Pradesh in 1991 was similar to what it was in Kerala and Tamil Nadu in 1971. The education and health conditions of the people at present in Kerala and Tamil Nadu are quite different from those in Uttar Pradesh and, therefore, the implications of the changing age distributions for the future would be quite different.

Differential Progress Made in Education and Health

Since the key determinants of fertility decline include infant mortality and female education, we have selected these indicators to show the progress made in the health and education sectors. In terms of education, we have focused on the percent of population aged 15 to 19 years which has completed primary level schooling. We have selected this age group because children would have ample time to complete primary level schooling by the age of 15 years even if they started schooling much later than the age of 5 years. Moreover, these ages mark the beginning of the reproductive period for women.

The infant mortality rate in all three states has declined during the last 20 years (see Table 5). However, IMR in Tamil Nadu in 1991 was about the same as it was in Kerala in 1971. IMR in Uttar Pradesh in 1991 was even higher than what it was in Kerala, but

TABLE 5. Infant Mortality Rate per 1000 Births for India and Selected States by Place of Residence and Gender, 1970-72 to 1990-92.

	Place of Residence				Gender		
PERIOD	Total	Rural	Urban	Residential Disparity (Rural/ Urban)	Male	Female	Gender Disparity (Male/ Female)
(1)	(2)	(3)	(4)	(5)	(6)	(7)	(8)
INDIA							
1970-72	132	141	86	55	131	134	3
1980-82	110	119	64	55	110	110	0
1990-92	80	86	52	34	81	80	-1
KERALA							
1970-72	58	61	44	17			
1980-82	36	38	27	11			
1990-92	17	17	15	2	17	16	-1
UTTAR PRADESH							
1970-72	174	184	116	68			
1980-82	152	160	98	62			
1990-92	98	103	73	30	95	100	5
TAMIL NADU							
1970-72	120	131	84	47			
1980-82	89	101	57	44			
1990-92	58	67	40	27	60	54	-6

Source: SRS

lower than what it was in Tamil Nadu 20 years ago. All three states have also made considerable progress in terms of education (see Table 6). Almost all persons (93 percent) in the 15-19 year age group in Kerala have completed primary level schooling in 1991 in comparison to 72 percent in Tamil Nadu and 56 percent in Uttar Pradesh. This level in Uttar Pradesh in 1991 was about the same as it was in Tamil Nadu, but lower than what it was in Kerala 20 years ago.

TABLE 6. Percent of Persons Aged 15-19 Years who have Completed at Least Primary Level Schooling for India and Selected States by Gender and Place of Residence, 1971-1992/93.

	Rural			Urban			Total		
PERIOD	Male	Female	Total	Male	Female	Total	Male	Female	Total
(1)	(2)	(3)	(4)	(5)	(6)	(7)	(8)	(9)	(10)
INDIA									
1971	49	23	36	76	62	70	55	31	44
1981	51	27	40	76	65	71	58	37	48
1992-93	68	40	54	84	75	80	73	50	61
KERALA									
1971	80	71	75	86	80	83	81	71	77
1981	88	84	87	91	89	90	89	85	87
1992-93	92	93	93	94	94	94	92	94	93
UTTAR PRADESH									
1971	45	13	31	66	50	59	51	19	37
1981	53	17	37	65	52	59	56	24	42
1992-93	70	32	51	76	66	71	71	40	56
TAMIL NADU									
1971	55	33	43	79	65	72	63	42	52
1981	71	49	60	81	70	75	75	56	65
1992-93	76	56	65	87	84	85	80	66	72

Source: Census for 1971 and 1981; NFHS for 1992/93

Disparities in these indicators of education and health are computed at three levels: regional, i.e., among states; residential, i.e., between rural and urban areas within a state; and gender, i.e., between male and female. Instead of or in addition to gender disparities at the individual level, one could have also considered class, or religion, or caste disparities in the achievement of good health and education. We have, however, selected gender to show the extent of disparity at the individual level because women have disproportionately borne the cost of fertility reduction in India. This

TABLE 7. Regional Disparities in Infant Mortality Rate and Education by Place of Residence, 1970-72 to 1990-92.

	Disparity in Infant Mortality Rate Place of Residence			Disparity in Education Place of Residence		
PERIOD (1)	Total (2)	Rural (3)	Urban (4)	Total (5)	Rural (6)	Urban (7)
	UTTAR PRADESH KERALA			**KERALA UTTAR PRADESH**		
1970-72	116	123	72	40	44	24
1980-82	116	122	71	45	40	31
1990-92	81	86	58	37	42	23
	TAMIL NADU KERALA			**KERALA TAMIL NADU**		
1970-72	62	70	40	25	32	11
1980-82	53	63	30	22	27	15
1990-92	41	50	25	21	28	9
	UTTAR PRADESH TAMIL NADU			**TAMIL NADU UTTAR PRADESH**		
1970-72	54	53	32	15	12	13
1980-82	63	59	41	23	13	16
1990-92	40	36	33	16	14	14

Source: Tables 5 and 6

is shown by the fact that out of 36.2 percent of couples who were using a modern method of contraception according to NFHS, only 5.8 percent were using a male method. The remaining 30.4 percent were using a female method — mainly female sterilisation (27.3 percent).

Regional disparity

The regional disparity is measured by the difference in the state level IMRs or primary school completion rates (see Table 7). While the regional disparities in IMR have declined over 20 years, disparities in education have remained about the same. For example,

TABLE 8. Gender and Residential Disparity in Primary Education Attainment for India and Selected States, 1971-1992/93.

	Gender Disparity Male/Female			Gender Disparity Male/Female	Combined Disparity Urban Male/ Rural Female
PERIOD	Rural	Urban	Total		
(1)	(2)	(3)	(4)	(5)	(6)
INDIA					
1971	26	14	24	34	53
1981	24	11	21	31	49
1992-93	28	9	23	26	44
KERALA					
1971	9	6	10	8	15
1981	4	2	4	3	7
1992-93	1	0	-2	1	1
UTTAR PRADESH					
1971	32	16	32	28	53
1981	36	13	32	21	48
1992-93	38	10	31	20	44
TAMIL NADU					
1971	22	14	21	29	46
1981	22	11	19	15	32
1992-93	20	3	14	20	31

Source: Table 6

the regional disparity in IMR between Uttar Pradesh and Kerala has declined from about 116 points in 1971 to 81 points in 1991 and between Uttar Pradesh and Tamil Nadu it has declined from 54 to 40 points. The regional disparity in education has remained around 40 points between Uttar Pradesh and Kerala and around 15 points between Uttar Pradesh and Tamil Nadu. It is possible that a reduction in regional disparities in IMR reflects the fact that interventions to reduce IMR like the UIP got impetus under the centrally sponsored schemes like Maternal and Child Health (MCH) and Child Survival and Safe Motherhood (CSSM) programmes. It is possible that these programmes disproportionately focused on states with high infant and child mortality and, thus, minimised the effect of biases in the allocation of state resources to primary health care. No such central scheme is active to universalise primary education.

Residential disparity

The rural-urban disparity in IMR in Kerala has virtually disappeared during the last 20 years (see Column 5 in Table 5). It has declined quite considerably in both Tamil Nadu (from 47 points in 1971 to 27 points in 1991) and Uttar Pradesh (from 68 points in 1971 to 30 points in 1991). The rural-urban disparity in education also follows the same pattern (see Column 5 in Table 8). It has completely disappeared in Kerala and has declined in both Tamil Nadu (from 29 points to 20 points) and Uttar Pradesh (from 28 points to 20 points) during the past 20 years. Thus, it appears that the potential benefits of fertility decline in terms of improved health and education are being shared with people living in rural areas. This, however, is not case with gender differences.

Gender disparity

Rapid population growth can affect gender disparity because of a gender bias in allocation of government's resources and because of a gender bias within the family. Large family size is assumed to adversely effect the allocation of parental resources for health and education of children within the family. It is, therefore, logical to expect that a decline in family size would improve parental allocation of financial and other resources per child. Are these benefits shared equally between male and female children?

There is very little information on this subject. Das Gupta and Bhat (1995) show intensification of gender bias in terms of sex selected abortions as a result of fertility decline during the 1980s.

Jejeebhoy (1993) showed that female children in rural Maharashtra do not benefit as a consequence of a decrease in family size, whereas male children do. Her study raises "the alarming possibility that with the increasing prevalence of small families, gender disparities in outcomes for children will widen". To counteract these adverse consequences of fertility decline on gender disparities, formulation and implementation of gender sensitive public policies in education, health and other spheres would be required.

Male infant mortality, in the absence of gender bias, should be slightly higher than female infant mortality. While IMR has declined over the last twenty years, the decline at the all-India level has been of the same order of magnitude for males as for females. Time trend data for gender-specific IMR for each state are not available. However, at present, the gender disparity in the risk of infant death has more or less disappeared in Andhra Pradesh, Karnataka and Orissa. The gender disparity in IMR remains quite pronounced in Bihar, Haryana, Punjab and Uttar Pradesh. In the remaining states, IMRs for males and females are about the same. While the effect of gender bias on the risk of infant death can be minimised through such public interventions as universal immunisation, this may not happen for the risk of death beyond the first year of life. During this period of life, the effect of behavioural factors such as neglect of female children (i.e., allocation of food and utilisation of health services), on their chances of survival may become more pronounced. However, while the age-specific death rate in 0-4 year age group has declined, the extent of gender bias in child survival at the all-India level has not changed much: the child mortality rates have remained about the same for both male and female children. In some states like Uttar Pradesh, the gender bias in child mortality has declined both in absolute and relative terms. The child mortality rate (0-4 age group) in Uttar Pradesh in the mid 1970s was about 65 for males and 97 for females. In early 1990s, these rates have declined to about 30 and 37, respectively. The effect of gender bias on child survival remains particularly serious in Bihar, Haryana, Madhya Pradesh, Punjab and Uttar Pradesh (SRS, 1993; Das Gupta and Bhat, 1995).

The gender differences in education tell quite an interesting story. The gender disparity in education is measured by the difference between the percent of males aged 15-19 years who have completed primary level schooling and the percent of females aged 15-19 years who have completed primary level schooling. The gender disparities in education are shown separately for rural and urban areas in Table 8. The gender disparity in education in Kerala was low to begin with. It has now completely disappeared from both the rural as well as urban areas. The overall gender disparity in education in Tamil Nadu has decreased from 21 points to 14 points over a period of 20 years. The decline appears to have been accelerated during the 1980s, which may have contributed to a faster fertility decline in Tamil Nadu during this period. However, almost all of this decline is accounted for by a decrease in gender disparity in urban areas of the state. In rural Tamil Nadu, the gender disparity in education has remained virtually constant around 20 points. The overall gender difference in Uttar Pradesh, on the other hand, has remained virtually constant at about 30 points, it has decreased in urban areas from 16 to 10 points, but has increased in rural areas from 32 to 38 points during 1971 and 1991. Thus, rural females in Uttar Pradesh have not done as well in education as rural males or urban females.

The joint effects of disadvantage due to the place of residence (urban - rural) and gender on the completion of primary school education can be measured by the difference between urban males (the most privileged) and rural females (the least privileged). The value of this index has declined from 15 points to 1 point for Kerala, from 46 to 31 points for Tamil Nadu, and from 53 to 44 points for Uttar Pradesh and the country as a whole. The regional disparities (differences among states) for male education is much lower than that for female education, especially in rural areas. Moreover, the regional disparities in education among rural females either has remained constant or increased somewhat during the last 20 years. In contrast, the regional disparity among rural males has declined over this period. Tamil Nadu, Uttar Pradesh, and perhaps all other major states have a long way to go to remove these disparities in female education. The removal of these disparities can be facilitated to some extent by changes in age distribution in Tamil Nadu but not too much in Uttar Pradesh. In addition, the removal of gender disparities in these and other states would require adoption and implementation of education policies that would disproportionately favour rural females and allocate adequate resources for this purpose.

Women's health

As mentioned earlier, women have disproportionately borne the cost of fertility regulation. Have they benefited in terms of better health?

Life expectancy at birth in India – one indicator of better health – has increased for both males and females from about 23 years at the beginning of this century to about 60 years at present. The life expectancy at birth for females is estimated to be about 61 years in comparison to 60 years for males. This is in contrast to countries in East Asia in which the life expectancy for females was estimated to be about 74 years in comparison to 70 years for males. Evidently, women in India are relatively disadvantaged as far as overall mortality is concerned.

High maternal morbidity and mortality are other indicators of low female health status and lack of their access to health resources in India. Information on these two indicators of maternal health is lacking. Recently, Bhat et al (1995) have estimated maternal mortality ratios by using indirect methods of estimation and using data from SRS. According to these estimates, the maternal mortality ratio for India is estimated to be 580 deaths per 100,000 live births for the 1982-86 period. The maternal mortality ratio is estimated to be higher in rural than in urban areas (638 vs. 389 deaths per 100,000 live births). There are some regional variations as well. For example, the state of Assam has an estimated 1,068 maternal deaths for this same period of time and 207 maternal deaths were recorded for Punjab, (both per 100,000 live births). Other states which show high maternal mortality are Uttar Pradesh, Bihar, Orissa and Rajasthan. Lower maternal mortality levels are reported for southern and western Indian states.

According to the NFHS conducted in 1992-93, the average maternal mortality ratio at the national level for the two-year period prior to the survey date is estimated to be 437 deaths per 100,000 live births. The rate for rural areas is estimated to be higher than for urban areas (448 vs. 397). The extent to which the difference between the indirect estimate derived by Bhat and his colleagues for 1982-86 and the NFHS estimate for 1990-91 reflects a real decline in the risk of maternal deaths between the two time periods cannot be ascertained.

In addition to the risk of maternal deaths, women also suffer a high risk of morbidity related to reproduction. However, the knowledge about reproductive morbidity and its determinants in India is virtually nonexistent. There are two studies which indicate a high level of reproductive morbidity among Indian women. Bang et al. (1989) found that 55 percent of women belonging to the Gond tribe in a Maharashtra village reported gynaecological complaints. Another recent study in Karnataka (Bhatia and Cleland, 1995) found that approximately one-third of all women reported at least one current symptom indicative of such morbidity conditions as anaemia, menstrual disorders, lower reproductive tract infection, and acute pelvic inflammatory disease.

While reproductive health in regions with low fertility may be better than in those regions with high fertility, the levels of maternal morbidity and mortality may still be unacceptably high. For example, according to Bhat et al (1995), the maternal mortality ratio even in the state of Kerala, with a slightly below replacement level fertility and very low infant mortality, is as high as 235 deaths per 100,000 births. It should be noted that other indicators of health care in terms of care received during the antenatal period and at the time of birth in Kerala are quite high (see Table 9), among births during 1988-89, i.e. four years prior to interview in NFHS, about 90 percent of mothers received antenatal care and about 90 percent of babies were born in medical institutions and/or attended by a health professional. The reasons of high maternal mortality in Kerala in

TABLE 9. Selected Indicators of Health Care for India and Selected States.

Indicators (1)	India (2)	Kerala (3)	Uttar Pradesh (4)	Tamil Nadu (5)
Percent of births during four years prior to NFHS to women who received:				
Antenatal Care	62.3	97.3	44.7	94.2
Two dosages of tetanus toxoid vaccine	53.8	89.8	37.4	90.1
Iron/Folic tablets	50.5	91.2	29.5	84.2
Percent of births four years prior to NFHS delivered in medical institutions	25.5	87.8	11.2	63.4
Percent of deliveries assisted by health professionals	34.2	89.7	17.2	71.2
Maternal mortality ratio per 100,000 births	580	247	920	372
Maternal death rate per 100,000 women	82	21	160	38

Source: NFHS for health care indicators; Bhat et al (1995) for maternal mortality.

spite of this good health care are not known. As expected, these indicators of health care in Uttar Pradesh are extremely low. Tamil Nadu seems to have made good progress in this regard.

While fertility decline would contribute to the improvements in women's health by eliminating high parity births and increasing intervals between subsequent births, additional interventions will also be required to improve women's health. This is especially important because women have disproportionately borne the cost of fertility reduction. These interventions should be oriented to reduce the risk of maternal mortality and morbidity during the gestation period and at the time of pregnancy termination, and to reduce maternal morbidity associated with the use of contraception. The average age at sterilisation among Indian women is close to 30 years, which means that they would remain exposed to the risk of disease for at least another 15 years of their reproductive life, but would have no contact with the health system which is currently oriented to provide contraceptive services to avoid pregnancies and to provide health services to mothers and children.

Conclusions

The rationale for reducing population growth through fertility reduction is to improve the social and economic conditions of people – referring both to level and distribution of socially valued outcomes. Thus, it is important to ascertain the extent to which the ongoing fertility transition has contributed to the reduction of disparities among people. To address this question, one must first demonstrate that there has been a reduction in disparities and then ascertain whether the reduction in disparities is a cause or consequence of fertility reduction.

We have found some significant disparities persisting or even increasing as fertility declines. In terms of disparities, we examined regional (between states), residential (between rural and urban), and gender disparities in infant and child mortality and education. The regional and residential disparities in the risk of infant and child death have declined over the past 20 years – alongside and to some extent as a function of fertility decline. The gender disparity in child mortality has declined in some states, but not in others. While rural-urban differences in education have declined, the regional disparity and educational attainment has remained the same and, with regard to gender, we find that girls in rural areas have not done as well as girls in urban areas or boys in rural areas.

It is very difficult to ascertain whether reduction in disparities is a cause or consequence of fertility reduction. Conditions

TABLE 10. Population Growth Rate and Female Literacy Rate in Kerala and Uttar Pradesh During 1941-91.

Period	Annual Exponential Population Growth Rate		Female Literacy	
	Kerala	Uttar Pradesh	Kerala	Uttar Pradesh
1941-51	2.08	1.12	32	4
1951-61	2.24	1.54	39	7
1961-71	2.26	1.79	54	11
1971-81	1.74	2.29	65	14
1981-91	1.34	2.27		

Note: Female literacy rates are shown for the ending year of each decade.

conducive to low fertility include low infant and child mortality and high female education at least up to the primary school level. The gender disparities in health and education are also low in states with low infant and child mortality and with high female education. A reduction in gender disparities in education and health, thus, could be included among the conditions conducive to fertility decline.

It should be noted that a tremendous progress in education was made in Kerala during the period of highest population growth rate. The annual exponential population growth rate in Kerala was over 2 percent during 1941-71 before it declined to 1.74 percent during 1971-81 (see Table 10). The female literacy rate increased from 32 percent in 1951 to 54 percent in 1971. In comparison, while the annual growth rate in Uttar Pradesh was low, it made very little progress in education. The annual exponential population growth rate in Uttar Pradesh was 1.12 percent during 1941-51, and it increased to 1.79 percent during 1961-71. The female literacy rate, however, increased from 4 percent in 1951 to 11 percent in 1971. The age distributions of population in both states were similar until 1971, but they made differential progress in improving female education. The progress made in education in Kerala, therefore, cannot be attributed to fertility decline and to changes in its age distribution. Kerala state allocated 35 percent of its resources to education and a bulk of it to primary school education, which was not the case in Uttar Pradesh. A decline in population growth rate in Uttar Pradesh, without concomitant changes in its education policies, therefore, is unlikely to improve conditions for females, especially for those living in rural areas[5].

The recent changes in the age distribution of the Indian population as a result of fertility decline should facilitate the efforts of the Government of India (GOI) to improve the well-being of the Indian people, releasing resources that might have been needed for a larger younger population. However, this demographic dividend will not translate into social justice without specific policies. Girls' education will especially suffer without rethinking how to transfer state-controlled resources from one state to another. With special measures, India has made good progress in reducing regional and urban-rural disparities in infant mortality. The changing age distribution is likely to further facilitate the reduction of these disparities, especially if centrally sponsored programmes like the MCH and CSSM direct a disproportionate share of resources to states with high infant mortality.

We are not optimistic that this levelling of may not be the case with female education. Changes in age structure are much more pronounced in states which already have achieved higher education and gender equality. For example, the potential saving in resources required for primary education is likely to be realised in states like Kerala which already have almost universal primary education. In contrast, the need for resources for primary education would continue to be high in states like Uttar Pradesh which have low levels of education and have shown very little change in the age

---

[5] The reasons why Uttar Pradesh does not allocate as much funds to education as does Kerala are quite complex and may be rooted in cultural differences between states. Low level of female education in Uttar Pradesh may not be simply a function of inadequate resources allocated to female education. Both may reflect the fact that females in Uttar Pradesh have a lower status and value than females in Kerala.

distribution. There are age as well as a gender "disparity issue" to consider. The welfare of children in the age group 0-4 is receiving some attention in all states through the centrally-sponsored health and nutrition programmes. However, in the absence of any centrally-sponsored scheme to universalise primary education, children aged 5 to 9 years do not get the same attention in all states in terms of their schooling needs. Investment in the education of this group, especially focused on girls living in rural areas would accelerate the ongoing fertility transition, and would contribute to the reduction of gender disparities. The achievement of both the goals of fertility transition as well as improvements in gender equality will, therefore, require the implementation of gender sensitive social policies in the areas of education and health.

References

Bhat, M.P. N., Nowaneetham K., and Irudaya Rajan S. 1995. Maternal Mortality in India: Estimates from a Regression Model. *Studies in Family Planning,* 26(4): 217-232.

Bhat, M.P. N. Forthcoming. Contours of Fertility Decline in India: As revealed by the 1991 Census.

Bhatia, J. C., and Cleland J. 1995. Self-reported Symptoms of Gynaecological Morbidity and their Treatment in South India. *Studies in Family Planning,* 26(4): 203-216.

Das Gupta, M., and Bhat M. P. N. 1995. Intensified Gender Bias in India: A Consequence of Fertility Decline. Working Paper No. 95-03. Center for Population and Development Studies. Harvard University. Cambridge, USA.

Dreze, J., and Sen A. 1995. India Economic Development and Social Opportunity. Oxford University Press.

Government of India, Planning Commission. 1992. Eighth Five Year Plan 1992-97 WC1. New Delhi, India.

Government of India, Registrar General, India. 1976. Census of India 1971: Social and Cultural Tables. Series 1, Part II-C (ii). New Delhi, India

Government of India, Registrar General, India. 1987. Census of India 1981: Social and Cultural Tables. Series 1, Part IV A, (Tables C1 to C6). New Delhi, India.

Government of India, Registrar General, India. 1962. Census of India 1961: Final Population Totals. Paper No. 1 of 1962. New Delhi, India.

Government of India, Registrar General, India. 1983. Census of India 1981: Key Population Statistics Based on 5 Percent Sample Data. Paper 2 of 1983. New Delhi, India.

Government of India, Registrar General, India. 1993. Sample Registration System: Fertility and Mortality Indicators. New Delhi, India.

Government of India, Registrar General, India. 1995. *Sample Registration Bulletin.* Vol. 29, No. 2. New Delhi, India.

Jain, K. 1981. The Effect of Female Education on Fertility: A Simple Explanation. *Demography,* 18 (4): 577-596.

Jain, K. 1982. Education Sector Policies, Educational Attainment and Fertility: A Case Study for India. In: R. Barlow (ed.). Case Studies in the Demographic Impact of Asian Development Projects, Ann Arbor, Michigan: University of Michigan's Center for Research on Economic Development.

Jejeebhoy, S. J. 1993. Family Size, Outcome for Children, and Gender Disparities: The Case of Rural Maharashtra. In: C. B. Lloyd, (ed.). Fertility, Family Size, and Structure: Consequences for Families and Children. New York: The Population Council.

Jejeebhoy, S. J., and Rama Rao, S. 1995. Unsafe Motherhood: A Review of Reproductive Health. In: M. Das Gupta, L. C. Chen, and T. N. Krishnan, (eds.). Women's Health in India: Risk and Vulnerability. Mumbai: Oxford University Press.

Krishnan, T. N. 1998. The Route to Social Development in Kerala. In: G. Martine, M. Das Gupta, and L. C. Chen (eds.). Reproductive Change in Brazil and India. Mumbai: Oxford University Press. Forthcoming.

International Institute of Population Sciences. 1995. National Family Health Survey 1992-93: India, and State Reports. Mumbai: India.

2

Target-Free Approach: Emerging Evidence

M. E. Khan and John W. Townsend

Introduction

The family welfare programme in India is currently passing through a transition in policy and programme organisation. During much of the last 30 years, the family welfare programme of the Ministry of Health and Family Welfare vigorously pursued a target approach to enhance contraceptive prevalence and to achieve the country's demographic goal of population stabilisation. Recently, the National Population Policy which is now tabled in Parliament, defines as its goals, among others, the achievement of a total fertility rate of 2.1 by the year 2010, and universal access to quality reproductive health care, including information and services, through the primary health care system, by the year 2015. Futhermore, it states that the *"system of setting method-wise contraceptive targets has already been replaced by decentralised participatory planning at the primary health centre level"* (MOHFW, 1997). Indeed, contraceptive targets were officially removed from the national family welfare programme in India in April 1996. Many questions remain, particularly how was this done and what have been its effects?

The target approach in India, which fixed method-specific numerical targets for contraceptive acceptance for each worker, was adopted as a management tool during the mid 1960s. Annually, the family planning performance of each state, district, primary health centre and its targets were set by the central government and passed on to the state government with limited discussion and certainly no participation at the community level. Targets for districts were allocated almost exclusively on the basis of population size, rather than existing contraceptive practice or level of unmet need. Furthermore, district magistrates were asked to involve rural development staff, unexperienced in family planning counselling or service provision, to recruit family planning users. Traditionally, half the district's target was allocated to non-health staff.

Target Approach and its Rationale

The target-based approach in India fixed method-specific quantitative targets for contraceptive acceptance for each worker. This approach was adopted as it was considered an effective tool for intensifying the level of effort of the programme, for assessing that the programme was moving in the desired direction, and placing pressure on the workers to increase the couple protection rate.

For many decades, the achievement of targets was stressed because it was quantitative, easy to monitor and because it was expected to have a direct link with reduction in fertility. However, over a period, it was observed that though the contraceptive prevalence rate was increasing (and targets were reportedly being met), the corresponding decline in fertility was lower than expected. This was attributed to acceptance of sterilisation predominantly by older and higher parity couples; poor promotion of the concept of birth spacing so that very few young, lower parity couples adopted contraception; and, inflated target achievements reported by the workers. A number of independent surveys and studies supported these findings (Jain, 1997; Khan and Cernada, 1996; Srinivasan, 1995; Visaria and Visaria, 1995).

It also became increasingly clear that in the zeal to achieve targets, inadequate attention was given to improving the quality of family planning services. Some of the major limitations of the programme that were repeatedly identified and reported, both in government policy documents and independent studies, included poor counselling, lack of informed choice for clients, and poor follow-up services for family planning acceptors. It was also observed that, target achievement had become an end in itself rather than a means to effective implementation and monitoring of the programme.

Experiences with the Target-Free Approach

Since the early 1980s, several states had been emphasising the maternal and child health approach, and giving lower priority to method-specific contraceptive targets. Notable among these localised initiatives to shift away from using targets is the experience in Tamil Nadu. In 1991-92, the Government of Tamil Nadu withdrew targets for non-health staff in two districts. By March 1992, it was clear that health department staff actually worked better without competition from other departments. In 1992-93, targets were abolished for all non-health staff. A review of annual results indicated no decline in the rates of sterilisation. However, service statistics for IUDs, pills, and condoms fell by 50 percent. State officials concluded that, when there were targets, service statistics for temporary methods were inflated (Ramasundaram, 1995).

Tamil Nadu achieved the targets fixed by the government during 1994-95 and began to effectively adopt the maternal and child health approach. This involved micro-level planning that established local targets based upon local needs, as opposed to macro-level target setting for contraceptive methods. For example, targets were set for early registration of every pregnancy, prenatal care, institutional delivery, immunisation of infants and children, and providing information, counselling and services for contraception according to each person's choice. Targets were established based on the population in the female worker's assigned area, the reproductive profile of the population and the available health infrastructure. State government officials concluded that when unhealthy competition from non-health staff was removed and targets were de-emphasised, health workers were able to provide maternal and child health care in their assigned areas more effectively (Ramasundaram, 1995).

In July 1993, the Government of India set up a committee under the chairmanship of Dr. M.S. Swaminathan to review the national family welfare programme and draft a new national population policy. The Swaminathan Committee report which was submitted in May 1994, four months before ICPD, contained far-reaching recommendations, including withdrawing the target-based approach, empowering women by increasing their opportunities to participate in the paid labour force, shifting programme emphasis from achieving national demographic targets to helping couples achieve their reproductive goals, and promoting male family planning methods to bring about a more equitable gender balance in the provision of family planning services. Many of these recommendations were reinforced by the ICPD Programme of Action.

Withdrawal of Family Planning Targets from Selected Districts in Each State

In April 1995, in an effort to a make the family welfare programme more need-based and client-oriented, the method-specific target approach was withdrawn on an experimental basis, from one or two districts in each state. The purpose of making selected districts target-free was to get empirical data on how the programme functioned without targets and to explore alternative programme management approaches. This effort was based on the premise that, if managed properly, the public system could deliver quality reproductive health and family planning services. It was hypothesised that quality services would eventually lead to greater demographic impact. Kerala and Tamil Nadu became the first two target-free states as they were already at or near achieving replacement level of fertility with crude birth rates of 17.8 and 19.2, respectively, (according to the SRS, 1996) and had experimented with alternative approaches.

A review of case studies on the implementation of the target-free approach in seven states and an analysis of programme performance, as reflected in service statistics, show that:

- In the absence of targets, district authorities as well as medical officers at primary health centres initially found it difficult to plan services and monitor the programme.
- Many strongly believed that targets were essential for getting the work done by grassroots workers. However, they subsequently realised the importance of shifting from a purely quantitative target-based approach to a client-centred, pregnancy-based approach.
- Lack of adequate infrastructure and supplies at subcentres and primary health centres continued to be a major bottleneck in improving the quality of services. It was argued that unless these facilities were improved, vacant positions of grassroots workers were filled, and the logistic support strengthened, the withdrawal of targets alone may not bring about any significant change in the access and quality of family welfare services. The need for additional financial support to improve the quality of clinical services was mentioned in various states.
- Supportive supervision was identified as a missing link in family planning services at all levels of the public service delivery system.
- Maternal and child health services in general improved in several districts after the removal of targets. However, the overall performance of family planning services dropped in most districts (Ramana, 1997; Salunke and Narvekar, 1997).
- In some states, even after declaring selected districts target-free, there was little change in the way the programme was implemented.

Introducing a Target-Free Approach at the State Level

Before the Ministry of Health and Family Welfare decided to withdraw targets in India, the experiences of districts that were made target-free during 1995-96 were reviewed. However, no lessons emerged from the review, except that in all the states the performance of the target-free districts had dropped. In the absence of coherent programme experience that was positive, views were divided on making the national programme target-free. Several states suggested the gradual withdrawal of targets over a five-year period. They argued that in the absence of proper preparatory work, the withdrawal of targets from an entire state would lead to a decline in performance, without any improvement in the quality of services. The government's decision on February 1, 1996, however, was to remove targets from the entire country beginning April 1, 1996. The states would now have to develop their own programme goals, guided by needs of the community and individual clients for quality services. Opinions were mixed regarding the government's declaration to get rid of the targets. For example, one official commented:

> *"The policy is a good idea. However, the unexpected announcement came too abruptly with little or no consultation or negotiation with states"* (Bondurant, 1997).

Another senior health administrator said:

> *"In none of the meetings the experience of target-free approach implemented in the selected districts in 1995-96 was analysed, reviewed and taken into consideration before making the entire country target-free"* (Salunke and Narvekar, 1997).

Efforts were made to sensitise state and district health authorities about the principles of the target-free approach and the procedure for assessing individual and community needs for family welfare services, and estimating expected workloads at the subcentre, primary health centre and district level. While targets were withdrawn in 1996, training of staff and other preparatory work was completed only in 1997-98. Suggestions for alternative indicators were proposed (Murthy, 1996; Satia and Subramanian,

1996; Townsend and Khan, 1996) but a widely accepted standardised set of indicators for monitoring programme performance had been elusive.

While many states had totally moved away from the target-based approach, a number of states continue to rely upon it in variant forms. For instance, in Andhra Pradesh, not only did method-specific targets continue to operate in 1996-97, but the targets changed three times during the same year. These revisions were made to meet the objective of the state population policy that replacement fertility level must be achieved by 2001. In other words, after nearly nine months had passed, the workers did not have self-determined levels of achievement for 1997-98 and were working towards a targeted level of achievement developed with the principal consideration of achieving demographic goals outlined in the state population policy (Ramana, 1997).

Similarly, in Maharashtra, district magistrates continued to closely monitor the performance of the programme. There is evidence that, based on their interest, the expected level of achievement actually increased to stimulate a higher level of performance in the family welfare programme. In Rajasthan, through a detailed survey of all the 31,000 villages, couples with an unmet need for contraception were identified. The survey also helped identify other health needs of the population. The main thrust had been on strict supervision and monitoring of the programme, issuing show cause notices to workers for not performing well and an aggressive information, education and communication campaign (Lubhaya, 1997).

Population Growth and the Target-Free Approach

The controversial decision to withdraw contraceptive targets continues to generate discussion. Some advocates of women's health have applauded the removal of targets. Others view the debate on targets as a distraction from more important issues of health financing and broader social development policy (Jain, 1997). Demographers have maintained that dispensing of targets is ineffective. In a review of policy directions, the Population Foundation of India expresses the opinion that the family planning programme needs to evolve further before targets for sterilisation and other methods of contraception are removed. They suggest that every eligible couple and every adolescent boy and girl must be informed of modern methods of contraception and the basics of reproductive health care, particularly in view of the increasing risk of HIV/AIDS (Srinivasan, 1995). While parliamentarians and politicians still like to refer to India's war against the population explosion, increasingly their public discourse points to the need for greater investment in education and the empowerment of women (Heptulla, 1997).

There has, however, been considerable concern about the detrimental effects on the population under the target-free approach. In three of the least developed states (Bihar, Madhya Pradesh and Uttar Pradesh), population control was reported to have suffered set-backs as a result of the target-free approach (Rai, 1997). In Bihar and Uttar Pradesh, it was suggested that this might have been due to the fact that the administration had been unstable and bureaucrats were constantly being shuffled. Another reason was that the efficiency of health workers and medical officers under the target-free approach was the same as it was before targets were removed.

Many have criticised both the state and central governments for their lack of vision and political will to address the larger issues of population growth and social development (Sahay, 1997). Some condemn poor performing states for not effectively using resources from the centre to support the basic minimum needs programme. However, public debate rarely advocates a return to targets; most call for better implementation of action plans (Regunathan, 1998).

In November 1997, the Population Council in collaboration with Futures Group International, the Government of Uttar Pradesh and USAID organised a national workshop to review the implementation of the target-free approach in the country. Case studies from seven states – Andhra Pradesh, Gujarat, Madhya Pradesh, Maharashtra, Rajasthan, Uttar Pradesh and West Bengal – were prepared by top programme managers in these states. These seven states taken together constitute about 60 percent of the national population. The workshop was attended by senior administrators, senior programme managers and scientists from national and international organisations. The presentations highlighted the following points:

- The process of implementing a target-free approach varied considerably across the country. In some states a target-oriented approach in some form was still in place.
- Most of the states would have preferred a gradual withdrawal of targets. It was strongly felt that states should be given more independence in planning and implementing development programmes.
- The initial 18 months of implementation (April 1996 to October 1997) was a transitional phase during which staff were not sure of the content of the target-free approach or how to monitor the programme.
- In most states, district collectors and magistrates no longer monitored the programme and as a result many health workers were not fully contributing to programme activities. However, in some states, these district administrators continued to play a key role in monitoring and implementation of the programme. The use of non-health staff for recruiting family planning cases, had, however, been discontinued.
- Declining service statistics were thought to reflect reduced pressure to inflate figures of family planning acceptors which had been observed under the target-based approach.
- The process of sensitising different levels of staff at the district and primary health centres had been completed in all states. Medical officers and workers were more conscious of the concept of quality, the importance of informed choice, the need for follow-up, continuation of contraception and reaching lower parity couples.

Improvement in maternal and child health care, early registration of pregnant women and increase in delivery by trained personnel were reported by many states (Maharashtra, Gujarat and Uttar Pradesh).

A change in the mindset of public sector workers whether district authorities, medical officers of primary health centres or grassroots workers requires time and constant effort. As grassroots workers and district and primary health centre doctors had started to appreciate the philosophy behind the target-free approach, they would hardly want to see the targets reinstated. Recommendations from the workshop drafted by senior bureaucrats from the seven states are presented in the Box on the facing page. Emerging from these recommendations is a consensus that the target-free approach should continue, and that its implementation should be a priority.

Emerging Evidence on the Effect of a Target-Free Approach

This section highlights the emerging evidence on the impact of a target-free approach on the family welfare programme[1]. Information from diverse sources suggests that it is premature to be overly concerned about the initial drop in service statistics in the absence of more reliable information from independent sources. National and state level programme managers must, however, continue to closely monitor the performance of the programme.

---

[1] Four major sources have been used: information on birth rates from the Sample Registration System (SRS) maintained by the Office of the Registrar General of India, service statistics compiled by Ministry of Health and Family Welfare, two cross sectional surveys conducted by the Population Council in Uttar Pradesh – in 1995 and 1997, and qualitative research conducted by Centre for Operations Research and Training (CORT), an independent institution and the observations of officials in different states.

Recommendations of the National Seminar on the Target-Free Approach, Lucknow, November 1997

- Monitoring indicators for the target-free approach at the national, state and district level should be continued in the present form. Information elicited should be used for corrective management action. Concurrent monitoring systems should be established.

- Decentralisation of financial powers at the state and district levels should be encouraged to facilitate the improvement of client-focussed services.

- The needs of under-served populations in urban areas must be addressed in the context of local government initiatives, introduced through a constitutional amendment.

- Resources of the private and commercial sectors should be used to provide health services to the satisfaction of the clients so that services at an affordable cost can be ensured.

- States should be encouraged to remodel service delivery structures to maximise the reach of client-centred services under the RCH programme.

- A reappraisal of the implementation of the target- free approach and its complementary RCH programme should be conducted after the experience of a full year (1997-98) is available. The discussion on related policy issues should continue between the Ministry of Health and Family Welfare, the states and other research and service organisations.

- Opinion makers, including political and social leaders, must be sensitised to the philosophy of the target-free approach.

- Long-term goals and short-term plans for improving family welfare services should be clearly stated and action plans in each state prepared accordingly. District-level discussions should be included in the development of state action plans and strategies.

Data on the birth rate from the Sample Registration System

The sample registration system (SRS) reports show that the crude birth rate continued to decline at the national level (from 28.3 in 1995 to 27.5 in 1996 and 27.2 in 1997). A review of the decline in the birth rate during the last 10 years shows that the drop in the birth rate during 1996-97 (0.9) was the highest since 1988 (Figure 1). This decline continued during 1997. A continued decline was reported even in areas of persistent high fertility, like Uttar Pradesh, from 34.8 in 1995 to 34.0 in 1996 and 33.5 in 1997 (SRS, 1998). While, total fertility is a function of the age structure, marital patterns and abortion as well as contraception, the trend is remarkable in its consistent downward direction since 1984.

FIGURE 1: Estimates of Birth Rates in India: 1981-1997 (Rate per 100 Population Per Annum)

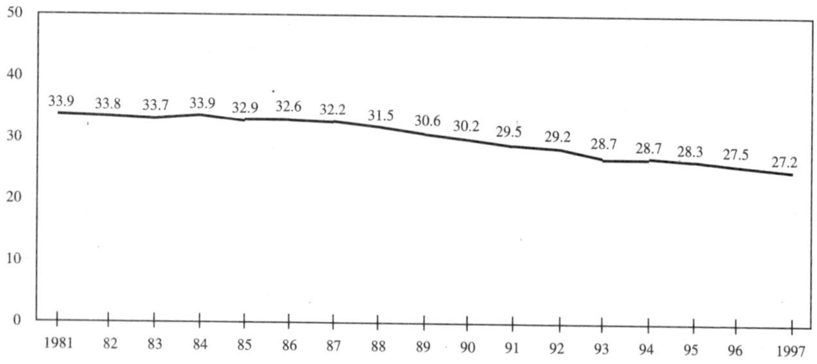

Service statistics from the Ministry of Health and Family Welfare

Recent service statistics from the Ministry of Health and Family Welfare demonstrate a reversal in the declining trend in family planning performance since the introduction of the target-free approach. Table 1 shows that while sterilisation and IUD acceptors increased in 1997-98 compared to the previous year, the number was still marginally lower (7-11 percent) than in 1995-96 (the year prior to the withdrawal of the target-based approach). Given the fact that family planning performance numbers under the target-based approach were inflated, these differences are modest. The

TABLE 1: Achievements during April-March, 1995-96, 1996-97, 1997-98

Year	Sterilisation		IUD	
	Total	% variation over 1995-96*	Total	% variation over 1995-96*
1997-98	4083,372	-7.6	6087,920	-11.1
1996-97	3861,473	-12.6	5673,537	-17.1
1995-96	4420026	—	6850524	—

Year	Oral Pills		Condom	
	Total	% variation over 1995-96*	Total	% variation over 1995-96*
1997-98	6241,211	+22.6	13858,393	-24.0
1996-97	5177,237	+1.7	13889,002	-19.6
1995-96	5088931	—	17282082	—

Source: MIES, Ministry of Health and Family Welfare

*The year after which targets were withdrawn

use of oral pills actually increased compared to 1995-96. In contrast, reported condom use continued to decline. During 1997-98 the free distribution of condoms declined by 8 percent as compared to 1996-97 and by 24 percent compared to 1995-96. However, this decline may also have something to do with the Ministry of Health and Family Welfare withdrawing support for free condom distribution. It is, however, encouraging that during 1997-98 the commercial distribution of condoms registered a 23 percent increase.

An analysis of family planning performance from 1992-93 to 1997-98 provides interesting results. In Table 2, over a period of time, the performance of all methods showed a reduction in pace and direction of change. During 1993-94, there was almost a 5 percent increase in sterilisation over the previous year (1992-93).

During the next year it was only a 1.8 percent increase. In 1995-96, a year before the country was made target-free, sterilisations registered a decline over the previous year (1994-95), and further declined by 13 percent in the first year of the target-free approach. This trend was reversed in the second year of the target-free approach by registering an increase of almost 6 percent, though it remained about 8 percent less than in 1995-96.

A similar but more obvious pattern can be seen for IUDs and pills. Condom acceptance showed a declining trend much before

TABLE 2: Trends in Family Planning Performance: 1993-94 to 1997-98 (April-March)

Year	Sterilisation		IUD	
	% variation over previous year	No. ('000)	% variation over previous year	No. ('000)
!992-93	–	4286	–	4740
1993-94	4.9	4496	26.8	6013
1994-95	1.8	4579	11.4	6702
1995-96	-3.4	4420	2.2	6851
1996-97*	-12.6	3861	-17.1	5673
1997-98*	+5.7	4083	+7.3	6088

Year	Oral Pills		Condom	
	% variation over previous year	No. ('000)	% variation over previous year	No. ('000)
!992-93	–	3001	–	15004
1993-94	43.2	4299	15.1	17283
1994-95	13.3	4873	2.4	17707
1995-96	4.4	5089	-2.4	17282
1996-97*	1.7	5177	-19.6	13889
1997-98*	+20.6	62413	-0.2	13858

Source: MIES, Ministry of Health and Family Welfare

*First and second year of target-free approach

targets were withdrawn. These data suggest that the existing delivery system was not meeting clients' expectations. Programme performance had plateaued and begun to decline, and any further increases in performance would have been difficult even if the target-based approach was continued. Clearly, the national programme was in need of major revamping to change its focus to quality care and to adopt strategies to reach couples with unmet need, particularly those living in remote rural areas.

The hasty introduction of the target-free approach contributed to a greater decline in performance than expected. However, it is encouraging to note that the declining trend has apparently been reversed.

The analysis also shows that, in absolute numbers more than three-fourths (76-82 percent) of the decline in acceptors of contraceptive methods (like sterilisation and IUD) in the first year of the target-free approach was contributed by Bihar, Madhya Pradesh and Uttar Pradesh (three of the four backward states). In terms of condom use, they contributed around 40 percent to the total national decline. Uttar Pradesh made the largest contribution to the decline in acceptors followed by Bihar and Madhya Pradesh (Table 3). Rajasthan, the fourth backward state, actually registered an increase in use for all methods.

In 1997-98, the second year of the target-free approach, the statistics showed a similar pattern. The sterilisation performance was better than the previous year (1996-97). Yet, the total number of sterilisations conducted during 1997-98 was 7.6 percent less than 1995-96.

A similar analysis of the four backward states showed that in absolute numbers, the drop in the number of sterilisations in Uttar Pradesh and Bihar taken together was more than the total drop at the national level. This indicates that these two states together contributed a major proportion of the decline in sterilisation in the country. The family planning performance of the 17 major states of India during the last three years and the percent variation in their performance during the target-free approach compared to 1995-96 are presented in Annexure I.

TABLE 3: Decline in Family Planning Performance During the First and Second Year of the Target-Free Approach Compared to 1995-96: India and Selected States.

	Decline in the First Year of the Target-Free Approach (1996-97) compared to 1995-96			
	Sterilisation	IUD	Pills	Condom
India	-558553	-1176987	+88,306	-3393080
Bihar	-183,786 (32.9)	-113,703 (9.6)	-23632	-91,360 (2.7)
Madhya Pradesh	-12,611 (-2.3)	-175,469 (14.9)	-17092	-229,473 (6.7)
Rajasthan	+32,466	+36,526	+79,053	+247,410
Uttar Pradesh	-262,905 (47.1)	-601,189 (51.0)	-50418	-1008,835 (29.26)
Three states (Bihar, M.P., U.P.)	-459302	-890361	-91142	-1329668
Four states (Bihar, M.P., U.P., Rajasthan	-426836	-853835	-12089	-1082258
Contribution of three states to national decline in performance	-82.2	-75.6		-39.1
Contribution of four states to national decline in performance	-76.4	-72.5		-31.8

	Decline in the Second Year of the Target-Free Approach (1997-98) compared to 1995-96			
	Sterilisation	IUD	Pills	Condom
India	+336654	-762604	+1152,280	-3423689
Bihar	-155,263 (46.1)	-113,132 (14.8)	-26848	-140,429 (4.1)
Madhya Pradesh	-17,745 (5.2)	-157,484 (20.6)	+40,890	-308,159 (9.0)
Rajasthan	+55,808	+55,077	+176,110	+361,793
Uttar Pradesh	-221,782 (65.8)	-229,842 (30.1)	+170,666	-741,192 (21.6)
Three states (Bihar, M.P., U.P.)	-394790	-500458	+184,708	-1189780
Four states (Bihar, M.P., U.P., Rajasthan	-338982	-445381	+360,818	-827987
Contribution of three states to national decline in performance	-117.2	-65.6	+16.0	-34.7
Contribution of four states to national decline in performance	-100.7	-58.4	+31.2	-24.2

Source: MIES, Ministry of Health and Family Welfare

Note: Figures in brackets indicate the contribution of the respective states to the total national decline in the use of specific methods.

Thus, while service statistics support the fact that the declining trend in performance has been reversed at the national level, they also indicate that some states need special attention to strengthen reproductive health services. In terms of sterilisation, the states with the greatest decline in performance were Uttar Pradesh, Bihar, Madhya Pradesh and Gujarat.

Comparison of District Level Survey Results in Uttar Pradesh

In 1995-96, Agra and Sitapur in Uttar Pradesh were the first two districts that were made target-free. Prior to this, the State Innovations in Family Planning Service Agency (SIFPSA), with technical assistance from the Population Council, conducted a detailed community-based survey in which 2,500 eligible couples randomly selected from the entire district were interviewed. Between November 1996 and January 1997, the Population Council, under its Asia Near-East Operations Research/ Technical Assistance project, supported a repeat survey in these two districts. A comparison of the survey findings showed no evidence of any reduction in contraceptive prevalence under the target-free approach. In fact, the results suggested that improvements in the quality of services may be taking place. For example, there was evidence of a modest increase in household visits by grassroots workers, an increase in family planning use among younger couples, and an improvement in prenatal care and immunisation of children. The total fertility rate in both districts had also declined (Table 4).

Indications of improvement in the quality of services was evident from the fact that grassroots workers were now giving clients a broader choice of contraceptives. As Table 4 shows, compared to 1995, a larger proportion of women were given information about various family planning methods including male contraceptives and traditional methods in 1997. Similarly, more clients were informed

TABLE 4: Selected Indicators in Family Welfare Activities in Rural Agra and Rural Sitapur

Indicator	Agra		Sitapur	
	1995	1997	1994	1997
A. Accessibility and Coverage				
Households visited by health worker in last 3 months	9.6	15.8	7.5	11.8
Pregnant women receiving Iron Folic Acid tablets	23.0	27.9	18.3	32.2
Pregnant women receiving tetanus toxoid injections	34.2	41.2	33.3	37.3
Children aged 12 - 23 months receiving:				
BCG	41.9	55.8	47.3	52.1
DPT - 3 doses	29.6	32.2	36.3	36.8
Polio - 3 doses	29.0	43.2	36.6	44.3
Percent of currently married women aged 13 - 49 currently using any family planning method (4 years)	30.5	33.6	21.0	21.1
13 - 24	11.0	17.1	11.3	8.4
25 - 39	37.0	47.9	21.8	28.2
40 - 49	48.2	48.6	38.1	34.5
Current use by method				
Male sterilisation	0.5	0.4	0.6	0.4
Female sterilisation	14.1	14.4	8.8	9.1
IUD	0.5	0.4	0.5	1.2
Pills	0.9	0.9	1.0	0.6
Condoms	4.3	2.8	2.4	1.9
Other methods	10.2	14.7	7.7	7.9
B. Quality of Care				
Percent of currently married women who had been counselled by a health worker and mentioned a particular method:				
Vasectomy	13.2	42.3	22.1	31.9
Tubectomy	70.5	64.7	79.4	69.6
IUD	34.5	36.3	27.4	47.5
Pill	31.7	52.3	27.4	78.1
Condom	37.8	62.9	28.8	63.8
Withdrawal	2.8	8.6	2.7	1.8
Safe period	2.5	15.8	3.3	6.5
C. Demand				
Unmet need for spacing	17.8	15.6	19.7	23.5
Unmet need for limiting	22.3	23.7	23.3	21.3
Total unmet need	40.1	39.3	43.0	44.8
D. Impact				
Total fertility rate per women	5.4	5.1	5.8	5.6

Source: Baseline and Endline Surveys in Agra and Sitapur District, Population Council

about how the method works and from where it can be obtained (83-93 percent in 1997 compared to 22-73 percent in 1995). While the results from these two districts are well below the desired standard, for quality, they do suggest that the changes that have occurred since 1995 are in the right direction.

Qualitative Data from Other Sources

Qualitative studies conducted in Agra district of Uttar Pradesh, and the Valsad district of Gujarat (CORT, 1998) showed that the medical officers in charge of primary health centres and grassroots workers were supportive of the target-free approach. According to them, the quality of the family planning programme had improved since the targets were abolished, particularly in terms of the coverage and care of pregnant women. Since grassroots workers were providing maternal and child health services and not merely chasing women for sterilisation, their credibility in the community had improved. The following quotes from focus group discussions with auxiliary nurse midwives reflect the general perceptions about the target-free approach and its impact on the family welfare programme.

> *"Previously, duplicate [fake] cases were made, which is not so now. Earlier, operations (sterilisations) were conducted on mothers with 4-5 children for the sake of targets, but today different family planning methods are offered to couples. Now more young couples are being contacted."* (auxiliary nurse midwife, Gujarat).

> *"Earlier (with the target approach) to achieve sterilisation targets we used to recruit several cases from outside the geographical boundary of our work area. Now in the target-free approach, we concentrate in our work area only. Earlier we had to run a lot to chase such cases. We were wasting our time for getting sterilisation case at the cost of other services.*

The target-free approach has made our work much easier. We can give our time for other services also [referring to maternal and child health]." (auxiliary nurse midwife, Uttar Pradesh).

"In the target approach, the stress was on sterilisation only, while the target-free approach is concerned with all services. Target approach used to be based on population, while target-free appoach is need-based. Now we conduct surveys to know who needs what?" (auxiliary nurse midwife, Gujarat).

"Earlier the villagers refused to talk to us. Now they themselves ask for family planning methods."(auxiliary nurse midwife, Uttar Pradesh).

Although there was no significant improvement in the quality of services provided, both doctors and workers were at least more sensitive to the need for improving the quality of the services. A senior health functionary from the Agra district said:

"It (target-free approach) is client-centred. The workers first identify community needs and then plan their work activities. Quality is given more importance than numbers."

Qualitative interviews with the community members suggested that outreach services of grassroots workers had not increased significantly, particularly in remote villages. As one woman said:

"She (auxiliary nurse midwife) is doing the same as she used to do previously."

Women informants, who reported an increase in the frequency of visits by the auxiliary nurse midwives, said:

"There is special change, they used to talk about only one thing previously (probably referring to sterilisation), now they talk about many things. They go from home to home. She is

here regularly, tells about operation, talks about operation camps. Previously someone else was coming, she never mentioned anything like this. She takes us to the doctor if there is any problem."

Over the past few years, there had also been a growing interest among donors and family planning managers to better understand the dynamics of implementation of innovations, including the target-free approach at the district level. Available data suggest that as new interventions are introduced, districts usually experience a drop of about 10-15 percent in the number of sterilisation cases. However, most see an encouraging increase in maternal and child health indicators and in the number of younger and lower parity couples served by the programme (Murthy, 1996).

Discussion and Future Challenges

Given the management tradition of more than 30 years and the current state of public sector services, is it possible to have a successful target-free programme in India? Does a target-free approach ultimately lead to poorer performance? While much remains to be done to improve the coverage and quality of family welfare services, it appears that the programme is moving in the right direction. All these findings come from independent sources, increasing the confidence in the conclusions drawn. Firmer evidence on the impact of the target-free approach will be available following the next round of the National Family Health Survey in 1998-99 and the district level surveys that are being conducted under the reproductive and child health programme in 1998. At the same time, there is an urgent need for developing, field testing and implementing new performance indicators which focus on the process and quality of services and the coverage of all components of the reproductive and child health programme.

From the earlier review, four elements emerge which merit further discussion. The first is the **background** to this particular issue. Since the first International Conference on Population and Development in Bucharest in 1974, India has been a leader in the world community in recognising the rights of individuals and couples to decide freely the number and timing of the births of their children and the means to achieve these reproductive goals. This right was reaffirmed at the ICPD in 1994 and at other international fora. The ICPD (1994) was different from previous meetings of this type in that it represented a paradigm shift away from "population control" toward a more holistic focus on community participation, the need for education, the empowerment of women, and better reproductive health for all. India was a leader in this process and this perspective is reflected in its policy documents and programme planning at the national and state levels. It should also be better reflected in implementation at the client level.

The second issue is **conceptual**. What is the difference between goals and targets? How can a state function without targets? Goals are expressions of desired achievement and they are absolutely necessary for individuals as well as for governments. They focus attention on priority issues, assist in mobilising resources, direct action to priorities and provide a standard against which progress can be measured. National and international goals for stabilising population growth are legitimate and consistent with other national goals, e.g., of universal access to primary education, reductions in infant and child mortality, access to safe water, adequate housing and security. The goals reflected in the National Population Policy are consistent with the ICPD Programme of Action and are important for giving a focus to the paradigm shift. While population stabilisation is significant globally, the ultimate goal of all development, including family welfare services, has to be the improvement of the quality of life of present and future generations. Targets, from this perspective, particularly targets for specific family planning methods, are to be viewed only as one management tool, among many, for achieving these shared goals. They are dispensable if other strategies for programme management which respond more closely to clients' needs are adopted.

The third comment has to do with **strategy**. India is undergoing profound changes in its economic structure. The country is moving from a centrally planned economy where expert committees, based upon the best available data, set the agenda for production and consumption, to a more market based economy, where clients' needs and clients' demands define the nature of goods and services. This secular economic process is accompanied by a move towards greater decentralisation in government. This shifts decision making on many issues of national importance from the centre to the states and then to the *panchayats*, and ultimately to the family and individuals. This process of decentralisation in planning and implementation is not limited to the family welfare sector, but is seen in other sectors as well.

Within this context of liberalisation, the government still plays many important roles. Government must define national goals, design service strategies, and establish standards for quality, and must be vigilant to ensure that these standards are met by public and private service providers of all types. At the same time, the government has to ensure that individuals and communities receive the benefits of development, and that all have access to the basic services they need and to which they have a right. Thus, the strategy the government selects for any programme, whether it is water and sanitation, primary education or family welfare, must be effective and responsive to individuals' needs. In this market driven context, where the client and not the service provider, defines need, assigning uniform targets to grassroots workers on how many couples in a village should use a condom or accept sterilisation services seems somewhat out of date and certainly out of touch.

But quality public services are not produced through wishful thinking or fine public pronouncements. They require **good governance and strong leadership** at all levels. Good governance demands the effective use of resources and vigilance to ensure that all the elements needed for a quality service are present, when a client seeks a service. Just as a good water system requires more than an abundant source and a thirsty population so, also, basic health and family welfare services require more than contraceptive supplies and a population with unmet needs. Good governance ensures that all the intermediate steps required for a quality service are there: accessible and well maintained facilities, competent trained staff, adequate information for clients to make decisions, counselling on how to best use the methods selected and follow up. Good governance demands local planning, continuous upgrading of facilities and services, and supervision of implementation. Good governance demands strong leadership at all levels to guarantee that resources provided by the state are directed to those who need and demand care. A renewed focus on the client, on quality and on resolving the systemic issues in implementation are clearly the key for the future of India.

Recommendations

Specifically, the following recommendations are suggested for policy makers and programme managers based upon the analysis presented above:

1) The target-free approach should continue to be implemented as a fundamental component of the reproductive and child health programme. Less than three years have passed since the introduction of the target-free approach nationwide and only about 14 months since the launch of the reproductive and child health programme, so time must be given to allow for adequate implementation. Much of the first 18 months of the target-free approach was devoted to preparatory work at the state level. Given this process, the centre should give more autonomy to the states in planning and implementation to better reflect local needs and priorities. However, states which seek to revert to the target-based approach should be assisted to move to more client-centred approaches.

2) The focus of the debate in the next few years should be on improving the processes involved in quality of information and care within client-centred target-free systems. Systemic improvements

in quality have been identified for the past 10 years as critical for both expanding the acceptability and coverage of care within the family welfare programme. Improving the quality of implementation must be the next step.

3) Investments must continue to be made in basic infrastructure, supplies and transportation. The trends in service statistics reflect a much broader problem, that is, the lack of adequate investment in the public service delivery system by many states. Unless adequate supplies of contraceptives, transportation to facilitate client-provider contact and supervision, and basic facilities are ensured, it is unlikely that the current system will be able to meet the needs of increasing numbers of men and women demanding family planning services in the future. Simultaneous efforts to incorporate private practitioners and the commercial sector will contribute significantly to the financial sustainability and impact of the programme.

Responsibility for the relative success or failure of the target-free approach should not be that of the local health workers only. Senior programme managers and middle level bureaucrats must also be accountable for its implementation. Supportive supervision is critical for maintaining the focus on quality and establishing good management practices. District magistrates should ensure that client-centred services are available in their districts.

In order to change the measures of performance, better client-centred indicators are required. The key for the next few years will be to implement sets of these indicators in one or more districts to see how they function as variables, and how they are used by health system managers to improve services. Impact of policy changes on demographic indicators like birth rate, maternal mortality rate and contraceptive prevalence rate may take some time but during the transitional period, intermediate variables need to be carefully monitored.

Process Indicators for Measuring Improvements in Quality of Services

- Increase in client-provider contact
- Increase in access and choice of contraceptives
- Improvement in counselling
- Establishing mechanisms to identify couples with an unmet need for contraception
- Increased follow-up of acceptors
- Improved supportive supervision at all levels
- Better logistics and contraceptive supply
- Change in method-mix
- Efforts made to involve NGOs and private sector

References

Asian Age. 1995. Consumer-oriented Policy for Better Family Planning. December 22.

Bondurant, T. 1997. The Introduction of Target Free Approach in West Bengal: A Case Study. Paper presented at the National Workshop on Performance of Family Welfare Programme under Target Free Approach, organised by Ministry of Health & Family Welfare, Government of Uttar Pradesh in collaboration with the Population Council and Policy Project, November 24-25. Lucknow, India.

Centre for Operations Research and Training (CORT). 1998. Preliminary Report on the Implementation of the Target-Free Approach in Two Districts. Baroda, India.

Expert Group on Population Policy. 1994. Draft National Population Policy. Submitted to Ministry of Health and Family Welfare, Government of India, New Delhi, India. May 21, 1994 (Unpublished Document).

Ghasura, N.D., Patel, B.C., and Khan, M.E. 1997. Implementing Target Free Approach in Gujarat. Paper presented at the National Workshop on Performance of Family Welfare Programme under Target Free Approach, organised by Ministry of Health & Family Welfare, Government of Uttar Pradesh in collaboration with the Population Council and Policy Project, November 24-25. Lucknow, India.

Government of India. 1997. Statement on National Population Policy, Department of Family Welfare, Ministry of Health and Family Welfare. New Delhi, India.

Heptulla, N. 1997. Role of Empowerment of Women in Population Stabilization. The Population Foundation of India, November 29. New Delhi, India.

International Institute for Population Sciences. 1994. National Family Health Survey, India 1992-93. Mumbai, India.

Jain, A. 1997. Consistency between Contraceptive Use and Fertility in India. *Demography India.* Vol. 26, No.1.

Jain, D. 1997. Population Control: Social Development is the Key. *Times of India*, New Delhi, India. September 3.

Khan, M. E., and Cernada, G. 1996. Promoting Spacing: A Step towards Paradigm Shift. In: M. E. Khan, and C. George (eds.). Spacing as an Alternative Strategy: India's Family Welfare Programme. Delhi: R. B. Publishing Corporation.

Khan, M. E. 1993. Unmet Need for Family Planning in India – Voices from the Field of Family Planning: Meeting Challenges: Promoting Choices. UK: The Pathenon Publishing Group.

Khan, M. E., and Townsend, J. W. 1998. Impact of Changes in Population Policy on the Family Welfare Programme in India. Paper presented at American Public Health Association(APHA) Conference, November 16-19. Washington D.C., USA.

Kothari, D., Maru, R., Khanna, A., Krishnan,V. K., Paliwal, S., and Abbasi, S. 1997. Vikalp: Managing Family Planning in the Post-ICPD Era, An Experiment in Rajasthan, India. Indian Institute of Health Management Research, Jaipur, India.

Lubhaya, R. 1997. Target-Free Approach for Family Welfare. A Review of Experiences in Rajasthan. Paper presented at the National Workshop on Performance of Family Welfare Programme under Target-Free Approach, organised by Ministry of Health & Family Welfare, Government of Uttar Pradesh in collaboration with the Population Council and Policy Project, November 24-25. Lucknow, India.

Measham, A., and Heaver, M. 1996. Summary of the Family Welfare Sector Assessment. The World Bank, New Delhi, India.

Mehrotra, P. K., Muralidhar, V., Khan, M. E., and Kole, S. K. 1997. Implementing Target-Free Approach in Madhya Pradesh. Paper presented at the National Workshop on Performance of Family Welfare Programme under Target-free Approach, organised by Ministry of Health & Family Welfare, Government of Uttar Pradesh in collaboration with the Population Council and Policy Project, November 24-25, Lucknow, India.

Murthy, N. 1996. Report of a Workshop on Districts Implementing Innovations in Reproductive Health. Ahmednagar, Maharashtra, India

Parekh, A. 1995. One District in Major States Exempted from FP Target. *Indian Express*. New Delhi, India. April 5.

Poornalingam, R. 1995. Family Welfare Program – MCH Approach Adoption during 1995-96. Department of Health and Family Welfare, Government of Tamil Nadu. Chennai, India.

Population Council. 1998. *UPDATES* 1-13, New Delhi, India.

Rai, U. 1997. Baby Boom May Follow Target-Free Approach. *Hindustan Times*. New Delhi, India. September 23.

Ramana, V. 1997. Target Free Approach for Family Welfare: A Review of Experiences in Andhra Pradesh. Paper presented at the National Workshop on Performance of Family Welfare Programme under Target Free Approach, organised by Ministry of Health & Family Welfare, Government of Uttar Pradesh in collaboration with the Population Council and Policy Project, November 24-25. Lucknow, India.

Ramasundaram, S. 1995. End of the Target Era. *Voices*, Vol. III, No. 2. Bangalore, India.

Regunathan, S. 1998. Doing Away with Targets. *The Hindustan Times,* New Delhi, India. March 20.

Sahay, K.B. 1997. Ghost of Malthus: On the Continuing Boom. *Asian Age*. New Delhi, India. July 11.

Salunke, S., and Narvekar, S. 1997. Target-Free Approach to Family Welfare: A Review of Experiences in Maharashtra. Paper presented at the National Workshop on Performance of Family Welfare Programme under Target-Free Approach, organised by Ministry of Health & Family Welfare, Government of Uttar Pradesh in collaboration with the Population Council and Policy Project, November 24-25. Lucknow, India.

Satia, J., and Subramanian, S. S. 1996. Suggested Indicators for the RCH Programme, International Council on Management of Population Programmes, Malaysia, and United Nations Population Fund, India.

Srinivasan, K. 1995. (ed.) Regulating Reproduction in India: Efforts, Results and Recommendations. New Delhi: Sage Publications.

Townsend, J.W., and Khan, M.E. 1993. Target Setting in Family Planning Programme: Problems and Potential Alternatives. *Demography India,* Vol. 22, No. 1: 113-125.

Townsend, J.W., and Khan, M.E. 1996. Indicators and a Management Information and Evaluation System for a Reproductive and Child Health Approach. In: A. Measham, and M. Heaver, (eds.). India's Family Welfare Program: Moving to a RCH Approach. The World Bank, Washington, D.C., USA.

Verma, L., Gupta, R. B., Khan, M. E., and Townsend, J. W. 1997. Implementing Target-Free Approach in Uttar Pradesh. Paper presented at the National Workshop on Performance of Family Welfare Programme under Target-Free Approach, organised by Ministry of Health & Family Welfare, Government of Uttar Pradesh in collaboration with the Population Council and Policy Project, November 24-25. Lucknow, India.

Visaria, L., Visaria, P., and Jain, A. K. 1994. Estimate of Contraceptive Prevalence Based on Service Statistics and Surveys in Gujarat State, India. *Studies in Family Planning.* Vol 25, No. 5: 293-303.

Visaria, L., and Visaria, P. 1995. India's Population in Transition. *Population Bulletin*. Vol. 50, No. 3. Population Reference Bureau, Washington D.C., USA.

Visaria, P., and Charu, V. 1998. India's Population Policy and Family Planning Programme: Yesterday, Today and Tomorrow. In: A. Jain (ed.). Do Population Policies Matter : Fertility and Politics in Egypt, India, Kenya and Mexico. New York: Population Council.

Annexure I: Performance of Family Planning Programme in Major States During 1997-98, 96-97, 95-96

	STERILISATION			IUD			ORAL PILLS			CONDOM		
Major States	1997-98	1996-97	1995-96	1997-98	1996-97	1995-96	1997-98	1996-97	1995-96	1997-98	1996-97	1995-96
Andhra Pradesh	600,324	513,726	520,552	293,872	298,127	282,933	254,499	242,987	242,262	599,873	613,013	820,164
Assam	11,431	16,243	23,866	36,277	32,853	34,964	31,009	18,948	24,059	29,320	33,054	49,767
Bihar	110,944	82,421	266,207	156,757	156,186	269,889	40,366	43,582	67,214	50,876	99,945	192,305
Gujarat	242,364	142,949	280,054	401,736	409,248	452,077	161,910	160,118	172,985	823,404	1015,432	1106,050
Haryana	92,722	100,292	101,257	160,862	158,450	164,010	58,713	57,392	52,869	405,447	474,862	510,813
Karnataka	395,123	384,056	381,571	368,565	376,247	345,937	154,102	157,060	150,685	323,099	358,62822	374,695
Kerala	129,408	125,126	121,539	75,931	75,372	81,613	31,182	34,614	35,806	198,636	3,511	258,728
Madhya Pradesh	366,597	371,731	384,342	615,997	598,012	797,548	552,178	494,196	511,290	1685,834	1764,520	2004,812
Maharashtra	571,189	518,897	566,168	432,681	447,598	470,580	373,441	375,534	435,341	585,988	964,771	1361,344
Orissa	123,448	134,818	146,713	240,167	192,205	206,310	106,689	108,329	99,733	252,769	379,979	437,530
Punjab	108,625	107,917	114,075	372,731	395,343	583,402	98,402	98,613	111,458	538,313	556,844	609,035
Rajasthan	224,053	200,711	168,245	223,316	204,765	168,239	301,340	204,283	125,230	837,065	722,682	519,049
Tamil Nadu	332,707	316,018	309,927	405,869	383,938	401,965	191,234	168,281	216,340	186,546	208,328	276,288
Uttar Pradesh	307,473	266,350	529,255	2035,368	1664,021	2265,210	749,015	527,931	578,349	2037,260	1769,617	2520,143
West Bengal	308,342	326,398	331,060	95,694	113,053	129,544	294,103	290,786	259,195	369,621	402,363	446,407
Himachal Pradesh	32,474	31,609	35,856	40,474	37,797	47,562	23,264	21,944	23,308	65,049	67,672	78,484
J & K	8,073	9,812	15,714	8,458	6,641	9,518	2,957	2,836	3,138	8,510	6,907	10,285
Delhi	35,050	33,178	37,833	68,000	65,711	75,480	9,615	8,522	10,258	208,075	279,038	330,650
Total Free distribution	4083372	3861473	4420026	6087920	5673537	6850524	3481534	3060314	3161162	9371587	10232752	12250832
Commercial distribution	—	—	—	—	—	—	2759677	2116923	1927769	4486806	3656250	5031250
Grand Total	4083372	3861473	4420026	6087920	5673537	6850524	6241211	5177237	5088931	13858393	13889002	17282082

Source: Year Book 1995-96 and MIES, Ministry of Health and Family Welfare

Annexture II: A Framework for Structuring Reproductive Health Indicators

Area of Measurement Level in Health System	Inputs	Coverage	Quality	Outcome Impact
Subcentre	5 6	11 13 12 13	2	–
PHC	5 7 8 16 6 9	4 12 9 13 10	2 10 15	–
District	7 8 16 9	4 11	1 10 15	3
State	7 8 16 9	4 11	1 10 15	3
Centre	7 8 16 9	4 11	1 10 15	3

Source: Townsend, J. W. and Khan, M. E. Indicators and Management Information and Evaluation System for a Reproductive and Child Health Program. In A. R. Measham and R. A. Heaver (eds). Supplement to India's Family Welfare Program: Moving to a Reproductive and Child Health Approach. World Bank 1997.

Health Services Indicators – Legend

1. Percent users provided with contraceptive choice
2. Percent users of clinical methods receiving follow-up by ANM
3. Percent couples achieving reproductive intentions
4. Percent male partners using modern contraception
5. Frequency of contact with client by health workers/functionaries
6. Stock of contraceptive supply position
7. Percent functionaries in positions filled in
8. Percent service deliveries points attended by competent personnel
9. Percent service points covered by mobile units
10. Percent IUD users screened for RTIs
11. Percent coverage of children by vaccination by type and dose
12. Percent children with growth monitoring charts
13. Proportion of pregnant women receiving 3 antenatal visits
14. Percent pregnant women receiving iron and folic acid supplement
15. Percent high risk pregnancies diagnosed and referred/serviced
16. Existence of district-level quality assurance mechanisms for MTP

3

Field Level Reflections of Policy Change

Leela Visaria and Pravin Visaria

An earlier version of his paper was first published as
'Reproductive Health in Policy and Practice: India'
by Leela and Pravin Visaria. Population Reference Bureau, January 1998.

Introduction

India has tried various ways over the past 45 years to alter the child-bearing behaviour of its people, but with limited success. However, many observers have given the country high marks for attempting a major shift in the orientation of its family planning programme since the International Conference on Population Development (ICPD). Temporal sequence does not necessarily reflect causal association. Therefore, it is important to identify the forces leading to the observed changes. While precise identification of the processes is difficult (if not impossible), and one is forced to rely on interpretation of evidence, an attempt can nevertheless be made to arrive at a tentative assessment. The primary objective of this study is to review whether and how central elements of the Programme of Action of the ICPD, 1994 are being translated into action in India.

Time constraints have forced us to focus mainly on the situation at the all India or the central government level, where the shifts in policy are most clearly articulated. At the implementation level, the study focuses on one northern state (Rajasthan), and one southern state (Tamil Nadu). The two states are at different stages of demographic transition; but they together accounted for a population of 100 million in 1991 (around 114 million as of October 1, 1998).

Annexure I reflects the diversity of situations in the two states. Within the two states, we held discussions with state level decision-makers as well as district level officers in charge of the family planning programme in two districts each. These discussions were supplemented by visits to two primary health centres in each district, as well as focus group discussions, and in-depth interviews with the service delivery personnel, and with the clients or potential users of the services in two subcentre villages within each primary health centre area. The total number of districts and primary health centres visited was four and eight, respectively. We conducted 22 focus group discussions and 21 in-depth interviews. Annexure II details the data collection work and explains the differences between the focus group discussions conducted in the two states, as well as the criteria adopted for the selection of the districts in the two states. While this study has relied on qualitative data, it is grounded in the broad familiarity of the authors with the overall situation.

Background

In 1952, India became the first country in the developing world to initiate a state-sponsored family planning programme to lower the country's birth and population growth rates. Over the past 28 years, the birth rate has declined throughout the country, albeit at a varying pace in different regions. India's birth rate has declined from about 40 per 1,000 population in the 1960s, to 28 in 1995-96. On the other hand, the population has continued to grow at, or around 2 percent per annum since the 1960s, because of the decline in the death rate. The population has more than doubled from 439 million in 1961 to an estimated 930 million in 1996, and could well be over 1.5 billion before it eventually stabilises some time during 2056-61.

Since the mid-1960s, attempts have been made to integrate the Indian family planning programme with other programmes, such as minimum needs, maternal and child health, and child survival and safe motherhood. The minimum needs programme, initiated in the early 1970s, sought to link family welfare and primary health care with efforts to alleviate poverty in the country. The maternal and child health programme received a boost after the adoption of the National Health Policy by Parliament in 1983. As part of the overall strategy for reducing infant and child mortality, the universal immunisation programme was launched in 1985-86 to control vaccine preventable diseases. The child survival and safe motherhood programme was begun in 1992 to accelerate the decline in infant and child mortality and reduce maternal mortality. Around the same time, an effort was initiated to pay special attention to 80 districts, where the 1981 census data had indicated relatively high levels of fertility through the social safety net programme. Despite these efforts to integrate family planning with health and family welfare programmes, the demographically driven goals of reducing the birth rate and the rate of population growth have continued to dominate monitoring and assessment.

In fact, the national goal of achieving a birth rate of 25 per 1,000 population was translated into number of acceptors of different contraceptive methods to be enrolled in different states, districts, towns and even villages. The pursuit of targets largely overlooked the 'cafeteria' approach of the programme, or the concern for client choice, and the provision of a wide range of services to suit the needs and preferences of the people.

Impetus to Reorient the Family Planning Programme

Since the late 1970s and early 1980s, programme managers have recognised the need to reorient the family planning programme in favour of reversible methods. Despite the substantial increase in the reported number of users of reversible methods in several states of the country, the birth rate did not seem to decline. As a result, there was some rethinking regarding the quality of both the data on the number of acceptors of different methods of family planning, and gradually, on the demographically driven goals themselves. There was mounting concern about the quality of the services provided to the people, which evolved into a commitment to provide more comprehensive reproductive and child health services. The shift in emphasis was marked by the abolition, in April 1996, of method specific family planning targets throughout the country.[2]

Several factors, such as the recognition of the very slow decline in the birth rate in most states, lack of motivation at all levels in the delivery of family planning services, concerns raised by women's groups and other non-governmental organisations regarding the narrow range of services offered, the programme becoming target-driven with little concern for women's needs, and the climate created by the ICPD, have all been to a greater or lesser extent responsible for bringing about the shift in India's approach. In addition, after the 1991 Census, the government also set up two independent committees to review the population situation and advise it on policy changes. The first commission was headed by Mr. K. Karunakaran, the Chief Minister of Kerala. The second, was an expert group chaired by Dr. M.S. Swaminathan. The government may not have officially acknowledged their recommendations, but some have found their way into the reoriented family planning programme.

Changes Introduced in the Indian Family Welfare Programme Since 1995

Target-free approach

In April 1995, the Department of Family Welfare proposed making one or two districts from each of the major states target-free on an experimental basis. The states selected the districts to be freed from

---

[2] During the previous year, targets were removed from one or two districts in most of the major states and from all the districts in the two southern states of Kerala and Tamil Nadu, where fertility had come down to replacement level.

method specific targets in consultation with officials from the centre; in most states, the districts performing better were selected. A year later, in April 1996, the government decided that the entire nation would become target free. There were apprehensions that this decision was made without adequate discussion on the strategies that would replace the old system, or an assessment of the experience of the selected target-free districts.

At the policy level, the shift to the target free approach and decentralised planning was recognised as necessary first steps to improve the quality of services. There was, however, a great deal of skepticism and confusion about the target-free approach, especially among programme implementers. Questions remained: If no targets were to be imposed, how would worker performance be evaluated? What would happen if family planning performance declined?

Because of these concerns, during 1996-97, many states imposed targets, using the previous year's centrally assigned targets as a base. The only change was that the target setting exercise emanated from the state, or the district level, rather than from the centre. In the next section, we shall examine in some detail the extent and the manner in which the target-free approach is now being implemented in the states of Rajasthan and Tamil Nadu.

Shift to Reproductive and Child Health

The removal of targets was a precursor to the effort to provide the services of a gynaecologist at some of the district or subdistrict hospitals, which are designated as the first referral units, so that broader health problems of women would get addressed. The village level health workers are expected to direct women needing examination and health care to the subdistrict or district level hospitals. There is, however, a scarcity of trained gynaecologists, willing to work in *taluka* (block level) towns. Efforts are being made to implement the idea through the reproductive and child health programme formally launched in October 1997. There are also plans to enlist private sector gynaecologists who will be contracted to visit designated primary health centres on specified days.

The reproductive and child health programme envisages changes not only at the policy level, but also at the management and implementation levels. These include: (a) encouraging states to remove, in a phased manner, the incentive payments to both providers and acceptors of certain family planning methods; (b) shifting financial priorities from building more infrastructure to increasing sustainability and utilisation of existing facilities; and, (c) expanding service access by encouraging NGOs and the private sector to fill gaps in the public sector services.

Programme level changes include: (a) district-level planning and monitoring that is more responsive to local needs; (b) improved quality of care and increased client focus; (c) expanded community involvement and responsibility for female health workers, through the decentralised system of governance (*panchayats*); and, (d) an improved referral system for health care seekers. At the service delivery level, the changes include revitalisation of the existing network of rural health facilities through better supplies of drugs and equipment, training and information and counselling for clients and communities (World Bank, 1997).

While efforts such as information, education and communication, training and programme monitoring are nationwide, other interventions are only in selected districts, based on the existing institutional capacity and reproductive health needs of the population in the blocks or subdistrict units.[3] In addition, focused interventions are planned in 24 districts or cities identified as having weak social indicators, in order to increase access to health care, for disadvantaged groups such as scheduled castes and tribes and the urban poor.

Besides addressing the issues of quality and informed choice, the reproductive and child health programme provides 'a vehicle

---

[3] The draft outline of the Fifth Five Year Plan (1974-79) attributed the failure to attain the targeted decline in the birth rate largely to the highly ambitious targets set earlier.

for continued policy dialogue; continuing evaluation and reviews; and significant flexibility for implementing recommendations of the evaluations and reviews through annual and state-specific modifications to implementation plans.' While the details of the programme can be debated, it does address several issues that were neglected in the family welfare programme.

It is too early to assess the impact of the activities initiated under the programme. However, while examining its implementation in Rajasthan and Tamil Nadu, we have considered not only the actual changes which have been brought about, or new activities that have been launched, but also the processes which have been initiated for introducing changes in the programme and strengthening ongoing activities.

Family Welfare Programme in Rajasthan and Tamil Nadu

In order to assess the impact of the 'paradigm shift', we have tried to understand the changes that have occurred, or have been initiated, in Rajasthan and Tamil Nadu. Our focus has been on two major changes – the target-free approach and the introduction of the reproductive child health programme.

Implementation of the Target-Free Approach

While the target free approach is a welcome first step in India's shift to a comprehensive reproductive and child health programme, changes till date appear unclear. In order to understand how the target free approach works on the ground, we looked at: 1) how the work load of the health workers is decided; 2) how records are maintained; 3) what activities receive emphasis during the review meetings at all levels; 4) what are the perceptions of the health workers about the shift in focus; and, 5) what changes have the clients perceived in the quality and range of services.

The target-free approach was introduced in the entire country in 1996, and the absolute number of acceptors of all methods of family planning (except oral pills) declined during 1996-97. The decline was most evident in the reported number of condom users, and to a lesser extent, in the number of new IUD acceptors, presumably because the pressure to distort the statistics had disappeared. However, during 1997-98, the acceptance of all methods improved, thereby allaying the fears of many skeptics that contraceptive prevalence will decline if targets are removed.

Interestingly, no decline was registered in the number of acceptors in Rajasthan, where removal of targets made little difference to the steady increase in the annual acceptors of all methods of family planning. In Tamil Nadu, even though couples are reportedly highly motivated to accept family planning after two or three children, the number of acceptors of all methods of family planning declined between 1995 and 1997.

Shift in Focus of Programme

Following the introduction of the target-free approach, the experience of some states and districts suggests that efforts are indeed being made to change the focus of the family planning programme. In Tamil Nadu, emphasis is on providing more comprehensive health care to couples. In the past seven to eight years, immunisation services, antenatal check ups, visits of the health workers to the villages, and mothers' meetings to discuss issues ranging from benefits of balanced diet during pregnancy, to advantages and disadvantages of various contraceptive methods have all increased significantly. As was noted by a respondent during an in-depth interview:

> *"There has been a tremendous change. Earlier, people used to be scared of using contraceptives, but now, the nurse informs and explains to us in detail about them during the mothers' meetings, so people are no longer scared to use them. Earlier, even the government neglected this aspect and did not care about explaining the methods."*

On the other hand, discussions with health workers and other officials in the primary health centres in Rajasthan suggest that the last quarter of 1996-97 accounted for a much larger number of acceptors of sterilisation than other quarters. It is unclear whether this reflects the needs of the workers to fulfil annual targets, or the fact that women are free from agricultural work at this time, or that women prefer to get sterilised in the winter months. It is likely that all these factors have contributed to some extent.

At the same time, other health needs of women, such as gynaecological problems and safe abortions, are yet to be addressed by the programme. Health workers in both Rajasthan and Tamil Nadu reported that some women do seek help from them for problems of excessive bleeding during menstruation or white discharge, but they invariably asked the women to go to the government hospitals. Some auxiliary nurse midwives gave iron and folic acid tablets to these women although these are unlikely to cure infections. During a focus group discussion in Rajasthan, one woman said:

> *"Women who have a problem of excessive white discharge, also complain of ache/pain in arms and legs and of headache. They also experience excessive bleeding during the periods and feel weak. When village women experience such problems, and cannot cope any longer, then they go to private doctors because the nurse has no medicines to treat such problems."*

Abortion services are available only at the district hospitals in Rajasthan. In Tamil Nadu, some of the upgraded primary health centres do provide abortion services but women continue to depend primarily on the private sector.

Basis for Deciding the Workload of Grassroots Health Workers

During our discussions, it was quite evident that in both the states, family planning targets are not prescribed from the centre, but are determined at the local level, with the help of an improved version of the former Eligible Couples Register. As an auxiliary nurse midwife from Rajasthan said during a focus group discussion:

> *"First, we survey the village to prepare the survey register with all the information about the women, their name, age, number of children, etc. We also find out about their unmet need for family planning. If we find that they already have at least one girl and one boy, then we suggest they accept the operation (sterilisation). For those who have only one small child, we suggest copper-T."*

The new Community Needs Assessment Manual provided to the health workers is expected to help identify the unmet need for family planning, to segment the couples in terms of parity and the number of surviving children, and to determine the requirements of different contraceptives and medicines or drugs. It also provides a basis to monitor the performance of the health worker. Instead of giving uniform targets to each worker, the targets are determined on the basis of actual information. An auxiliary nurse midwife in Rajasthan reported:

> *"The programme is not target free. The targets are still there, except that we set the targets ourselves. We set them based on the unmet need of our area."*

However, the information collected varied considerably in the two states. Since 1996, Rajasthan has adopted a survey format, designed by the Indian Institute of Health Management Research (IIHMR), Jaipur, in which information is collected on the unmet need and other ancillary characteristics. The primary health centres in each district used this information to determine the method specific contraceptive targets for the health workers.

In Tamil Nadu, the district-specific estimate of the current birth rate (based on a 1995 survey, with a sample large enough to provide district-level estimates) was applied to the subcentre population covered by the village health worker, to arrive at the number of births likely to take place in her area. This provided a basis for the number of pregnancies that the health worker would have to register in a year. While providing services to pregnant mothers, the health worker was expected to inquire about the number of children born, and surviving, to determine the method best suited for her, and to encourage her to accept that method. An auxiliary nurse midwife from the state, during a focus group discussion said:

> *"When we enumerate the eligible couples in our population, we ask a question about the number of living children, and on that basis, we advise women with one child to use a temporary method, and those who have more children, to undergo sterilisation."*

The family planning workload of the health workers is determined differently in both states, but the workload is translated into targets, and the health workers are expected to achieve them. The health workers' own involvement in determining the workload is minimal. Client segmentation is done on the basis of the number of surviving children.

Record Keeping

The target free approach manual suggested formats which were expected to simplify record keeping. However, in both states, most health workers seemed to be preoccupied with keeping their records updated and faced difficulties in doing so. One auxiliary nurse midwife in Rajasthan complained:

> *"there is so much of record keeping work, that we do not get any time for our practical (field) work."*

They seemed more confused and found record keeping more difficult than before. It is likely, that they had become used to maintaining the records designed for the target-oriented approach. In both Rajasthan and Tamil Nadu, the health workers indicated that: (1) the number of registers had increased; (2) there was a lot of duplication; and, (3) they had to seek help of other more educated family members, or their supervisors. In their opinion, the information that they were required to collect had little relevance to understanding the needs of the clients or planning their own schedule of work. Most health workers, therefore, felt that record keeping was a waste of their time. An auxiliary nurse midwife from Rajasthan said:

> *"During training we were taught about malaria and how to give injections. Now, we are expected to do statistical work. If we knew before hand, what this job was all about, perhaps we would not have come for it. A middle school pass (upper primary level) auxiliary nurse midwife does not know how to calculate percentages, and tally other statistics, but we have to somehow manage."*

In Bharatpur district of Rajasthan, health workers reported that they were not able to cope with the 'paper work'. In Dausa district, record keeping is computerised by IIHMR, but health workers seem to be equally confused and found the task too complex. We were told that some workers had stopped using the computerised records and had gone back to the old manual system.

Health workers in both the districts of Tamil Nadu also complained about the increase in the paper work. However, they reported that they could do the work on their own. Perhaps, the higher average number of years of schooling, and longer work experience might explain why health workers in Tamil Nadu faced fewer difficulties in maintaining records. All the same, they found little time for statistical work during week days. A nurse stated:

> *"We do it (record maintenance work) mostly on Sundays. Family members complain about it, saying that even on holidays we are busy with paper work. But during the week days, we have many other duties. We also have to attend to the delivery cases."*

Monitoring and Supervision

The experiences of Tamil Nadu and Rajasthan also varied in the frequency of contact between the health workers and their superiors, the emphasis on various activities and the evaluation of their performance.

Health workers in Tamil Nadu met the medical officers, on an average, six times in a month, either at the primary health centres or when the doctors visited the field. The state government was concerned about the relatively high infant mortality and therefore monitored infant deaths very closely. Consequently, pregnancy care through antenatal visits, immunisation, etc. were greatly emphasised.

In Rajasthan, meetings between health workers and the medical officers were held once a month as in the past, and the auxiliary nurse midwives were asked about sterilisation performance and spacing methods, especially IUD. The emphasis continued to be on family planning performance. However, in one district, concurrent evaluation was being carried out, and so the performance of the workers was monitored quite regularly.

Overall, targets continue to be assigned, although they are now determined at the district, or the primary health centre level. Clients' needs are rarely considered. Also, the health workers' involvement in determining the targets is minimal. All the same, the workers feel that they are now given 'correct' or realistic targets. Strategies to involve village level groups, women's groups and *panchayat* representatives are yet to be evolved and implemented. Discussions with functionaries at various levels as well as observations during the visits to the subcentres and primary health centres do suggest that attempts are being made to redress several limitations of the old approach. Efforts are also being made to broaden the range of services, and each service is viewed as important.

In Tamil Nadu, the training in these new approaches was initiated for workers of both the primary health centres and the subcentres, and included neglected topics such as quality of care, informed choice, assessment of community needs, and participatory learning and awareness building. Most auxiliary nurse midwives in both the districts of Tamil Nadu went through the training and seemed quite happy with the range of issues covered in the six-day training course.

In Rajasthan, efforts are underway to organise training programmes. An agency has been identified to coordinate the training activities and the modules are being prepared in the local language.

Provision of Reproductive Health Services

While the need for providing comprehensive reproductive health services is recognised, there are few replicable models for providing such services. Doubts have been raised that implementation of the reproductive and child health approach requires skills and training beyond the present capacity; that the upgradation of facilities and services at the peripheral level is unrealistically high under the current conditions in rural India; and that contraceptive needs will be ignored. Further, some estimates made of the likely costs of expanding services suggest that they will be formidable (Rama Rao, Townsend, and Khan, 1996).[4]

Our focus group discussions with health workers and the clients centred around four major components of reproductive health: family planning, maternal care, abortion services and treatment for reproductive tract infections (RTI). Understandably, the perceptions of the health workers and the clients differed on certain issues.

Family Planning Services

We tried to ascertain from the health care providers and the potential acceptors, whether the choice and range of contraceptives available now was different compared to when method-specific targets were laid down for the workers. In both Rajasthan and Tamil Nadu, the

---

[4] Rama Rao, et al. have worked out the cost of RTI case management under the alternative load of infection and level of utilisation scenarios. Even under the low infection scenario, with the lowest level of utilisation, the estimated annual cost at the block PHC level, worked out to a minimum of Rs 1.8 million (or US $ 51,000). The costs are staggering, and we need to think of ways to reduce costs without sacrificing quality of care (Rama Rao, op.cit).

workers indicated that they followed the client segmentation approach, and motivated women who have two or more children to accept sterilisation. In Rajasthan, women with one surviving child were encouraged to accept IUD, oral pills or condoms, in that order. If women did not like to use the IUD, they were offered a choice of oral pills, and then condoms. During one of the focus group discussions with clients in Rajasthan, we heard conflicting views. We have reason to believe, however, that when the relationship between the villagers and the auxiliary nurse midwife was not cordial, both sides accused each other:

> *"There are no contraceptives available in the village – not even with the nurse. She does not tell us anything about spacing methods."*

> *"We have even heard that the nurse sells the condoms and the pills that she gets for free distribution from the government to a shopkeeper."*

In Tamil Nadu, the workers reported that for the past four or five years, they did not have to motivate couples or women to accept family planning. They came on their own to seek postpartum sterilisation. During a focus group discussion with clients in Tamil Nadu, one woman said:

> *"We make a decision (to get sterilised) ourselves. My husband did not want me to get sterilised. I asked the nurse for her views and suggestions. She advised me to go in for sterilisation since I did not want to have any more children, and I went in for it."*

Sometimes, women with only female children, or with just one child, wanted sterilisation and the health workers had to dissuade them. During the weekly mothers' meetings in the village, the health workers reportedly spent a few hours discussing and describing the various methods of contraception that are available through the programme, their relative advantages and shortcomings. Women seek information about methods such as rhythm, injectables and traditional methods that they may have heard about from other sources. Many clients in Tamil Nadu were quite positive about the services provided by the health workers in their area:

> *"The nurses insert loop, give tablets. They advise us to accept a family planning method. They also tell us about the advantage and side effects of each method."*

Rajasthan and Tamil Nadu have adopted very different approaches regarding incentive payment, or the compensation scheme, as it is called. The scheme of cash compensation for the loss of wages to the acceptors of sterilisation and IUDs was modified in 1996-97 and gave flexibility to the states to apportion this amount among various items of expenditure incurred for providing the services. As a result, Rajasthan completely withdrew cash payment and the provision of free transport and other services to the acceptors. Instead, it used the money to meet the expenditure on transport and paying the private doctors who performed sterilisations, as well as on drugs and dressing material, etc. The acceptors of sterilisation complained about not receiving the cash payments. At the same time, they were categorical that they would accept sterilisation with or without payment. In a focus group discussion held in Rajasthan, one woman noted:

> *"Earlier, the women who got operated upon (sterilised) were given some cash which helped them during recuperation. But now, nothing is given, and the poor women can't take care of their post-operative requirements of more nutritious food or medicines."*

Tamil Nadu, on the contrary, decided to continue cash compensation to the acceptors of sterilisation, the rationale being that the amount would be used to buy more nutritious food after the surgery. The state government also continues to provide transport after the operation. Officials feel that the government cannot abruptly withdraw payment or the facilities that it has provided for so many years. As one village health nurse put it:

> *"It is good that the incentive payment is continuing. In fact, it should be increased. Rich people do not need, and expect, cash payment, but poor people expect money. If it is increased for the poor families, it will be good."*

Maternal Care

On paper, maternal care has for long been an integral part of the family welfare programme. Yet, only very minimal services, such as tetanus toxoid injections and iron and folic acid tablets are provided during pregnancy. Health workers in Tamil Nadu reported that in the past, the monthly family planning targets did not allow them to concentrate on maternal child health services, because they were always busy motivating clients to accept family planning. As one of them said:

> *"But now the pressure is off, and we are able to inquire about women's health, their children's health. We are also better accepted in the community. People do not identify us only as family planning workers, but consult us about ailments of all family members."*

Health workers in the state follow the pregnancy based approach and are now able to register pregnancies quite early. Many women report the pregnancy during the third month on their own to the health worker, and inquire about tetanus toxoid injections and iron and folic acid tablets. The health worker checks their nails, hands, eyes etc. to diagnose anaemia and starts giving the tablets from the fifth month, or even earlier. On an average, women contact the health worker six to seven times during their pregnancy. Women also report that the health worker gives them dietary advice. Only a few health workers reported having weighing scales in working condition, and having used these to measure weight gain during pregnancy. Other services, like checking the blood pressure or haemoglobin, etc. are not yet available.

During a focus group discussion in Tamil Nadu, clients reported a significant change in the quality of services:

> *"Earlier the health workers used to advise us not to feed the baby soon after delivery. They also did not allow [us] to wash the baby soon after birth. They did not weigh the child. But now they ask us to feed the baby immediately after birth, wash it, and the baby is kept besides the mother. It is also weighed. Now baby care and mother care is much better than before."*

Health workers in Tamil Nadu are aware of the fact that there is a drive in the state to lower infant mortality and that they, therefore, have to attend to pregnant women and also provide the required immunisation to the infants. A high degree of concern for lowering maternal mortality is also visible at all levels. Health workers encourage every pregnant woman to deliver in an institution rather than at home.

The situation in Rajasthan is somewhat different. There is an overall feeling among both health workers and clients that the coverage of antenatal services has improved as compared to the past when the percentage of women receiving tetanus toxoid injections was reportedly quite low. The workers of the integrated child development services scheme help health workers identify pregnant women in the community. The supply of iron and folic acid tablets has improved but it is, however, unclear as to how many women actually take the tablets. During one of the focus group discussions, a client said:

> *"When it is convenient to her, the nurse gives us the red iron tablets. Some women eat them, and some carry them home, and put them away."*

The majority of deliveries in Rajasthan take place at home. Health workers have been distributing safe delivery kits to pregnant women but the women gave somewhat conflicting reports about their use. According to some women, the traditional birth attendant is expected to bring the kits when she comes for the delivery but they could not remember whether they received the kit or where they kept it. It appears that the traditional birth attendant rarely brought the kit.

Abortion Services

Safe abortion services are not available either in Rajasthan or Tamil Nadu because these services require a trained gynaecologist. Specialists are not easily available to work in public sector hospitals or health centres in rural areas or even small towns. Consequently, most women who want an abortion go to private practitioners in district towns as is clear from the following quote:

> *"There is no facility for abortion in our village. If any woman wants to get an abortion done, she has to go to the private hospital in Bharatpur, where they charge Rs 1,000 (approximately US$ 25) for it. This facility is not available even in the block-level hospital."*

Women in Tamil Nadu report that the charges for abortion services tend to be quite high and depend upon the duration of pregnancy. According to some women, the fees are determined at the rate of Rs 300 ($7.50) for every month of pregnancy. However, Tamil Nadu has a good public transport network and women can return the same day after undergoing an abortion in a nearby town. The situation in Rajasthan is different. Even when women can afford to pay a private practitioner, access to services is a problem.

In Tamil Nadu, according to state officials, nearly 40 percent of the doctors in the primary health centres are women, who provide abortion services at a very reasonable cost. We could not verify this report, but these doctors are permitted private practice after their official duty hours. Although they cannot officially set up private nursing homes, some of them may have set up private clinics at home or may be using the facilities of the primary health centre, such as labour rooms or operation theaters, to perform abortions. A client in Tamil Nadu reported:

> *"Government doctors perform abortions at their private clinics. Once, when I went to a government hospital, the doctor asked me to come to her home. She said that she will not perform the abortion in the government hospital. I, therefore, had to go to her house. She charged me Rs 300. We cannot afford to spend that much."*

Also, according to some women, if a pregnant woman tells the health worker that she wants an abortion, the health worker offers to take her to a private doctor, provided that she accepts some method of family planning. Again, it is difficult to verify such statements and whether they reflect the past, or the present, or both.

Services for Reproductive Tract Infections

Very few public sector institutions in India offer treatment for reproductive tract infections. Our discussions with the women, and the health workers indicated that many women do seek help from the health workers and complain about some of their obvious problems, such as white discharge and excessive bleeding. Apart from advising them to go to a private practitioner in the town nearby, the health workers are unable to do much. One client in Tamil Nadu said: *"The nurse does not help us with such problems and does not have medicines for them (RTIs). She just gives medicine to the children."*

Comment

The primary objective of this study was to review whether and how the central elements of the 1994 ICPD Programme of Action were being translated into action in India. Such an assessment, less than four years after the ICPD, is in one sense somewhat premature, particularly for a country like India where the family planning programme has been operating since 1952. It is not at all easy to revamp an extensive and elaborate infrastructure that has been built up to provide maternal care, child health, and family planning, services. Yet, India has recognised that a major shift is needed in the family planning programme to rid it of the target-oriented approach and base it on the needs of the clients. The in-depth interviews and focus group discussions held with programme officials, as well as with clients in Rajasthan and Tamil Nadu, do indicate that efforts are underway to initiate programmes and processes to change the focus of the programme.

The study has examined issues such as how the work load of the health workers is determined; whether the programme has become more responsive to the needs of the clients; and whether the range and quality of services have improved. The focus group discussions held with the service providers indicate that the family planning work load of the grassroots level workers, in the post-target-free period, is decided on the basis of the number of living children of the couples. Both states follow a 'client segmentation' approach to determine the health workers' work load. As a general rule, workers encourage couples with two or more children to accept sterilisation and those with fewer children, or no children, to accept reversible contraceptive methods. Also, the health workers still have to report their performance in quantitative terms, but they say they are no longer reprimanded for not meeting the targets. The clients also perceive that the pressure to accept sterilisation has lessened, and that the health workers inform and encourage couples to accept reversible methods.

Further, interviews and focus group discussions with the clients indicated that in Tamil Nadu, immunisation services, prenatal check-ups, visits of health workers to the villages, and mother's meetings to discuss wide-ranging issues have all significantly increased in the last seven or eight years, and health workers also enjoy a better status. In Rajasthan, improvements have begun, but at a slower pace than in Tamil Nadu.

Facilities for abortions, (although legal in India since 1972) and for the treatment of reproductive tract infections are yet to be initiated in primary health centres in both states. Safe abortion services require trained doctors who are usually not available in small towns and rural areas. As a result, most women seeking abortion go to private practitioners who charge high fees. Similarly, very few public health centres offer screening or treatment of reproductive tract infections. If women complain of symptoms, nurses can only advise them to go to private practitioners. Provision of these services at the primary health centres will require training of the grassroots level workers, and resources to set up clinical and other support systems and assured referral services. The tasks are immense but a beginning seems to have been made.

Resource Flows for the Indian Family Welfare Programme

An important issue relevant to the implementation of the ICPD Programme of Action is the extent to which the government has committed additional resources for the reproductive and child health programme.

In evaluating any data on the subject, one must remember that resource allocation is also a function of the extent of buoyancy in government revenues and its tax-raising capacity at any given time. As opposed to the concept of the welfare state, there is today greater reliance on market forces and a greater role for the private sector in achieving more cost effective solutions without increasing the size of the bureaucracy. However, the need for effective interventions to improve the performance of the social sector, education and health, and restrain the rate of population growth is widely recognised as being critical to the success of any measures aimed at strengthening the economy. Accordingly, efforts are being made to mobilise resources from within and outside the country to upgrade social sector institutions both in the public sector, as well as in the private, or the NGO sector.

Data from the Ministry of Health and Family Welfare

The family welfare programme has always been a centrally sponsored programme where the central government is expected to meet the cost of all the (approved) initiatives to achieve its goals. Accordingly, we have focused first on the total expenditure disbursed on the programme as reported by the Department of Family Welfare, Ministry of Health and Family Welfare. These data, summarised in Annexure III, reportedly also include expenditure by state governments and union territories.

The five year plans broadly lay down the financial allocations for each sector of development. Within the plan period, the actual budgetary allocation is influenced by the need to calibrate the resource allocations for strengthening the performance of different sectors in the light of internal and external developments. During the Eighth Plan period (1992-97), against a plan allocation of Rs 65 billion (1.5 percent of the total proposed outlay of Rs 4,341 billion), the actual expenditure (Rs 82.67 billion) exceeded the allocated amount by 27 percent in nominal terms. Expenditure on family welfare reported by the Ministry thus constituted between 0.18 and 0.21 percent of the total GDP of India.

During 1993-94, the Department of Family Welfare had succeeded in raising the per capita expenditure on its activities by almost 26 percent; subsequently, this pace could not be maintained. The central government's budget allocation for the family welfare programme for 1998-99 (Rs 24,894 million) exceeded the budget allocation for 1997-98 (Rs 18,294 million) by 36 percent.

The increase in the budget allocation for the Department of Family Welfare during 1998-99 is possible probably because of the successful negotiation of external assistance of the order of US $960 million for the reproductive and child health programme from the World Bank (about $490 million), the European Community ($250 million), United Nations Population Fund ($100 million), United Nations Children's Fund ($121.5 million), and other bilateral donors including the USAID.

For the Ninth Plan period (1997-2002) the Department of Family Welfare has asked the Planning Commission for an allocation of Rs 167.5 billion from domestic budgetary support and Rs 53 billion from external assistance. If this request is accepted, the resources available for family welfare (Rs 220.5 billion) will exceed the actual expenditure of Rs 76.75 billion during the Eighth Plan period (1992-97) by 187 percent.

Ministry data on expenditure on family welfare are separately available for sub-programmes or activities. These data provide an indication of the shift in the emphasis on different elements of the family welfare programme. However, before examining these details, it is appropriate to note here that data from this Ministry seem to differ from that compiled by the Department of Economic Affairs, Ministry of Finance. These data have also been summarised in Annexure III.

Data from the Ministry of Finance

Each year, the Ministry of Finance also compiles a comprehensive summary of the revenue, sources of revenue and capital expenditure of the central government, state government and union territories. While family welfare is identified as a separate social service, expenditure on medical services, public health, water supply and sanitation are grouped together. In view of the close links between water supply and sanitation on the one hand, and public health and need for medical services on the other, the combined head is a good approximation to the total health expenditure by the government. Unfortunately, the expenditure by institutions of local self-government are excluded; but this is believed to be relatively small.

The juxtaposition of the Finance Ministry estimates of family welfare expenditure with the corresponding estimates of the Ministry of Health and Family Welfare, highlights some interesting differences. For the three years 1992-93 to 1994-95, the estimates are quite close. For 1995-96, however, the Finance Ministry estimate exceeds the other. For 1996-97, the Finance Ministry relied only on

exceeds the other. For 1996-97, the Finance Ministry relied only on the revised estimates and not on the audited figures of actual expenditure.

The advantage of Finance Ministry data lies in the basis they provide for estimating total expenditure on health and family welfare. Family welfare expenditure formed between 11 to 13 percent of the total expenditure on health and family welfare. More importantly, however, these data suggest that over the five year period between 1992-93 and 1996-97, the per capita expenditure on health and family welfare together had risen by 70 percent, faster than the average annual rate of inflation (8.4 percent). In dollar terms, it rose from $ 3.49 during 1992-93 to $ 5.13 during 1996-97 or by 47 percent (partly because of a very slow depreciation of the Indian rupee). These figures have been presented here mainly for international comparisons despite the known differences in the purchasing power of different currencies.

Expenditure on Family Welfare by Programme or Activity

The preceding discussion has focused on the aggregate expenditure on the family planning programme. To understand the extent to which the pattern of expenditure on different components of the family welfare programme has changed over the last five years, when the emphasis gradually shifted to the reproductive and child health approach, expenditures on different sub-programmes or activities are presented.

Annexure IV, V and VI consider 19 different activities and group them into three distinct categories according to whether the expenditure had (i) increased in real terms (i.e., faster than the rate of inflation, estimated at 40 percent); (ii) decreased in real terms but not in nominal terms; and, (iii) decreased in nominal terms as well over the five year period 1992-93 to 1996-97. The sub-programmes are listed according to the percentage increase (or decrease) in expenditure during the last year of the Eighth Plan as compared to the first year of the Plan period.

Activities for which expenditure increased in real terms

According to the data presented in Annexure IV, expenditure on 10 sub-programmes or activities increased (69 percent over the five-year period) in real terms. These include area projects, rural and urban family welfare centres, training and postpartum programme where expenditure has increased by 58 to 140 percent over the five year period. The expenditure on maternal and child health, which accounted for one-seventh of the total expenditure on family welfare, shows an increase of 334 percent over the five year period.

The Family Planning Services Project in Uttar Pradesh State funded by the USAID, had barely begun in 1992-93, and the expenditure for the project during 1996-97 was 29 times that in the earlier year. Expenditure on 'involving voluntary organisations in the family planning programme' had risen by 481 percent, although it was still a very small part of the total expenditure.

Expenditure on 'direction and administration' (increased by 46 percent) and on the free distribution of contraceptives (increased by 44 percent) accounted for about 9.5 percent of the total. The expenditure on IUDs and oral pills had risen by 117 and 427 percent, partly because of the import content but also because of the rise in their off-take. Expenditure on condoms had risen less than the rate of inflation, probably because their production by Hindustan Latex Ltd., a public sector firm, helped to ensure that their prices had remained virtually unchanged. The decline in the popularity of laparoscopies contributed to an absolute decline in the expenditure on laparoscopes by 60 percent.

Activities for which expenditure declined in real terms

Five sub-programs on which expenditure had declined in real terms, though not in nominal terms (Annexure V) were: sterilisation beds; information, education and communication activities; research and evaluation activities; India's contribution to international organisations; and, the amount spent as compensation to acceptors.

The last of these budget heads presumably reflected the implementation of the policy to de-emphasise the incentives for demographic targets. The decline in the real expenditure on 'research and evaluation' seems most unfortunate. Policy-makers appear to be skeptical about the benefits of research undertaken by the scholarly community and about the gains from information, education and communication expenditures. Those engaged in these activities are caught in a vicious circle. They do not have the requisite basic infrastructure to fulfill expectations and, as a result, they get a rough deal from the decision-makers.

Activities for which expenditure declined in nominal terms as well

As shown in Annexure VI, the special input for the 90 backward districts had declined sharply, presumably because of the uncertain returns from the investments. The expenditure to involve other departments in family welfare work was also brought down through efforts to persuade those departments to make the necessary additional provisions. The Village Health Guide Scheme, introduced in 1978 after the revocation of the emergency, has gradually lost its purpose and it is being wound down. The fourth scheme in this category was the commercial distribution of contraceptives: condoms and oral pills; the expenditure on oral pills had more than doubled, but that on condoms dropped considerably, with some sharp annual fluctuations. The new scheme of social marketing of contraceptives is likely to prove an improvement over the earlier one. It is likely that the data under this head are not comparable over time.

Overall, the expenditure data confirm an impression of a marked reallocation of expenditures in favour of strengthening the network to deliver the family welfare services both in rural and urban areas and to support maternal and child health services.

Expenditure for Family Welfare in Rajasthan and Tamil Nadu

Annexures VII and VIII present the available data relating to expenditure on family welfare in Rajasthan and Tamil Nadu. Annexure V presents the total expenditure on 'medical education, public health and family welfare' in Rajasthan with the breakdown between revenue and capital account. It makes the point that the expenditure on capital account formed only a small part of the total expenditure on health and family welfare during 1986-87 to 1990-91 but thereafter, its share increased to about 7 percent as funds became available for the construction of primary health centres and subcentre buildings.

There is a marked difference between the state government figures of the expenditure on family welfare, and those provided by the central government. The latter are substantially below the state estimates. Their use in any analysis understates the actual expenditure by between 13 to 41 percent in Rajasthan (except in 1991-92, when the two sets of number converged closely) and by between 28 to 112 percent for Tamil Nadu. The problem of arrears only partly explains the divergence between the two sets of data. Among other things, the central government since April, 1970 has covered the salary cost of auxiliary nurse midwives employed by each state. Those employed earlier continue to be paid by the state governments from their own funds. Some other items of expenditure incurred by state governments may not be covered by the central government scheme.

Overall, the annual per capita expenditure on family welfare in the two states was nearly the same around Rs 7-8 during 1986-89; but it increased to Rs 21-24 during 1994-98 in Rajasthan, and to Rs 17-21 in Tamil Nadu during the same period. As noted earlier, fertility decline has been much faster in Tamil Nadu than in Rajasthan, despite the relatively lower level of expenditure which illustrates the need to examine the other correlates of social and demographic change, including the dispersal of population, the state of infrastructure and the level of development in the areas under study. Such analysis needs to continue.

Private Expenditure on Health and Family Welfare

The preceding discussion has focused on public sector expenditure on health and family welfare. In addition, individual households also spend on these services. According to the National Family Health Survey conducted during 1992-93, 62 percent of the urban users and 87 percent of the rural users received modern contraceptive methods from public sector sources. The private medical sector met the needs of about 26 percent of the urban and 10 percent of the rural users of contraceptives. About 11 percent of urban users, and 3 percent of rural users reported other sources for the services, mainly shops and husbands for the supply of condoms, and shops and friends for the supply of oral pills (IIPS, 1995). With respect to curative care, the public sector facilities met the needs of 43-44 percent persons seeking out patient treatment in hospitals and 80-81 percent of those seeking hospital care, between 1995-96 in both rural and urban areas.

According to a nation wide survey of the level and pattern of consumption expenditure during 1993-94, annual medical expenditure (institutional as well as non-institutional) added up to Rs 183 billion, approximately 68 percent more than that incurred by the central and state governments together. Such private expenditures formed about 2.5 percent of the GDP of the country. For family welfare also, private expenditure is likely to exceed the percent of users relying on private medical and other sources, because of the relatively high fees charged by the private hospitals, clinics and doctors as well as pharmacies and drug stores for providing the services of sterilisation, IUD insertion and supply of oral pills. However, quantification of these expenditures is not feasible without detailed research.

Between 1993-94, Private health expenditure is estimated at Rs 183 billion or $5.8 billion (@Rs 31.40 per dollar) in aggregate terms, and works out to $6.53 per capita (with an estimated population of 892 million on January 1, 1994). One might round it up roughly to $7.00 or $8.00, if allowance is to be made for the apparent understatement of family planning expenditure at the state level and the private expenditure. (The figure of $16 shown in the World Development Report of 1993 appears to be unduly high).

Conclusions

There are clear signs of a shift in the orientation of the public sector functionaries engaged in the task of promoting family planning and lowering of fertility. Since the family planning programme effectively began more than 25 years ago, a high proportion of the male and female health workers are now in their late 40s or early 50s. A shift of gears is not likely to be an easy task for these workers. However, there is reason to believe that since senior policy makers recognise the importance of broadening the reach and the scope of services, there have been some efforts to modify the training of the grassroots level workers and provide backup support of well trained senior health care providers. Given the size and diversity of the country, this is a Herculean task and the resources required for the purpose will be immense.

As noted above, India appears to have succeeded in securing external assistance of the order of US$ 1.2 billion for the reproductive and child health programme[5]. A similar effort is being made to secure World Bank credits and loans for strengthening health services in several states of the country. Health reform projects have already been launched in Andhra Pradesh, Karnataka

[5] The RCH initiative is financed by credit from the World Bank's International Development Agency (IDA). The two-part financing arrangement that is worked out consists of overlapping five-year projects covering an eight-year period.

and West Bengal and negotiations are at an advanced stage for Maharashtra, Orissa and Madhya Pradesh. Both Rajasthan and Tamil Nadu, studied by us, expect that external assistance will help to raise the expenditures on family welfare significantly. The challenge nevertheless seems to lie in raising the productivity of the large manpower, through more effective training and more responsive administration, so that the credibility of the programme among the people could be raised through a more holistic and empathetic approach and concern for clients and their problems.

Higher life expectancy levels, lower morbidity rates and current fertility levels, will require a substantial step-up of investment in the health infrastructure. While external assistance to achieve this would be welcome, in the long run, sustainability of the system will necessitate a sizable mobilisation of domestic resources.

References

Coale, A.J., and Hoover, E.M. 1958. Population Growth and Development in Low Income Countries, Princeton: Princeton University Press.

Government of India. 1996. Manual on Target Free Approach in Family Welfare Programme. Ministry of Health and Family Welfare. New Delhi, India.

Government of India. 1998. Manual on Community Needs Assessment Approach in Family Welfare Programme. Ministry of Health and Family Welfare. New Delhi, India.

Government of India. 1998. Annual Report of the Ministry of Health and Family Welfare, 1997-98. Ministry of Health and Family Welfare. New Delhi, India.

Government of India. 1992. The Eighth Five Year Plan 1992-97. Planning Commission. New Delhi, India.

International Institute for Population Sciences. 1995. India: National Family Health Survey, 1992-93. Mumbai, India.

Operations Research Group. 1990. Family Planning Practices in India: Third All-India Survey. Baroda, India.

Ramachandran. V. 1996. NGOs in the Time of Globalisation. *Seminar*, 447.

Rama Rao, S., Townsend, J.W., and Khan, M.E. 1996. A Model Costs of RTI Case Management Services in Uttar Pradesh.Technical Paper. Population Council, New Delhi

Ramasundaram, S., Rangarajan, T., and Muthuramalingam, S. 1997. The Role of Political Will and Official Commitment in Tamil Nadu's Fertility Decline. Studies of Human Development in India. Discussion Paper Series, No. 24. Centre for Development Studies, Trivandrum, India.

Satia J.K., and Giridhar, G. 1991. Supply Aspects of Meeting Demand for Family Planning. In: J.K. Satia and S. J. Jejeebhoy (eds.). The Demographic Challenges: A Study of Four Large Indian States, 114-148. Mumbai: Oxford University Press.

Singh, P.1994. Women, Health and Population in India: An NGO Perspective - A Synthesis of Reports of Regional Meetings in the Context of ICPD – 1994. United Nations Population Fund. New Delhi, India.

Visaria, L., Visaria, P., and Jain, A. 1994. Estimates of Contraceptive Prevalence Based on Service and Surveys in Gujarat State, India. *Studies in Family Planning,* 25(5): 293-303.

World Bank. 1997. India: Reproductive and Child Health Project. Project Appraisal Document, Report No. 16393-IN. World Bank, Washington D.C., USA.

Annexure I

Selected Demographic Statistics for Rajasthan and Tamil Nadu

Item	India	Rajasthan	Tamil Nadu
Population			
1981 (mill.)	683.3	34.2	48.4
1991 (mill.)	846.3	44.0	55.8
1998 (mill. estimated)	975.0	52.7	61.0
% Increase,1981-91	23.8	28.4	15.3
Area ('000 kms.)	3,287	342	130
Sex Ratio (Males per 1000 females)			
1981	1071	1088	1024
1991	1079	1095	1029
Density (Persons per sq km)			
1981	273	129	429
1991	230	100	372
Percent of Urban Population			
1981	23.7	21.0	32.9
1991	26.1	22.8	34.1
Daily per capita calorie intake 1993-94			
Rural Areas	2153	2470	1884
Urban areas	2071	2184	1992
Vital Rates			
Birth Rate			
1991-93	29.1	34.6	20.3
1994-96	28.1	33.1	19.5
Death Rate			
1991-93	9.7	9.9	8.4
1994-96	9.0	8.6	7.9
Total Fertility			
1990-92	3.6	4.5	2.2
1995	3.5	4.4	2.2
% of deliveries taking place in Institutions, 1995			
All Area	25.2	7.6	64.2
Rural	17.4	4.0	51.7
Urban	59.6	28.6	92.4

Annexure I contd...

	India		Rajasthan		Tamil Nadu	
	Males	**Females**	**Males**	**Females**	**Males**	**Females**
1991						
All Areas	25.2	19.6	24.5	19.0	27.0	21.3
Rural Areas	24.5	18.0	22.0	17.1	27.0	20.8
Urban Areas	27.0	21.3	24.0	19.2	28.4	22.1
Literacy Among Persons aged 7 and over (%)						
Males						
1981	56.5	29.8	44.8	14.0	68.0	40.4
1991	64.1	39.1	55.0	20.4	73.7	51.3

Annexure II

Criteria Adopted for Selection of the Districts and for Conducting Focus Group Discussions in Rajasthan and Tamil Nadu, India

Based on discussions with the state officials and also with some faculty members of the research institutes within the states, we selected one of the two districts in each state where family planning targets had been removed in 1995 before they were removed from the entire country in 1996 (the better performing districts within their respective states). The second district selected for our study both in Rajasthan and Tamil Nadu was a relatively backward district.

Rajasthan

In Rajasthan, targets were removed from Dausa and Tonk districts in 1995. We selected Dausa, located at a distance of about 65 km from the state capital, Jaipur. The other selected district, Bharatpur, is located at some distance from Jaipur, and has fewer infrastructural facilities such as a poor road network, and relatively poor family planning performance.

Within each district, in consultation with the district officials, we selected two primary health centres, on the basis of their performance, both in family planning and other health services. A good and a poor performing primary health centre was selected. Within each centre area, covering a population of about 30,000, there are generally six subcentres each functioning with an auxiliary nurse midwife (ANM) and providing services to a population of 5,000. Two subcentre villages were selected for focus group discussions (FGD) with women or clients. A team of two assistant professors, one moderator and two team assistants from IIHMR assisted in conducting the focus group discussions and in-depth interviews in both the districts of Rajasthan.

Tamil Nadu

In 1995, all the districts in Tamil Nadu were made target free. The experiment of removing method-specific family planning targets was initiated in 1992 in the district of North Arcot (Ramasundaram et al, 1996). We therefore, decided to include this district in our present study. The other district selected for the study is Salem, where both the birth and death rates, according to the statistics for the past three years, have been higher than the state average. Salem district is also part of the contiguous region where some communities have been reported to be practising female infanticide.

The same criteria were applied for selection of primary health centres and sub-centres in Tamil Nadu as were used in Rajasthan. A team of three Ph.D. candidates, under the supervision of a professor in the Population Studies Department of the Bharathiar University in Coimbatore conducted the focus group discussions and the in-depth interviews in the two districts.

Rajasthan Dausa	Bharatpur	Tamil Nadu North Arcot	Salem
5 FGDs with Clients (43)	4 FGDs with Clients (33)	4 FGDs with Clients (45)	4 FGDs with Clients (38)
1 FGD with ANMs (6)	1 FGD with ANMs (5)	2 FGD with ANMs (12)	2 FGD with ANMs (10)
In-depth interviews (5)	In-depth interviews (7)	In-depth interviews (2)	In-depth interviews (8)

Annexure III

Expenditure on Family Welfare During the Eighth Plan Period, 1992-93 to 1996-97 According to the Ministry of Health and Family Welfare and the Ministry of Finance

(in ten million Rupees)

Activity	1992-93	1993-94	1994-95	1995-96	1996-97	Total of Eighth Plan
Data from the Ministry of Health and Family Welfare						
Total expenditure (FW)	1190.40	1521.80	1714.88	1781.35	2059.26	8267.29
Total expenditure on FW as % of GDP	0.19	0.21	0.20	0.18	0.18	0.19
Data from the Ministry of Finance						
Total expenditure on medical & public health, water supply & sanitation (MPHWSS)	8265	9536	11091	12453	15029@	56374
(a) Exp. on Family Welfare (FW)	1055	1343	1489	1827	1985@	7699
(b) FW as % of MPHWSS +FW	11.3	12.3	11.8	12.8	11.7	12.0
(a) Exp. on MPHWSS + FW	9320	10879	12580	14280	17014@	64073
(b) 5(a) as % of GDP	1.5	1.5	1.4	1.4	1.5	1.5
Mid-year Population (million)	872	888	904	920	937	—

Activity	1992-93	1993-94	1994-95	1995-96	1996-97	Total of Eighth Plan
Per capita annual expenditure on MPHWSS + FW						
(a) Rupees	107	122	139	155	182	142
(b) Dollars	3.49	3.89	4.43	4.63	5.13	4.31
(c) Exchange rate (Rs per $)	30.65	31.37	31.40	33.45	35.50	—

Note: Average exchange rates are taken from : Ministry of Finance, 1998. Economic Survey, 1997-98, New Delhi, p.s-78.

@ Revised estimates, subject to further revision after audit.

Source: Data from the Ministry of Finance cover both revenue and capital expenditure by the centre and the state governments. They are taken from : Indian Public Finance Statistics, 1997 published by the Economic Division of the Department of Economic Affairs, Ministry of Finance, Government of India, 1997. p.1.

Annexure IV

Programmes on which expenditure increased in real terms i.e. by more than 40 percent (the rate of inflation) between 1992-93 and 1996-97

Nature of the Scheme	1992-93	1993-94	1994-95	1995-96	1996-97	Total of Eighth Plan	% Increase 1992-93 to 1996-97
Family Planning Services Project in U.P.	1.00	5.00	30.00	20.50	29.16	85.56	+2810.0
Involvement of Voluntary Organisations	1.36	4.35	8.14	8.50	7.90	30.25	+480.9
Maternity and Child Health	100.00	142.78	241.41	280.65	434.21	1199.05	+334.2
Area Projects	73.65	149.08	148.31	172.42	176.90	720.87	+140.1
Rural FW Services	429.60	502.73	568.37	626.46	726.07	2862.23	+69.0
Urban FW Services	30.39	37.62	43.77	36.40	50.07	198.25	+64.8
Training	26.81	26.80	33.25	36.51	42.76	165.63	+61.3
Post Partum Programme	57.00	66.71	74.51	80.15	90.20	368.67	+58.2
Direction and Administration	51.42	58.23	61.53	62.10	75.13	308.41	+46.1
Free Distribution of Conventional Contraceptives	67.93	98.37	129.24	85.46	97.88	478.38	+44.1

Annexure V

Programmes on which expenditure declined in real terms but not in nominal terms

Nature of the Scheme	1992-93	1993-94	1994-95	1995-96	1996-97	Total of Eighth Plan	% Increase 1992-93 to 1996-97
Sterilisation Beds	1.35	1.22	1.63	1.93	1.84	7.87	+35.3
Information, Education and Communication	18.86	22.95	23.48	28.78	24.21	118.27	+28.4
Research and Evaluation	13.29	13.36	17.12	14.93	16.10	74.79	+21.1
India's Contribution to International Organisations	0.90	0.79	1.08	0.97	0.98	4.72	+8.9
Payment as compensation to acceptors	90.00	92.40	96.05	87.36	90.21	456.02	Negligible

Annexure VI

Programmes on which expenditure declined between 1992-93 and 1996-97 in absolute terms

Nature of the Scheme	1992-93	1993-94	1994-95	1995-96	1996-97	Total of Eighth Plan	% Increase 1992-93 to 1996-97
Special Inputs for 90 Backward Districts	45.00	31.01	19.80	5.26	4.03	105.10	-91.2
Involvement of Other Departments in Family Welfare	5.89	5.09	1.29	1.20	0.76	14.23	-89.0
Health Guides Scheme	21.00	13.93	12.98	16.09	11.12	75.12	-47.0
Commercial Distribution of Contraceptives	34.32	18.69	26.37	16.10	30.67	127.15	-10.6

Annexure VII

Rajasthan: Revenue Expenditure on Family Welfare, 1986-87 to 1998-99, According to the State Sources and the Central Government Reports

Year	State Sources	Central Govt. Reports	State Estimates as % of Central	Percent Increase State Sources	Percent Increase Central Reports	Per Capita Expenditure @ (Rs.)	Per Capita Expenditure @ % Change
1986-87	262.0	214.1	+122.4	—	—	6.6	—
1987-88	302.6	268.2	+112.8	+15.5	+25.3	7.5	+13.6
1988-89	316.8	255.9	+123.8	+ 4.7	- 4.6	7.6	+ 1.3
1989-90	398.0	322.0	+123.6	+25.6	+25.8	9.4	+23.7
1990-91	464.5	406.8	+114.2	+16.7	+26.3	10.7	+13.8
1991-92	538.6	536.0	+100.5	+16.0	+31.8	12.1	+13.1
1992-93	629.8	500.2	+125.9	+16.9	- 6.7	13.9	+14.9
1993-94	766.3	543.9	+140.9	+21.7	+ 8.7	16.3	+17.3
1994-95	1022.1	—	—	+33.4	—	21.3	+30.7
1995-96	1068.1	—	—	+ 4.5	—	21.7	+ 1.9
1996-97	1190.1	—	—	+11.4	—	23.6	+ 8.8
1997-98#	1252.7	—	—	+ 5.3	—	24.3	+ 3.0
1998-99*	1071.9	—	—	-14.4	—	20.3	-16.5

Revised estimated presented in the budget for 1998-99.

* Budget estimates approved by the State Legislature for the year beginning April 1, 1998.

@ Figures are based on the state budget estimates of expenditure on family welfare.

Annexure VIII

Tamil Nadu: Expenditure on Family Welfare, 1986-87 to 1998-99, According to the State Sources and the Central Government Reports

Year	State Sources	Central Govt. Reports	State Estimates as % of Central	Percent Increase		Per Capita Expenditure @	
				State Sources	Central Reports	(Rs.)	% Change
1986-87	335.2	239.7	+139.8	—	—	6.4	—
1987-88	356.8	278.4	+128.2	+6.4	+16.1	6.7	+5.0
1988-89	435.5	287.6	+151.4	+22.1	+3.3	8.1	+20.3
1989-90	566.5	361.2	+156.8	+30.1	+25.6	10.4	+28.3
1990-91	630.8	378.4	+166.7	+11.4	+4.8	11.4	+9.8
1991-92	768.4	398.4	+192.9	+21.8	+5.3	13.7	+20.2
1992-93	871.4	492.9	+176.8	+13.4	+23.7	15.3	+12.0
1993-94	1016.1	479.0	+212.1	+16.6	-2.8	17.6	+15.3
1994-95	1160.2	—	—	+8.9	—	19.6	+7.7
1995-96	1223.6	—	—	+10.6	—	20.8	+9.3
1996-97	1033.9	—	—	+15.5	—	17.3	-16.5
1997-98#	1193.4	—	—	+15.4	—	19.8	+14.1
1998-99*	1408.8	—	—	+18.0	—	23.1	+16.7

Note: Figures for years up to 1996-97 show reported actual expenditure during the year. Change in per capita expenditure on family welfare over successive years has been calculated with more detailed figures than are presented in this Table.

Revised estimated presented in the budget for 1998-99.

* Budget estimates approved by the State Legislature for the year beginning April 1, 1998.

@ Figures are based on the state budget estimates of expenditure on family welfare.

4

Decentralised Participative Planning and Monitoring

Nirmala Murthy

Introduction

The International Conference on Population and Development (ICPD) held in Cairo, in 1994, urged participating countries to make reproductive health services available through their primary health care systems. The Government of India supported this approach and committed itself to providing a package of reproductive health services through its family welfare programme. The package included services for contraception, safe delivery, antenatal, postnatal and infant care, abortion, management of reproductive tract infections (RTIs) and sexually transmitted infections (STIs), and counselling on sexuality, reproductive health and responsible parenthood. Some of these services were already in place; others needed strengthening; and some were to be introduced in the family welfare programme.

Most importantly, the programme needed a change in focus – from population control – to meeting the reproductive health needs of the people. This change also implied a change in policy – of moving away from the achievement of contraceptive targets – towards providing a range of reproductive health services of acceptable quality to the client (Pachauri, 1998).

Following the ICPD, the government decided to make this policy shift. Its first decision was to convert the family welfare programme into a Reproductive and Child Health programme to adopt a target free approach for providing contraceptive services. Target free approach not only meant freedom from the practice of setting contraceptive targets centrally, but also meant promoting the practice of local planning, providing quality services and improving client satisfaction (World Bank, 1997).

The government's decision to introduce the reproductive and child health programme was partly a result of many years of lobbying and sustained dialogue among different stakeholders – service providers, women's advocates and programme administrators. These consultations suggested that the resources required for the new programme might exist within the current government structure but that efforts to change the mindsets of service providers and of clients might require substantial additional inputs. The service providers, used to viewing women merely as 'family planning cases', needed to change that orientation and view women as clients who had a right to demand services of acceptable quality delivered in a gender sensitive manner. Clients, on their part, needed to learn about reproductive health problems, overcome the sense of shame and fear associated with these problems and demand improved services (Jejeebhoy, 1997).

Scenario before ICPD

A review of India's family welfare programme carried out in 1995 identified three constraints in implementing the new programme (World Bank, 1995). These were: many services were either not available or were of poor quality; primary health centres were not properly equipped and staffed; and gender bias and low status of women affected service provision.

Assessment of the services showed that antenatal care was minimal, consisting mainly of registration of pregnancies and of giving women tetanus toxoid and 100 tablets of iron and folic acid. Most women were not screened for contraindications before they were provided with contraceptives. Women were not told about possible side effects. Follow-up and after-care for side effects was nearly non-existent (Murthy and Barua,1998).

Such quality issues were identified as critical for improving the performance of the programme but were never addressed systematically for a variety of reasons. Quality improvement is a slow process, requiring patience and hard work, both of which are generally lacking in the government system. Health providers are usually not given on-the-job training nor do they have the motivation to improve service quality. Effective supervision, crucial to ensuring quality standards is also lacking. Field experiments have shown that supervisors are reluctant to use quality checklists when there is no pressure on them to improve quality. A study carried out in south India on service providers' perspective on quality of care showed that while clients appreciated quality improvements, administrative commitment to quality was minimal (Ramasundaram, 1994).

One frequently noted reason for poor quality of services was the pressure exerted on workers and doctors to achieve sterilisation and other contraceptive targets. The system of setting method specific targets was adopted as a management tool during the mid 1960s, essentially in an attempt to bring down the birth rate rapidly. The central government determined the targets for each state. These targets were based on several criteria such as population size, birth rate, education levels, past performance, and proportions of poor and disadvantaged populations. Targets below the state level were allocated on the basis of population numbers.

The Planning Commission, Government of India, decided to set targets for the first time during the Fourth Five-Year Plan (1969-74) with the goal of achieving a contraceptive prevalence rate of 60 percent and a net reproduction rate of 1 by 1974. This goal remains the same in the Ninth Plan, but the achievement year has changed to 2002 or even later. In the eagerness to achieve this goal, two irrational practices crept into the process of target setting. One was that the Department of Family Welfare kept increasing the targets each year to make up for the backlog of previous years. Another practice was to further increase the targets for better performing states because the poorly performing states were not contributing enough to the national goal: thus, the pressure on well-performing states kept increasing to meet higher and higher targets.

To make matters worse, the Ministry of Health and Family Welfare introduced a 'carrot and stick' approach to keep this pressure on. Apart from giving incentives to acceptors, states gave attractive awards for the best performance in meeting contraceptive targets. States began to co-opt staff of other departments such as revenue, rural development, and agriculture – who had nothing to do with either health or family planning – to recruit for family planning acceptors. Such practices led to the neglect of the quality of family planning and other health services such as maternal and child health services. Health staff were told, directly or indirectly, to concentrate only on family planning. They could ignore other health services with complete immunity. They were encouraged to 'somehow catch a case and fulfil the target'. Their methods could include giving women additional incentives, giving them false promises, pressurising village leaders, or sometimes even reporting false numbers.

Therefore, it came as no surprise to anyone when the target system did not produce the desired results. Although the reported contraceptive prevalence rate was increasing, the fertility rate did not decline correspondingly (Jain, 1997). Population experts played a major role in highlighting the dysfunctional aspects of method-specific targets. They argued that targets were more harmful than beneficial because the programme was neglecting low-parity couples who were not candidates for sterilisation; the department was encouraging over reporting of achievement; and the large sterilisation camps organised to achieve the targets were detrimental to service quality. Over time, contraceptive targets and the target setting process came under so much criticism and ridicule that removing them seemed to be the only way to improve the quality and effectiveness of the family welfare services (The Policy Project, 1998).

Efforts to replace the target-based system

In April 1996, the Government of India implemented the target free approach. This was a major paradigm shift for the policy makers who now had to promulgate the view that the government's goal was not to achieve fertility reduction but to help couples make reproductive choices by providing information and enhancing access to health services. This shift also implied a change in the orientation of the programme, from one of meeting targets to that of improving service quality, access and client satisfaction. Service quality was defined as a combination of technical competence and quality of the physical environment where services are provided. Client satisfaction was defined as service access, quality and usefulness from the clients' perspective. To implement this new approach, efforts were needed at three levels – at the policy, programme and grassroots levels.

Policy level changes

The first policy level change was the government's declaration that family planning was not a public investment programme that aimed at reducing fertility but one that aimed at safeguarding the health and reproductive rights. There was concern, however, that such a programme may actually slow down the fertility decline, which India could ill afford. Several state secretaries criticised the government's decision to remove contraceptive targets.

However, this decision was neither sudden nor arbitrary. Data from the National Family Health Survey carried out in 1992-93 had shown that there was a large unmet need for contraception (20 percent of couples) which, if tapped, could reduce the birth rate without resorting to targets. There were some field experiences to support this. During 1990-1996, urban family welfare programmes in the slums of Mumbai and Chennai had achieved a substantial decline in fertility and under-five mortality by giving less priority to contraceptive targets and more to maternal and child health (Measham and Heaver, 1996). Tamil Nadu had demonstrated that by setting targets for maternal and child health services, it was possible to improve performance without affecting the family planning performance (Ramasundaram, 1995).

Based on these experiences, in April 1995, the government decided initially to withdraw contraceptive targets on an experimental basis from one district each in the six largest states. At the end of one year, all states involved in this experiment informed the centre that some sort of targets were essential to get any work done by the health workers. Also, removing the targets was not enough to improve quality and access to services. Additional resources and strong supervision were needed to achieve those two objectives. States did, however, report improved performance in maternal and child health services although family planning performance dropped from 10 to 50 percent.

Most states, therefore, recommended a gradual withdrawal of targets over a period of about five years. They also voiced their apprehension about the term 'target free approach' which to many meant a 'work-free' approach. Notwithstanding these recommendations, in April 1996 the government decided to withdraw targets nationwide. The target system was replaced with a system of decentralised planning which would determine the work load locally.

State-level workshops were organised and a target free approach manual was prepared to provide guidelines on how to prepare decentralised plans. The existing monitoring system was modified to focus on coverage, quality and client satisfaction. The new monitoring system consisted of regular reporting of service statistics and regular household surveys to enable programme managers to get a realistic picture of ground realities.

Programme level changes

The message conveyed at the programme level was that the reproductive and child health package of services did not require substantial additional resources but that services should be integrated. This meant that service providers must not see a client as an antenatal case or a family planning case, but as a woman needing reproductive health care of a quality acceptable to her and that the service must be delivered in a manner that will enhance her appreciation for the public system.

At the programme level, these objectives were to be achieved by providing integrated training and modifying the monitoring system. Training and monitoring systems were re-designed to inform health staff as to what services they should provide, how they should deliver these services from a technical point of view and how they should be sensitive to clients' needs. The monitoring system used three tools: (1) activity reports by the workers; (2) technical assessment reports on service quality; and (3) client's reports of access, quality and attitudes of service providers. Data from these three tools were to be used to monitor the programme, instead of the target based monitoring system practised earlier.

Grassroots level changes

At the grassroots level, an attempt was made to direct service providers' attention to client needs and client satisfaction. The concept of clients' needs was to be built into the decentralised plans by undertaking needs assessment surveys and community level consultations. The concept of client satisfaction was somewhat difficult to build in to the day-to-day activities at the grassroots level. The most widely accepted theory of client satisfaction defines it as meeting, or exceeding clients' expectations (Parasuraman et al, 1988). Programme managers rightly argued that in terms of health care, clients do not have clear expectations and are not able to evaluate service quality. Therefore, the concept of client satisfaction in the reproductive and child health programme was defined on the basis of research which showed that client satisfaction is determined by the effectiveness of the treatment, availability of staff and medicines, the health centres' accessibility, quality of client-staff interaction, and the information given to the client (Ruben, 1993). Data are to be collected on all these aspects to enable health staff to take corrective actions to improve client satisfaction.

Progress in implementing target free approach

Simultaneously with the implementation of the target free approach, the government also initiated the decentralised planning process to replace the target-based system. This transition was difficult for two reasons. First, the term decentralised planning was interpreted in many different ways (Gilson et al, 1994), expectations were much higher than what the government had intended and resulted in disappointment. Second, the scope for planning under the reproductive and child health programme was limited. It only allowed health workers to estimate their work load for those services that were included in the programme. The community was not given the freedom to express their 'felt needs'. People had to choose from 15 services to start with (see Table 1). This number is expected to increase with time, as the programme matures.

TABLE 1: RCH Services for which Client Needs are Assessed

Services
Registration of antenatal cases
Early registration of antenatal cases
Referral of high risk antenatal cases
Anaemic antenatal mothers given therapeutic dose
Pregnant women given 2 tetanus toxoid doses
Pregnant women completing 3 visits to health centre for check-up
Institutional deliveries
Home delivery attended by midwifery trained person
New-born babies weighed
High risk new-borns referred for medical examination
Infant received full immunisation
Children given vitamin A prophylaxis
Diarrhoea episodes treated with oral rehydration therapy
Acute respiratory infection episodes treated by doctor
Couples provided sterilisation service
Couples provided spacing methods of contraception

Many researchers and health activists were quick to observe that this method of planning was nothing but an attempt to push target calculations down to the health worker level. The approach was called decentralised planning simply because the exercise started at the sub-centre level. Data were collated at the primary health centre and district levels to form the district plan.

The government's guidelines on decentralised planing were:

> *"work out the (service) requirement by conducting a household survey, validate the estimate of requirement through discussion with anganwadi workers, members of mahila swasthay sangha, panchayat members etc, relate this estimate with the birth rate of the area and with the achievements in the previous years to ensure that the estimates of requirement are realistic."* (Government of India, 1998).

This planning method was the second disappointment. Although the government had tried to simplify the methodology by eliminating formulae and calculations (Government of India, 1996), only six states developed plans in 1997-98. Others were not sure of how to assess community needs and described guidelines as 'not clear enough', 'process too complicated', or 'too time consuming'. Some states carried out the needs assessment surveys through the health workers and found that needs were underestimated up to 30 percent compared to what they would have been if calculated normatively. As a result, different states decided to adopt different approaches to planning. In all states, the target for maternal and child health services was uniformly set at 100 percent of expected pregnancies (based on the birth rate). But targets for family planning were decided differentially. For example, in Assam and Uttar Pradesh, workers were asked to set family planning targets equal to the average performance of the previous three years. In Rajasthan, workers actually obtained information on clients' needs for family planning through surveys and could use this information to decide their targets with one condition – the 'need' must not be less than 1 percent of the population.

In Karnataka, clients' needs were estimated for the 15 reproductive and child health services (see Table 1), based on a survey of 100 women per sub-centre. These data were collated and analysed at the primary health centre, where the workers were helped by their supervisors to make the calculations. The estimated targets were similar to those under the target-based system. The only difference was that the workers said that they knew how to calculate them and felt that they had a role in decision-making.

In Andhra Pradesh, health workers were asked to list all married women with two or more children and then guess how many were likely to accept sterilisation (if they had not already done so), or any other method. These 'guess-estimates' were discussed at the primary health centre level. If these were too low or too high compared to the previous year's performance, workers were asked to revise them. In Maharashtra, for the first year, workers were asked to estimate their own targets using the formula, '7 acceptors per 1000 population'. The following year, the workers calculated their targets as an average of three years' performance. But in one district, when the needs assessment methodology was pilot tested by surveying all the women in the area, it was found that the survey had substantially underestimated the need for family planning. The actual performance was almost double the estimated need.

In Tamil Nadu, workers used a normative approach to determine contraceptive targets, based on the birth-order distribution observed the year before. It was assumed that all women who delivered and had three or more children, and 50 percent of those with two children needed sterilisation. The remaining women were assumed to need spacing methods. This formula linked family planning targets with the number of births and the birth-order distribution in the area. A district which had a higher birth rate and more high-order births would have a higher contraceptive target. The logic built into this formula was acceptable to the workers.

From all these variations in implementing the target free approach, the lessons that emerged were:

1. A census of women to assess service needs is a time consuming process and is likely to underestimate needs. A sample survey would take less time and might yield better information.

2. Needs assessment exercises have some advantages over the normative approach. Health workers become more client-oriented; their communication with clients improves; and they are able to identify specific health education needs in their areas.

3. Involving health workers in analysing their own data stimulates them intellectually because they feel responsible for meeting those needs. *"If done in groups at PHCs, these exercises are not burdensome but enjoyable,"* said the workers.

Monitoring system for the target free approach

The programme has a long tradition of recording and reporting elaborate service statistics and maintaining numerous registers. Under the reproductive and child health programme, an attempt was made to integrate related information, spread over different reports, into one report. This system, which was developed in response to the government's concern regarding 'how to monitor a programme which has no targets', was a step towards conceptual integration of reproductive and child health service delivery.

The government constituted a small committee to recommend an alternative system of monitoring with quality indicators. The committee studied the monitoring systems in Tamil Nadu, Maharashtra, Rajasthan and Uttar Pradesh, states that had introduced innovative features in their systems. The idea was to combine the best features of all systems. Thus, quality indicators from Tamil Nadu, technical assessments from Maharashtra, client needs assessments from Rajasthan and concurrent evaluations of health facilities from Uttar Pradesh were combined into the new monitoring system. The plan for the new system was presented at a two-day workshop in New Delhi where over 50 participants including the programme managers, researchers, NGO representatives, women activists, and representatives from donor agencies hotly debated each item of information and approved the new monitoring system.

The new system incorporates data on quality aspects such as postpartum complications, IUD discontinuation, and complicated deliveries, which the earlier system had not included. Another feature of the new monitoring system is regular household and facility surveys to be undertaken by independent agencies. Programme performance had always been monitored through internally generated programme statistics. Large scale surveys were rare and were carried out only when foreign funding was available. The government did not sponsor many such surveys. The reproductive and child health programme built rapid surveys into the monitoring system to provide district level estimates of service coverage, quality and client satisfaction.

Thus, household surveys will be undertaken in 50 percent of the districts each year. The sample for each survey consists of 1,000 households in each district. All married women of reproductive age in these households and women who have given birth in the previous three years will be included. Information will be collected on maternity care received, immunisation status of children, and need and use of family planning and other reproductive health services. Information about the use of public health services and the perception of service quality will also be obtained from the sampled households.

These surveys would not only provide managerially useful information, but would also give the clients a 'voice' to express their views about the services. This is a highly recommended tool in the literature for improving the accountability of the public health system and is a key to improving service delivery. These surveys are also expected to improve the process of decentralised planning as the planners in each district would have information on the views of their own clients.

Effect of the target free approach to reproductive and child health

In November 1997, the Population Council in collaboration with the Futures Group International, organised a national workshop to review the effect of the target free approach. At this workshop, seven states presented their experiences. The positive outcomes noted by all states were: (1) there is now no pressure to report inflated performance figures; (2) there are improvements in maternal and child health care; and, (3) younger and lower parity couples seem to be accepting contraceptive methods. Studies in these states showed that close supervision was the key to the success of the target free approach. Some states reported improvements in household visits by health workers (Khan and Townsend, 1998).

The government has since identified critical outcome and impact indicators to monitor progress (see Table 2). The choice of these indicators confirms the government's intention to strike a healthy balance between family planning and other reproductive health services. Of the ten critical indicators, three monitor family planning and seven, other services. There are two new indicators:

Number of district plans developed based on community need assessments –

This indicator assesses the extent to which the policy of decentralised planning has been implemented. So far, about 60-70 districts (15 percent) have reportedly developed their plans. Additional districts are likely to carry out this exercise in 1999.

Percentage of safe deliveries –

Safe delivery is defined as a delivery conducted at private or public institutions or at home and assisted by a person trained in midwifery. It does not include delivery conducted by trained traditional birth attendants. The government is committed to increasing safe deliveries from 30 percent in 1996 to 40 percent in 2002.

TABLE 2: Critical Indicators for Monitoring

Service Coverage

% safe deliveries conducted by midwifery trained persons
% pregnant women received "full" antenatal care
% children "fully" immunised below 2 years of age
% couples using contraception
% households visited by health worker

Service Quality

Early registration of pregnancy for antenatal care (before 16 weeks)
Children fully immunised before they reach age one
Contraceptive acceptors report no health problems
Men/Women having essential knowledge of reproductive health risks
Number of contraceptive side effects detected and treated

Clients Reporting Satisfaction

Doctors/ nurses/ medicines available when needed
Staff is friendly and helpful
Treatment given at SC/PHC/FRU is effective
Health centres are conveniently located and function regularly

Service Effectiveness in terms of Reduction

Birth rates, neonatal, infant and maternal mortality rates
High risk pregnancies
Low birth weight babies
Unmet need for family planning

Implementation experience and lessons learned

The target free approach is almost 30 months old and therefore it may not be out of place to ask: Has this policy change had any impact on field operations?

Some of the changes observed at the field level are:

Reduced pressure of target

One positive outcome noted in many states is there that there is now 'no target pressure'. Even though the states have some form of targets, their style of implementation has changed because of the government's insistence on the target free approach. Almost all states report an improvement of prenatal care. Acceptance of spacing methods among younger and high fertility couples is increasing in all states. The extent of decline in sterilisation acceptance differs between states but has declined in all states compared to the pre-target free approach level.

In the first year, this decline was alarming. It ranged from 10 to 50 percent. The states with the lowest decline attributed it to less false reporting. Those with a very high drop attributed it to health staff thinking that 'no target means no work'. Some states reacted to the setbacks by imposing some form of targets. But in 1997-98 the trend was reversed. Family planning performance improved further in 1998-99. Did this happen because the states abandoned the target free approach approach? We think not.

The target free approach has contributed to some qualitative changes. Health workers have started appreciating the client-centred approach. There is a modest increase in their visits to households. Interviews with community members show that they, too, have perceived some changes in service delivery; about 20 percent were aware that the targets had been removed (Khan and Townsend, 1998).

Concern for quality and client satisfaction

The concern for quality and client satisfaction is slowly beginning to assume importance in the programme. By including quality indicators, such as contraceptive failure rates and side effects, the government has signalled that it is important to report these and that they cannot be ignored. Health staff get credit for identifying and treating side-effects. States like Tamil Nadu and Maharashtra have decided to use technical quality checklists to send the message down to the worker level. Although service quality may not improve for quite some time, until the required staff, training and equipment are in place, the checklists inform the worker about what they are expected to accomplish in terms of quality.

Specific skill training programmes have been planned to improve the technical competence of service providers. But the quality of training remains a concern. Aspects such as how to improve privacy and convenience in service delivery and how to increase clients' awareness about service quality need attention. The fact that more and more women go to private doctors in the hope of getting quality service indicates that there is a demand for such services. These issues need to be addressed.

Range of services provided

The target free approach has increased health workers' awareness of the range of services they should provide under the reproductive and child health programme. However, the programme has not yet started providing services for emergency obstetric care, safe abortion and treatment of RTIs/STIs and infertility.

Reflecting local needs through locally determined targets

Since the central government has stopped setting targets, states have stepped in to assume that role. This is an unexpected change. State governments had always regarded the family planning programme as the central government's programme and had bitterly complained about centrally determined targets. Now that the states are determining the targets, there is a wide variation in the priorities set by different states. Some states are focusing on increasing institutional delivery and emergency obstetric care while others want to improve the training of traditional birth attendants and set up facilities for deliveries at the village level.

The decentralised planning approach has also brought about some attitudinal changes among the health staff. Though for the most part planning is nothing more than applying a set of formulae decided by the state, health workers are happy that they understand the rationale of setting targets and that they can participate in the planning process. This process ensures that the numbers get decided at levels closer to the clients. By the end of 1998, results from client surveys will become available and will provide additional inputs for determining local needs. But we need a robust methodology to develop plans based on these needs. Without such a methodology, there is a risk that targets will again be imposed from above.

Critical next steps

The reproductive and child health programme has been implemented recently. Considerable field research is needed to ensure that the new approach is effective. There are several important research questions that should be addressed: What are the barriers that clients face in accessing services? What criteria do clients use in judging service quality? How do professionals view quality? The difference in the perceptions of providers and clients could have a direct impact on the quality of reproductive and child health services.

Another important issue that needs urgent attention is the private-public mix of service delivery. While the government is busy equipping public facilities to provide new and better services, even a cursory assessment of the programme shows that the pressure point is likely to be lack of manpower. Some states have found temporary solutions to this problem. They are asking young doctors to work under a one-year bond, and are appointing private doctors on contract. However, these arrangements will not improve service quality although they may improve service availability in remote areas. It is, therefore, important to know who provides reproductive health services at the community level and how people choose among the different service providers? How can the service providers be involved in the programme? Answers to these questions may help us find systemic solutions for improving service accessibility and quality.

Considerable attention is focused on how to assess clients' needs and on the methodology for decentralised planning, but we have yet to address issues regarding incentives for local health officials to promote decentralisation. So far, only the central government has let go of its prerogative to set targets. The states and districts have not. What will make the latter relinquish this responsibility to the lower levels, especially to the community? This is an issue that requires further research.

Finally, an issue that has received little attention is how to involve women in decision making. Involving women's groups or women *panchayat* members are some of the ideas being tried in the field. This works well when there is higher level support but falls apart when that support is withdrawn. A lasting solution is to improve women's status so that they can assert themselves in decision making. A study in Maharashtra showed that women participate in decision making if they are educated and when they understand reproductive health and where to seek treatment (Barua, 1998). Economic status is not a significant barrier especially if husbands support their wives' decisions. The husbands' support interestingly also depended on their level of education, their knowledge of reproductive health problems, and how they perceive their role in these matters. Such studies provide valuable insights for programmatic action to build women's capacity to demand services and to support men's involvement.

Concluding comments

Although method specific targets have been under attack for quite some time, the need for programme targets was never questioned even by the health workers themselves. There was all round agreement that targets were needed to clearly communicate what programme functionaries should do, and to help managers in programme monitoring. Therefore, even under the target free approach, there are targets – but different ones. These are targets not only for contraceptive methods but also for a broad range of reproductive and child health services. The targets are not decided centrally but by health workers and their supervisors and are based on their estimates of service needs and past performance. These self-determined targets are used to monitor programme performance. However, the programme is also monitored through client surveys that provide information on service coverage, improvement in service quality and client satisfaction.

Contrary to the earlier fear that 'no targets will mean no work', it is now becoming clear to all concerned that there is not just one target. Monitoring is more elaborate and involves the workers, their supervisors and the clients themselves. The workers report their actual performance against their planned work. Supervisors are expected to assess the technical capacity of the workers periodically. Independent agencies are expected to report on service coverage and client satisfaction.

However, the discussion around targets continues. Unfortunately, some see the target free approach as a result of pressure by donor agencies, especially the World Bank. Some see it as a move by donors to discourage sterilisation and promote spacing methods at a tremendous future cost to the country. Some express disapproval of the elaborate monitoring system introduced to facilitate the target free approach, which they fear is becoming an end in itself.

The government's preoccupation with the elaborate planning and monitoring system associated with the target free approach is, no doubt, overshadowing other programme concerns such as resource needs, the quality of training, and the health system's capacity to provide a range of services. These issues must be urgently addressed. If a balance is not restored soon, this unique opportunity to give a fundamental reorientation to the programme will be lost.

References

Barua, A. 1998. Use of Reproductive Health Services by Married Adolescent Females, Findings From a Study in Rural Maharashtra. Paper Presented at the ICRW Workshop, May 1998, Bangalore, India.

Gilson, L., Kilima, P., and Tanner, M. 1994. Local Government Decentralisation and the Health Sector in Tanzania. *Public Administration and Development*, 14: 451-477.

Government of India. 1996. Manual on Target Free Approach in Family Welfare Programme, 35-36. Ministry of Health and Family Welfare, New Delhi, India.

Government of India. 1998. Manual on Community Needs Assessment Approach. Department of Family Welfare, Ministry of Health and Family Welfare, New Delhi, India.

Jain, A. 1997. Consistency between Contraceptive Use and Fertility in India, *Demography India*, 26.

Jejeebhoy, S. 1997. Addressing Women's Reproductive Health Needs: Priorities for the Family Welfare Programme, *Economic & Political Weekly*, March 1-8.

Khan, M. E., and Townsend, J.W. 1998. Has the Indian Family Welfare Programme Lost Momentum Under the TFA? Emerging Evidence. Paper presented at the Workshop on the Target Free Approach, World Bank, New Delhi. April 2-3, 1998.

Measham, A.R., and Heaver, R.A. 1996. India's Family Welfare Programme: Moving to a Reproductive and Child Health Approach, Washington D.C: The World Bank.

Murthy, N., and Barua, A. 1998. Integrating Reproductive Health in Health Programmes in India. In: M. Krishnaraj et al. (ed.). Gender, Population and Development, 293. New Delhi: Oxford University Press.

Pachauri, S. 1998. Defining a Reproductive Health Package for India: A Proposed Framework, In: M. Krishnaraj et al.(eds.). Gender, Population and Development, 310- 339. New Delhi: Oxford University Press.

Parasuraman, A., Zeithaml, V., and Barry, L. 1988. SERVQUAL: Multi-item Scale for Measuring Consumer Perceptions of Service Quality. *Journal of Retailing*, 64(1): 2-40.

Ramasundaram, S. 1994. Quality of Care in Health and Family Welfare Programme. Paper presented at the Seminar on Quality of Care, Gujarat Institute of Development Research, Ahmedabad, India. April 28-29, 1994.

Ramasundaram, S. 1995. End of the Target Era. *Voices*, 3(2). Bangalore, India.

Ruben, B. 1993. What Patients Remember: A Content Analysis of Critical Incidence in Health Care. *Health Communications*, 5 (2): 99-112.

The Policy Project. 1998. Targets for Family Planning in India: An Analysis of Policy Change, Consequences, and Alternative Choices, 3. The Futures Group International, New Delhi, India.

The World Bank. 1995. India's Family Welfare Programme: Toward a Reproductive and Child Health Approach. Population and Human Resources Operations Division, South Asia Country Department II.

The World Bank. 1997. India: Reproductive and Child Health Project: Project Appraisal Document, 32-36. Population and Human Resources Operations Division, South Asia Region.

5

Monitoring and Evaluating New Systems

K. B. Pathak, F. Ram and Ravi K. Verma

Introduction

In keeping with the commitments made at the International Conference on Population and Development (ICPD) held at Cairo in 1994, the Government of India revamped the family welfare programme with an explicit focus on community needs assessment and enhancing quality of services and care (Government of India, 1998). The government's new strategy aims to address wide ranging issues within the overall reproductive health framework. A significant step in this direction was the removal of method specific targets on April 1, 1996. The removal of targets presented a unique challenge as well as an opportunity to try alternative strategies for monitoring and evaluation. A critical aspect of the new monitoring and evaluation strategy is to capture the nature of the paradigm shift proposed. The ICPD Programme of Action recognises the need for suitable indicators to assess and measure the quality and accessibility of care, in addition to gender and ethnicity specific information to enhance and monitor the sensitivity of the programme (ICPD Programme of Action, 1994).

This chapter describes the new system that has been designed to monitor and evaluate the reproductive and child health programme. We begin with briefly describing the system of monitoring and evaluation used in the past, and then present the current shift. Since the new system has been in operation for less than two years, it is not possible to assess its effectiveness. We therefore focus on describing the changes in the system and discussing issues that have emerged in the process of change.

Past System of Monitoring and Evaluation

Until recently, the family welfare programme was governed by 'population-control' concerns. During the first three decades, the policy goal was to reduce the birth rate, which in turn guided the monitoring and evaluation system. During the past two decades, the net reproductive rate has been the policy goal and the programme had become more comprehensive in its design.

The term target was first used in 1965 in relation to the IUD. In 1966, targets were set for all the methods. These targets were determined mainly in terms of the number of acceptors per 1,000 population. Until 1980, the crude birth rate continued to remain the single most important programme goal. In the1980s, targets were also set for maternal and child health activities. The programme aimed to achieve replacement level fertility using the net reproduction rate (NRR) of one as its policy goal. The concept of NRR was expected to enable the programme to move away from its exclusive family planning concerns to broader health concerns (Government of India, 1980). The crude death rate (CDR) and the infant mortality rate (IMR) became equally important indicators to measure programme impact.

In programmatic terms, however, the emphasis continued to remain on the achievement of method specific targets. Information on the latter was collected routinely from field workers and aggregated through the service system up to the state and the national levels. Method specific targets, determined at the national level, were distributed all the way down to the subcentre level. While the criteria for distributing targets to the states varied from year to year, the programme continued to place emphasis on past performance as an important criteria for allocating targets.

In the past, few indicators were used to monitor the family welfare programme at various levels of the service system. At the grassroots level, data were collected on either acceptance rates, i.e. acceptors of various methods per 1,000 population or percent target achieved for sterilisation and other spacing methods. In fact, the government relied heavily on target achievement for sterilisation to monitor performance. No attention was paid to the other service components of the programme and the health problems that acceptors may have because of contraceptive use. Until 1980, data on maternal and child health services were not published in the family planning yearbook, a government publication. In addition to the percent target achievement at district level, state level couple protection rates (CPR) were also used to monitor and evaluate programme performance. Thus, the monitoring system and the generation of data were guided by the sole objective of achieving fertility decline. Data on demographic characteristics of acceptors were considered as indicators of the quality of the programme.

The younger the age, and the lower the parity, the better the quality since it would have a greater impact on fertility. Thus programme monitoring was essentially based on service statistics which provided information on age, parity and religion.

Due to an over emphasis on targets, the quality of data reported from service statistics was always suspect. Many studies showed that performance data provided at all levels were unreliable, incomplete, and inadequate. There was general over-reporting of spacing methods, which increased over time due to the absence of any corrective measures and increased pressure for achieving targets. The Government of India was aware of this fact, and always discounted acceptor data before using these in the calculation of the CPR. The discounted rates varied between states. The government commissioned independent agencies to evaluate the process. Population research centres that are based within various university departments and non-governmental organisations played an active role in monitoring the programme on a regular basis. Population research centres carried out evaluative work in one or two districts in their respective states every year. These reports were sent directly to the central government. Because these studies depended entirely on the records of acceptors maintained at the primary health centres, they were considered less authentic by many researchers.

New System of Monitoring and Evaluation

The new monitoring and evaluation system is designed within the context of the community need assessment approach, which characterises the planning process of the reproductive and child health programme. With the help of the male multi-purpose worker, the auxiliary nurse mid-wife is expected to carry out a community needs assessment once at the beginning of each year according to the government's manual on community needs assessment approach. Primary health centre plans are aggregated to form a district plan and district plans are aggregated to form the state plan. Auxiliary nurse midwives at the subcentres are expected to assess community needs through discussions with *panchayat* members, trained birth attendants, *anganwadi* workers and others. The plan does not envisage the involvement of medical officers at the primary health centre level. It is expected that this assessment approach will help to define service coverage and expected quality of care and will lead to client satisfaction. There are three components in the revised monitoring system:

1. Monthly activity reports from the subcentre, primary health centre and first referral unit.

2. Technical assessment of subcentre level services by a lady health visitor.

3. Rapid household surveys and facility surveys by independent agencies.

Monthly Activity Reports from the Subcentre, the Primary Health Centre, and the First Referral Unit

Monthly activity reports are expected to reflect the annual plan that is based on the auxiliary nurse midwife's assessment of community needs. The manual on community needs assessment does not describe the concept of community needs. For example, it does not specify as to what constitutes community needs and what methodology should be used to assess community needs. Every month, activity reports of primary health centres are combined in a single format and sent from the district to the state level and then to the Evaluation and Intelligence Division of the Ministry of Health and Family Welfare.

Information is to be maintained at the subcentre level for all the indicators which were used for the earlier family planning, maternal and child health, and child survival and safe motherhood programmes. These monitoring indicators relate to antenatal, natal and postnatal care, pregnancy outcome, maternal deaths, immunisations, childhood diseases, infant and child deaths, contraceptive use and services and communicable diseases. Some of the new monitoring indicators that have been added are: complicated deliveries referred to the primary health centre/first referral unit, the number of high risk new born infants referred to the primary health centre/first referral unit, complications during postnatal care referred to the primary health centre/first referral unit, RTI/STI detected and referred, adverse reactions reported after child immunisation, specific childhood diseases referred to the primary health centre/first referral unit, and interaction and community meetings with the *panchayat* health committees, *mahila swasthya sanghs*, and *anganwadi* workers. These indicators are collected at the subcentre level. The new set of monitoring indicators are provided in Annexure I.

Technical Assessment of Subcentre Level Services by a Lady Health Visitor

Lady health visitors are expected to conduct technical assessment of subcentre level services by checking one subcentre every month. Some of the activities that they have to undertake in this technical assessment include: checking the accuracy of the auxiliary nurse midwife's records; observing the technical skills of auxiliary nurse midwives; check availability of equipment and supplies, and assessing clients' knowledge and perceptions of service delivery. This information is expected to identify training needs of auxiliary nurse midwives and to plan information, education and communication activities.

Rapid Household Surveys and Facility Surveys by Independent Agencies

In order to provide independent estimates that would also be useful for monitoring the programme at the district level, rapid household surveys by independent agencies are being undertaken. The International Institute for Population Sciences (IIPS) is the nodal agency to plan, supervise, and provide technical assistance to carry out rapid household surveys and facility surveys in selected districts of India. At present, 15 regional agencies are conducting household surveys and will prepare district and state level reports. The nodal agency will prepare the national report.

Rapid household surveys on service coverage, quality of care, health seeking behaviour and client satisfaction are being conducted in 50 percent of the districts in each state and union territory in 1998. All the districts in the state were alphabetically arranged and every alternate district was selected. In each district, 50 primary survey units consisting of villages and urban wards were selected following the probability proportional to size sampling method. The remaining 50 percent of the districts will be covered in 1999. These surveys will be repeated each year. This project is planned for five years.

In each primary survey unit, a complete listing of houses was carried out, if the population was about 1,500, to prepare the sampling frame for household selection. If the population was more than 1,500; then, after segmenting the village in two or more groups of equal size, one segment was selected randomly for house listing. After listing the houses, 22 households (including 10 percent over sampling for non-response) were selected by the systematic random sampling method.

Two sets of questionnaires were used for household surveys. In addition to service coverage, clients' perceptions about the government's services and questions on awareness about RTIs, STIs, HIV/AIDS were asked. The rapid household survey also included male respondents. Men 20-54 years of age (irrespective of their marital status) are asked about their perceptions of HIV/AIDS and RTIs/STIs, symptoms of STIs in men, their choice of family planning methods and their reasons for not choosing male methods. In addition, questions were also asked to assess adolescent girls' health problems and counselling needs.

The government has also provided support for concurrent evaluation and rapid household surveys that will be conducted by 18 population research centres and selected NGOs. These surveys will be conducted in one or two selected districts of the state each year to provide information on several monitoring and evaluation indicators. The surveys thus conducted, follow a standardised methodology, and a uniform time-frame to report results for all the 18 population research centres.

Facility surveys are being conducted in all the states and union territories by eight regional agencies. One district in each state is covered every month and reports are available by the 30th of each month. Institutions covered under the facility survey are the primary health centres, first referral units, sub-divisional hospitals, district hospitals and postpartum centres. The indicators for which information is collected include infrastructure facilities, staff positions, in-service training, the status of reproductive and child health services, equipment and cold chain maintenance, and availability of equipment supplied under the reproductive and child health programme. These surveys also provide information on the types of services offered at each facility level during the last quarter of the year, before the survey. These include RTI and STI cases treated at the primary health centres and referred.

Discussion

The new monitoring system is a marked departure from the earlier top-down approach of programme monitoring. However, the need to use targets to monitor the programme remains an important guiding principle in its design. The document on the community needs assessment, which lays out the basic monitoring and evaluation plan begins by stating that *"the target free regime does not mean the abolition of work targets for service providers"*. The document specifies the methodology of setting work targets by the workers themselves, after consultation with community leaders about the community's needs.

Two other binding criteria are past performance and general norms observed for each of the services at the community level. For example, the requirement for the coming year should always be 5-25 percent higher than the achievement in the previous year, for each of the services. In addition, the government's manual specifies an expected range of the number of clients requiring different services in a given population. For example, it is expected that there would be at least 50 percent anaemic cases among all registered antenatal women. Similarly, 50-70 percent of the registered antenatal cases would require RTI services. Five percent less and 25 percent more than the expected level would reflect poor performance of the worker. To what extent these expectations will affect the quality of services and provide real assessment of needs is a matter of concern. This is particularly true given the work ethos of government staff. There is obviously a need to build into the system process indicators and give greater freedom at the primary health centre level to plan strategy.

The strength of the current monitoring system lies in its ability to capture the extent to which community needs have been assessed and reflected in programme planning and implementation. Health workers, both male and female, have to work towards achieving community participation. It is not clear how the monitoring indicators will capture the community needs assessment process. How will workers detect RTI cases from the community? How will women who need abortion services, particularly adolescent girls or women going against the desire of their husbands access service? From the operational viewpoint, it is essential that the workers maintain an eligible client register based on a regular household survey conducted at a fixed time in the year. This would enable them to segment the population needing various services. Consultations with *panchayat* leaders, *anganwadi* workers and others in the village should not be considered a substitute for household surveys. While these consultations are important tools to assess the community's perceptions, and to design strategy at the community level, they cannot provide regular feedback to monitor the programme.

The removal of method specific targets is an important step in the direction of decentralised planning and monitoring. Through district and facility surveys, the new system should provide useful independent parameters to assess programme impact. The usefulness of monitoring indicators that are routinely collected from health workers and aggregated up to the state and the national level will have to be reviewed in the context of the district and facility surveys. The practice of routinely aggregating statistics on numbers of women needing different types of family planning and maternal and child health services may not be very useful in assessing impact. Instead, workers should be encouraged to offer integrated services to clients, and client's needs should be addressed at the primary health centre level. Indicators of the quality of services are needed only up to the primary health centre level for monitoring the performance of health workers.

The current shift is likely to lead to a situation where each state may work out different priorities and therefore emphasise different sets of indicators. For example, in states where HIV/AIDS is posing a most imminent threat, the programme may place greater emphasis on the prevention and treatment of the STIs. Indicators relating to the detection and treatment of STIs and addressing risky sexual behaviour would assume greater priority both in terms of implementation and monitoring. Similarly, states like Goa and Kerala, where the population has stabilised, there may not be a need to collect family planning related statistics routinely for monitoring purposes, as the priorities in these states have changed. There is obviously a need to develop a holistic system of monitoring, where information is collected on the needs of population subgroups including adolescents, newly married, pregnant and non pregnant women, and childless couples. Each group has special needs that should be addressed.

The policy of the government is a step in the right direction. Careful monitoring and evaluation will be needed to ensure that the programme is implemented well and that it achieves its objective of providing quality services to address clients' needs.

References

United Nations. 1994. International Conference on Population and Development. 1994. Plan of Action, Chapter XII, pp 62-63. New York: United Nations.

Government of India. 1980. Family Welfare Year Book, Ministry of Health and Family Welfare, New Delhi, India.

Government of India. 1998. Manual on Community Needs Assessment, Ministry of Health and Family Welfare, New Delhi, India.

Annexure 1

MONITORING INDICATORS

Antenatal Care
No. of pregnant women under treatment for anaemia
No. of pregnant women given prophylaxis for anaemia

Natal Care
Complicated deliveries referred to primary health centre/first referral unit

Pregnancy Outcome
Weight of the new born < 2.5kg
Number of new borns referred to primary health centre/first referral unit

Postnatal Care
Complications referred to primary health centre/first referral unit

Maternal Deaths
During pregnancy
During delivery
Within five weeks of delivery

RTIs/STIs
Detected
Referred

Immunisation and Vitamin A
Adverse reaction reported after immunisation
Vitamin A administration (9 months to 3 years)

Childhood Diseases

Vaccine preventable diseases

Detected

Treated

Referred

Acute Respirating Infection (ARI) under 5 years of age

Treated with Co-trimoxozole

Referred to primary health centre/first referral unit

Deaths

Acute diarrhoeal diseases under 5 years of age

Treated with ORS

Referred to primary health centre/first referral unit

Deaths

Infant and Child Deaths

Contraceptives Services

Complications and number of cases followed up for each method of contraception

Abortion

Referred to primary health centre/first referral unit

Follow up of complications

Communicable Diseases

Interaction with Community

Panchayats

Mahila Swasthya Sanghs

Anganwadi workers

Monthly Stock Position

Vaccine Received from the Primary Health Centre

6

From Population Control to Reproductive Health: The Role of Advocacy

Anjali Nayyar

Defining Advocacy

Advocacy comes from the word advocate – which means to argue your case. The Webster Dictionary defines advocacy as the act or process of advocating, supporting a cause or proposal to plead in favour of. Today, advocacy refers to a process that brings about change and ensures accountability within the system.

Coalition building, leadership development and extensive public participation form the foundation of successful advocacy initiatives. To succeed, these require a host of skills including long term strategic planning based on research and analysis, goal-setting, alliance building and coalition management, grassroots organising, lobbying techniques, fund raising and substantial media savvy.

Advocacy seeks to increase the power of individuals and groups to make systems more responsive to human needs. It attempts to enlarge the choices that people can have by increasing their power to define problems and solutions, and participate in the broader social and policy making arena.

Advocacy assumes that people have rights and that these rights can be enforced; it works best when it is focussed on something specific; it is primarily concerned with rights and benefits to which someone or some community is already entitled; and, is concerned that institutions should work the way they are supposed to (Amedei, 1991).

Keeping these characteristics in mind, the advocate's goal is to increase the capacity of the community to participate more fully in determining its own needs and developing and implementing strategies that best address these. The various mechanisms that can be used depend on goals and strategies and, include research, documentation, dissemination, networking, coalition building, campaigning, training and capacity building. Since skills and resources have to be developed, capacity building is a long term advocacy mechanism.

Advocacy Process Leading to the ICPD

The advocacy process, though not termed as such, began in India much before the International Conference on Population and Development (ICPD). Activists, NGOs and women's organisations advocated several issues through a wide range of mechanisms such as protests and legal actions but there was no clear conceptual framework and also little understanding of how to undertake advocacy.

Since the mid-1970s, women's organisations, social activists and community based organisations have raised their voices against the contradictory positions taken by the government on population and family planning. While on one hand, the Bucharest Conference espoused that *"development is the best contraceptive"*, back home family planning measures were intensified with women becoming the focus of sterilisation (Ramachandran, 1996). The first glimmer of doubt at the government level emerged in the 1980s when the approach paper to the Eighth Five-Year Plan stated *"in spite of massive efforts in the form of budgetary support and infrastructure development, the performance of the family welfare programme has not been commensurate with inputs."* By this time, many women activists and NGOs had either distanced themselves from the government's programme and the population control lobby or had begun to oppose it. There was little or no positive dialogue between them. The moderates, who argued for a more balanced view of population, women's health and poverty linkages, were either silent or found their campaign/advocacy ineffective (Ramachandran, 1996).

The efforts to identify human development indicators according to quality of life forced demographers and the population control lobby to rethink issues. By 1993, it was evident that a significant section of policy makers and administrators within the government was articulating the need to redesign the family welfare programme. With this background and the climate created pre-ICPD, women's groups, advocates of primary health care, demographers, family planning groups, environmentalists and other concerned activists came together to lobby for change.

During 1992-93, about 20 workshops were organised at the district and state levels, which were funded by the donor community in response to an expressed need. These workshops provided a forum for defining and prioritising key problems and concerns, to find common ground and to evolve practical ways of addressing problems. There was conflict and dissension on many issues but some common themes emerged. The consensus was that ethical considerations and quality of services cannot be compromised in the zealous pursuit of demographic goals.

Four key concerns were identified: the need for efficient management of the programme; ensuring quality of care; widening the scope of reproductive health; and, using communication and media for disseminating information (Singh, 1994). National level workshops were held on the first three themes during 1994, prior to the ICPD. These views were reflected internationally at the PREPCOM III and finally at ICPD. ***This bringing together of several diverse constituencies on a common platform, leading to a consensus reflected at the ICPD was an important milestone in the history of India's population and development advocacy process.***

Agreement on the central role of women was not even an issue at the ICPD. The debate focussed on woman's control over her own body, the need to empower women, provide them with more choices, expand their access to health services and education, skill development and employment, and ensure their full involvement in policy and decision-making at all levels. The ICPD Programme of Action facilitated reforms in population/family planning programmes wherein targets, incentives and coercion were no longer to be used. Integrated approaches, quality services and informed free choice in all matters related to sexual and reproductive life were upheld as core principles. Finally, in addition to the long-established basic right to family planning, the universal right to sexual and reproductive health was affirmed.

An important contribution of the ICPD was that it changed the language to include hitherto unmentioned words such as sexuality, reproductive and sexual health and reproductive rights. Experts replaced words such as 'population control' with 'population stabilisation' to stress the voluntary nature of actions sought. The terms 'reproductive and sexual health', women's rights', 'sustainable development', 'quality of life', 'quality of care' and 'informed choice', reflect the shift away from quantitative achievement to a holistic vision of individual well being.

The Need for Advocacy Post-ICPD

India had been experimenting with the removal of method-specific family planning targets even before the ICPD. The first Indian state to go target-free was Kerala, followed by its neighbour Tamil Nadu. In 1995, one or two districts from each of the other major states became target-free. In April 1996, the government took a bold decision by declaring the entire country target-free and launched an integrated, holistic reproductive and child health programme in October 1997.

In the absence of a clear understanding of the underlying philosophy, the proposed shift would remain a mere change in nomenclature without achieving the desired outcome in health and well being. It was, therefore, necessary that multiple stakeholders be informed and empowered to catalyse a process of networking so that the ideology and ethos of the paradigm shift could be internalised and programmes responsive to people's needs could be designed with the active involvement and participation of all (Pachauri, 1997). There was now an even greater need for advocacy to make the shift to a client-focussed, gender-sensitive approach.

Advocacy is being increasingly recognised as a concrete way to hold the government accountable to the commitments it made at the ICPD. Several individuals, groups and donors see advocacy as the need of the hour and there are some initiatives underway. For reproductive health advocacy to be effective, advocates must find answers to several questions:

- How do reproductive health experts in India understand advocacy?

- What is the scope of advocating for reproductive health in India?

- Should the priority areas for advocacy be selected from an infinite range of reproductive health needs or should priority reproductive health issues that have not been adequately looked at in the Indian context be highlighted?

- How can advocacy tools such as networking, training, media, research and legislation be effectively used for advancing the reproductive health agenda?

- Who are the key actors towards whom advocacy needs to be directed?

Some answers can be gleaned from the advocacy initiatives described in the following case studies. The methodology used, the successes achieved and constraints encountered could provide lessons for future programming.

Reproductive Health Advocacy Programme: Population Council

Rationale

The process of dialogue undertaken in India pre-ICPD provided an excellent base for continuing advocacy. The importance of community involvement, both in defining and articulating needs as well as in monitoring the quality of services, was widely acknowledged. Several questions had to be addressed: How can a reproductive health agenda be operationalised? What are the short and longer range priorities? What strategies should be designed to address the diverse needs of populations in different regions and states? And what, are the specific investments needed? For all these reasons there was an urgent need to organise an advocacy programme in India.

Objectives

The objectives of the programme were to: (1) re-orient the thinking of key constituencies involved with policy and programmes from a population control to a reproductive health approach; (2) develop mechanisms to bring about changes at the conceptual and operational levels; (3) find common ground through discussion and dialogue between constituencies, particularly those with polarised views; (4) develop the capacity of local institutions to undertake advocacy programmes; and, (5) promote networking with a growing number of organisations and groups to enhance the advocacy process.

Process

The first step in the process was to demystify the concepts, ideas, and perspectives in the reproductive health approach. This included focussing on issues related to sex and sexuality and the social context of reproductive decision-making, as well as gender and health needs.

The close inter-relationships between various sectors such as education, employment and productivity, the status of women and health, were examined. The benefits of adopting the reproductive health approach needed to be understood by all concerned constituents including politicians, policy makers, service providers, researchers and grassroots functionaries, not only in theory but also in terms of tangible programme activities. It was evident that to effect change, each constituency must have a clear idea of how this approach would be beneficial and how it could be adopted. The project aimed at taking the identified constituents through this process, recognising that it had to be a continuing effort that would require constant reinforcement and support.

The Population Council is engaged in advocacy efforts at the national, state, district and grassroots levels.

National level advocacy

Advocacy efforts at the national level aim to facilitate information exchange and understanding by all important constituencies such as population planners, demographers, researchers, service providers, health professionals, NGOs, women activists, and the media – all stakeholders who can play a leadership role to influence their respective constituencies. For example, obstetricians and gynaecologists who are important providers of reproductive health services and can also influence policy were targetted. Several workshops were organised with them to discuss the concept of reproductive health and explore what it meant in terms of policy and programmes. The project similarly targetted demographers who have for decades led the population field in India and in other countries.

Several meetings and small group discussions were held with the corporate sector. A 'Committee on Population and Development' has since been formed by the Confederation of Indian Industry, chaired by a member of Parliament and former finance minister.

In an effort to involve the political community and build political will and commitment for reproductive health issues, members of Parliament and party spokespersons were familiarised with the reproductive and child health programme and were urged to become involved in evaluating and monitoring its implementation in their respective constituencies. A core group comprising of committed parliamentarians, senior bureaucrats, researchers and media influencers has been formed to help in the advocacy process.

In addition, consultative meetings and briefings were held with various members of the donor community because even though most donors are committed to funding reproductive health programmes, their understanding of issues is often limited.

State and district level experiences

Since health is a state subject and the responsibility for implementing the reproductive and child health programme rests with state governments, project activities were focussed at the state level. In addition to working with the health sector, other government sectors were also involved, particularly those dealing with education, women and child development, rural development, human resource development and *panchayats*. Discussions were conducted at the grassroots, district and state levels on specific priority concerns within the state.

The Population Council's advocacy programme is being implemented in the states of West Bengal, Gujarat and Orissa. The encouragement and support of ministers, senior bureaucrats and professionals was important in the advocacy process. Such support gave the project legitimacy and acceptance, and greatly facilitated the process.

Some important strategies used were:

Linkages with partners

It was important to identify local partners at the state and district levels as it is they who would actually take the work forward. Logistic, linguistic and geographical considerations make local involvement imperative. Further, to be sustained, there must be local commitment, particularly if the advocacy project seeks to mobilise the people and strengthen local capacity.

Responding to local needs and opportunities

Needs and opportunities were different in each state. For example, explorations identified *panchayats* as important stakeholders in West Bengal. Therefore, workshops were organised for *panchayat* members, and specifically for women *panchayat* members. In Gujarat, the need was to build linkages between NGOs and the state government. Consequently, advocacy efforts focussed on the development of a process of interaction with key stakeholders and programme implementers in government programmes as well as NGOs, research and training institutions. A programme of workshops and consultations is underway. In Orissa, the strategy was to create a multi-disciplinary task force to collaborate and interface regularly with the state government. The task force will work with the government programme, identify areas of NGO activity and monitor the reproductive and child health programme at the grassroots level. The members of the task force represent multiple constituencies.

Documentation and dissemination

An extensive documentation and dissemination effort is underway to reach wider audiences. Workshop reports, case studies, statements expressing priorities, policy guidelines, emerging perspectives, as well as scientific papers and articles on reproductive health matters are disseminated to interested and influential individuals/ organisations.

Using media as an advocacy tool

Increasingly, the government and NGOs are realising that providing information to people in ways that they can understand and act upon, is an essential part of providing reproductive health services. The mass media's ability to influence the public agenda, amplify and lend legitimacy to the national debate on important issues renders it an essential catalyst for change. The Population Council, therefore, uses media advocacy as an integral part of its advocacy programme at the national and state level.

Mass media, used strategically, aggressively and effectively, can become a significant force in influencing public debate. It can put pressure on individuals/ institutions by increasing the volume of information on health issues, thereby increasing their visibility and importance. The innovative use of media along with advocacy initiatives, including coalition building, developing effective spokespersons and increasing public participation, supports the development of a healthy public policy .

The project aims to use available information and design accurate and appropriate messages that can be disseminated through various media channels. It also uses media influencers and experts as spokespersons to disseminate these messages. For example, mainstream politicians are sensitised and encouraged to write on reproductive health issues in leading newspapers and speak about them in various public fora.

The objectives are to: (1) sensitise the media at the national and state levels to the reproductive health concept and related issues for more regular, sensitive and factual reporting and analysis; (2) design messages that are at the centre of the reproductive health agenda; (3) reinforce these messages through a variety of channels on a regular basis to effect a change in mindset; (4) facilitate information exchange between the media, individuals and organisations to build a collective voice; and, (5) create a resource group of parliamentarians/legislators, media persons, media influencers and researchers who can help impact policy and programmes.

The strategies used to achieve these objectives are many. Some examples are analytical articles carried by national and regional dailies and magazines; health capsules and information sheets; eminent spokespersons who talk on reproductive health issues through the print and electronic media; fillers (sound bytes) for the electronic media; involving consultants and news services particularly at the state level, for placement of data, liaison with spokespersons and follow-up; and, documentation.

When the project started, there was considerable skepticism and little understanding about the reproductive health approach and the paradigm shift. Few media persons were aware of the government's reproductive and child health programme. A large section of political journalists felt that this was a soft issue and, therefore, not as important as issues related to economics and politics. It was this group that clearly had to be advocated to. With sustained interaction, through small informal meetings and workshops at the centre and state levels, many negative perceptions and confusions have been dispelled. In fact, many of the misconceptions were not due to insensitivity but rather to the lack of reader-friendly material. Sustained interaction and information dissemination actually led to senior political editors becoming a part of the Population Council's working group. There was an increasing demand for information on reproductive health and related issues such as women's legal rights, education, health and economic progress. It became clear that when information was accessible and presented in a reader-friendly, non-technical format, the media would use it. The Population Council is working with the media in several states.

Advocacy Through Networking: The Health Watch Experience

In 1994, a network of voluntary organisations, researchers, activists and concerned individuals formed a civil society organisation, Health Watch. This organisation is committed to monitoring post-ICPD action in the country. This was a significant development because for the first time, researchers worked together with activists on health matters, particularly those who had been working at the grassroots level with no access to research data. Along with other civil society organisations, and individual activists, Health Watch continued to put pressure on the government to remove method specific targets and adopt a holistic reproductive health approach. By establishing a dialogue with the highest level of government, it provided inputs to health and related policy matters.

Health Watch organised a regional consultation on the preparation of the manual for the target-free approach. Its members organised regional and state level meetings and at its request facilitated feedback on the draft manual to the government. In addition, Health Watch discussed the proposed reproductive and child health programme during these consultations. It lobbied with government officials, facilitated and organised orientation and training programmes, and accessed and disseminated information. These consultations led to several recommendations to strengthen reproductive and child health service delivery particularly for grassroots workers, auxiliary nurse midwives and male multi-purpose workers.

In a recent qualitative analysis (1998) in two states, Tamil Nadu in the south and Rajasthan in the north, Health Watch studied the work load of health functionaries, assessed whether programmes had become more responsive to the needs of the people, and whether the functioning of the programme had changed at the field level. These research results along with similar studies in other states have become a powerful tool for advocacy as they address skeptics who believe that the removal of targets would seriously affect programme performance. They also highlight existing gaps in the provision and implementation of services at the ground level and, offer solutions (Visaria, 1998).

The experience of Health Watch demonstrates how through advocacy, a network of NGOs can provide feedback to the government. Though NGOs in India provide a small proportion of health services, they are more concerned with improving the quality and outreach of public services. The government has been wary of activist NGOs and the relationship between the two has not always been smooth. By initiating a dialogue and using alternative advocacy strategies, Health Watch has shown that there are several areas of mutual collaboration. However, Health Watch needs to work at different levels to maintain its momentum of a continuing dialogue with the government so that it can influence health policy favourably (ICOMP, 1998).

Other Advocacy Efforts

Several groups, some of which are listed below, have used a variety of advocacy methods. These NGOs undertake specialised tasks such as training, research, media communication, publication and documentation. As the successful experiences of NGOs have enhanced their credibility with the government, NGO leaders have begun to interact with policy makers and to play a more important role in policy advocacy.

Centre for Health, Education, Training and Nutrition Awareness (CHETNA)

As a member of various national and international networks, CHETNA aims to promote holistic and gender-sensitive health programmes. It is a member of a national network, Women and Health, and has been actively involved in defining a role for NGOs in the implementation of the reproductive and child health programme in Gujarat. CHETNA sees its role as that of an enabling rather than an implementing agency. Thus, training is aimed at helping NGOs develop their skills so that they can organise holistic and gender-sensitive health programmes. Research and dissemination form an integral part of its advocacy programme. For example, CHETNA has prepared a manual on evolving gender-sensitive indicators for programmes such as abortion, infertility, reproductive tract infections, and adolescent reproductive health. This manual is used by NGOs and the government for monitoring and evaluation.

CHETNA has also developed a range of health education material for awareness generation and training. This includes a training kit for traditional birth attendants which incorporates traditional health practices, gender issues and technical aspects; and health education material for adolescents on topics like abortion, adolescent pregnancy, gender equality and sex determination presented in a culturally sensitive manner. This NGO has also initiated advocacy efforts with other stakeholders including the private sector, the corporate sector and the media.

Rural Women's Social Education Centre (RUWSEC)

Based in south India, this NGO aims to change women's health seeking behaviour. Through health education and awareness raising programmes, women are encouraged to initiate self-treatment or seek medical help when ill, and actively seek antenatal and delivery care. A unique feature of RUWSEC is that it has been able to combine action and service provision with research. It has succeeded in making the local people and the field staff a part of the research process. RUWSEC has brought out a number of pamphlets and booklets in the local language on a variety of topics including the human body, HIV/AIDS, condoms, diaphragms, and, essential medicines (Mamdani, 1997).

Urmul Rural Health, Research and Development Trust

This NGO is based in Rajasthan. It started with delivering maternal and child health and family planning services. Its focus is now shifting to strengthening and empowering village communities to demand services from government and non-government agencies. It has played an important role in shaping state policies on primary health care, primary education, women's development programmes and agriculture (Mamdani, 1997).

Women's Feature Services

This is an independent non-profit society, headquartered in New Delhi. It began in 1978 with the objective of bringing women's analysis, views and experiences to the mainstream media. Since then it has commissioned articles, procured and offered information to the mainstream media in India and in several countries. Post ICPD, this organisation has focussed its effort on the government's shift in policy in India.

Over the years, Women's Feature Services has closely followed development processes highlighted by the international United Nations conferences and since 1991, has sent a team of reporters to cover the conference proceedings and produce a daily tabloid.

Women's Feature Services did this at the ICPD as well. It has also conducted workshops for media professionals from Brazil, India, Nigeria and Mexico for the ICPD and for those from South and Southeast Asia for ICPD+5. In recent years, the organisation has begun to focus on political and economic empowerment, human rights, reproductive health and gender issues.

Media Advocacy Group

The work done by this organisation in setting up a viewers' forum that reflects the needs of all sections of society, is exemplary. The group believes that in a situation of socio-political transition, it is essential that the civil society respond to change. In the case of the media, the challenge is two-fold: (1) coping with the onslaught of images and new value systems and understanding and articulating responses to it; and, (2) putting in place appropriate checks and balances so that with changes in the media structure and ownership, marginal groups such as women, are not neglected. (Media Advocacy Group, 1997). In an innovative venture, the organisation has identified a core group of women in Mumbai, Delhi and Chennai to work with a cross-section of the community and deepen its involvement and responsibility with regard to the media.[1]

[1] Information about Women's Features Services, CHETNA and Media Advocacy Group has been provided by the organisations.

Lessons Learnt

Until recently advocacy was seen as an alien idea. The concept of reproductive health was also new so there were no models that could be emulated. However, it was clear that if a new policy was to be implemented in the spirit in which it had been conceptualised, advocacy was essential. Some of the lessons are:

Multiple constituencies must be informed and empowered
It is not enough to address each group individually. It is equally important to ensure that there is an interface between them so that they have a better understanding of each other's roles, perspectives and the constraints under which they function.

National level advocacy is essential
Even though health is a state subject, decision-makers at the national levels must send clear signals for policy change to the state level. Establishing a dialogue with the highest level of government is important to provide inputs to government policy.

Diversity between regions and states is challenging
India is a country with tremendous diversity and each state represents a different political, cultural and social context and different levels of development. The advocacy process must be tailored to suit local needs. For example, Population Council's advocacy strategy was formulated after state specific needs were identified through a dialogue with local partners.

Successful advocacy requires a clearly defined issue with identified goals and strategies
Reproductive health is an umbrella concept consisting of several distinct, yet related issues. Each element requires different advocacy goals and strategies, since the need differs in each case.

Advocacy must be based on a strong credible database
Data on the extent of the problem indicates the magnitude of the problem that justifies concerns and the social action required.

Detailed and defendable arguments to support advocacy work, based on information, data and testimony work well.

Involvement of partner institutions

Partners need to be involved not just by introducing them to the goals and objectives, but also by assigning each one a concrete role thereby promoting a sense of ownership in the advocacy process. This can be done by organising workshops, presenting key papers and identifying resource persons. Local partners are important as they can sustain the advocacy effort over a longer time frame.

Powerful constituencies and key decision makers can make a difference

Public encouragement and support from influential constituencies gives the advocacy process legitimacy and acceptance.

Networking for advocacy achieves better results if it involves all stakeholders

This process promotes sharing, lobbying and harmonising by developing a common platform for action. If stakeholders are well represented, it also provides an appropriate opportunity for adapting practices and upscaling.

Advocacy processes must evolve and change in response to changing needs

Immediately after the ICPD, advocacy was needed to bring about an understanding of the ethos and ideology underlying the reproductive health approach. With the launching of the reproductive and child health programme, new challenges have emerged which need to be addressed. Hence, advocacy strategies need to be reviewed and tailored to address these challenges.

Advocacy and dissemination activities should form an integral part of all reproductive health programmes

The reproductive health agenda deals with related areas, several of which have been neglected or totally ignored. Advocacy can play a key role in bringing these issues on the national agenda through discussion, debate and dissemination among policy planners, service providers, donors and other concerned stakeholders.

Dissemination and communication as advocacy mechanisms must ensure that the individual becomes an active rather than a passive receiver of information

Information has to be disseminated in a manner that is timely, relevant, accessible and tailored to the needs of the individuals receiving the information.

Media communications should be linked with advocacy initiatives

The purpose of media advocacy is to use the media strategically to apply pressure for policy change or for the effective implementation of existing policies. For this, an enlightened media that keeps issues alive in the public eye and generates debate and discussion, is essential. Appropriately and effectively used, the media forms a powerful advocacy tool.

Challenges Ahead

Several organisations have prepared the ground for advocacy to promote reproductive health. Advocacy is also increasingly being recognised as an important mechanism that can effect change and ensure accountability (Ford Foundation, 1998). The government has made strides at the policy level to make the paradigm shift towards reproductive health. In addition, the 73rd and 74th Amendments of the Constitution which ensure 33 percent reservation to women in *panchayats* and locally elected bodies, provide for a positive environment to make reproductive health rhetoric a reality. Efforts must now focus on enabling all stakeholders to catalyse a process of networking with a growing number of organisations and individuals to facilitate the process. Advocacy is essential both to understand the concepts on which policy is based and also to translate policy into concrete programmes.

While advocating for reproductive health, a key challenge is to bring on the agenda issues that have so far not received attention. Some examples are reproductive choice, sexuality and sexual health, gender violence and sexual abuse. Reproductive health is inextricably linked to the issue of reproductive rights and freedom and women's status and empowerment. Advocacy efforts should now begin to focus on these issues to enable clients to make informed choices; receive information and services for responsible and healthy sexuality; have access to safe abortion services; as well as services for the prevention and management of reproductive morbidity (Pachauri, 1998). The emergence of HIV/AIDS and the rising incidence of sexually transmitted infections pose new challenges. It is necessary to address the multiple medical, social, legal, ethical and policy dimensions of these problems and using suitable advocacy goals and strategies.

There is some acknowledgement of the need to involve men as responsible partners in reproductive and sexual health. However, there is little understanding on how this can actually be accomplished. Similarly, adolescent boys and girls have a need for information, counselling and services. Yet, efforts to address these needs are limited. Innovative advocacy programmes must be evolved to address these emerging challenges.

Finally, most advocacy efforts have so far focussed on advocating against an insensitive population policy. These efforts must now be complemented by constructive strategies to promote client-centred, gender-sensitive programmes with a sharp focus on individual well being.

References

International Council on Management of Population Programmes. 1998. Upscaling Reproductive Health Innovations: Enhancing The Role Of Civil Society. Report of an International Seminar. Malaysia.

Amidei, N. 1991. The Advocacy Connection. In: L. Wallack, L. Dorfa, D. Jernigan, and M. Themba. 1993. Media Advocacy and Public Health, 26-29. New Delhi: SAGE Publications.

Ford Foundation. 1997. Advocacy for Reproductive Health and Women's Empowerment in India – A Report. New Delhi, India.

Mamdani, M. 1997. Community-Based Programmes Addressing Reproductive Health Interventions in India. Ford Foundation Working Paper Series.

Media Advocacy Group. 1997. The Audience Speaks – Building a Consumer Forum. A Report. New Delhi.

Pachauri, S. 1997. Advocacy For Reproductive Health. Working Paper No.1. Society for Operations Research and Training, Baroda, India.

Pachauri, S. 1998. Reproductive Health Approach: Concept, Ideology and Ethos. Paper prepared for the Meeting on Media Advocacy for Reproductive Health, April. Population Council, New Delhi.

Ramachandran, V. 1996. NGOs in the Time of Globalisation. *Seminar* No. 447. November.

Singh P. 1994. Women Health and Population in India An NGO Perspective. A Synthesis of Reports of Regional Meetings in the Context of ICPD - 1994. United Nations Population Fund. New Delhi, India.

Visaria, L.1998. From Contraceptive Targets to Reproductive Health Services: Evolution of India's Policies and Programmes. Paper prepared for seminar on Gender Inequalities and Reproductive Health: Changing Priorities in an Era of Social Transformation & Globalization, Campos de Jordao, Brazil, November.

7

Human Resource Management: Issues and Challenges

Dileep V. Mavalankar

Introduction

The International Conference on Population and Development (ICPD) held at Cairo in 1994, was a land mark in the development of the reproductive health approach in India and other developing countries. While redefining health services delivery, the ICPD Programme of Action suggested that family planning programmes, rather than focussing on demographic objectives, should focus on the needs of individual couples across the range of reproductive health services from maternal and child health, to management of reproductive tract infections and sexually transmitted infections including HIV/AIDS. Reproductive health is seen in the Programme of Action as linked to reproductive rights which in turn are a part of basic human rights. The Programme of Action called upon all countries to strive to make reproductive health accessible through the primary health care system to all individuals (United Nations, 1995). This implied a substantial reorientation of the family planning and related health programmes in developing countries.

India has been in the forefront of various international movements in the health and population sectors. As a signatory to various international conventions on human rights, and a participant at the Primary Health Care Conference in Alma-Ata in 1978, India has accepted health as a basic right and primary health care as an approach to Health for All. Over the years, India has built a large and complex infrastructure within the government sector to provide maternal and child health, family planning and other health care services[1]. Following the ICPD, India has taken several steps to reorient its family planning programme to address the reproductive health needs of the community. A key step was launching the reproductive and child health programme in 1997. Given that the family planning programme, implemented through the primary health centre system has been highly top-down, selective, target-oriented, quantity focussed and centralised, reorienting it to become client-oriented, comprehensive, participative and sensitive to gender concerns and quality issues will be a challenging task. The key to making the paradigm shift will be to change the mindset of the staff involved and secure their commitment at all levels of the programme.

This paper reviews the status of human resource systems in primary health care before the ICPD, the problems faced, the policy changes in the family planning programme following ICPD, and efforts made to reorient staff to the policy and programmatic changes. As the process has just begun in India, there is a long way to go. Therefore, the paper also discusses key challenges for the future in this monumental effort to reorient the Indian family planning programme.

A Review of Human Resources Management in the Primary Health Care Sector

India has a mixed health care system where preventive and promotive programmes are dominated by the government run primary health care system while curative services are largely the domain of the

---

[1] In India, family planning, maternal and child health and immunisation are under one programme called Family Welfare and are fully funded by the central government and are managed by The Department of Family Welfare within the Ministry of Health and Family Welfare. Other health programmes such as specific disease control programmes for malaria, tuberculosis and leprosy are managed by the Department of Health.

private sector (formal and informal). Both the public and the private health care sectors are large and diversified and cover most of the country. The public health system has followed the three tier primary health care model with primary health centres, district health offices and hospitals and state level health services. The enormity of the government health care sector lies in its large numbers and wide reach. The public health system has more than 100 tertiary care teaching hospitals, more than 450 district level hospitals, about 21,000 primary health centres staffed by one or two doctors and paramedics, and around 130,000 sub-health centres, each staffed by an auxiliary nurse midwife[2] and a male multipurpose health worker.

This system has been in place for several years. Management has generally been top-down. The focus has been on family planning and a few major public health programmes such as immunisation, with little attention given to the other health needs of clients. This has lead to the alienation of people from the public health system. Other management problems further constrain the performance and effectiveness of the health system (Mavalankar, 1998a). To reorient this large system with thousands of doctors, and hundreds of thousands of paramedical workers is obviously not an easy task.

A major source of tension is the fact that key health policies are formulated by the national government which also funds major public health programmes, but the responsibility for implementation rests with state governments. Another complicating factor is the large private health sector over which neither the state nor the central government has effective control. The private sector has several times more providers than the government sector and these providers are not organised into any system.

---

[2] Auxiliary nurse midwives and male multipurpose health workers are the most peripheral health workers in India. One of each category are appointed for each sub-health centre covering a population of 5,000-7,000.

Key Human Resource Issues Limiting the Health System

The large public health infrastructure follows a more or less similar pattern across the states. This system faces several managerial problems which are well recognised and which limit its effectiveness. Some of the key problems related to the human resources are reviewed here.

Limited range of services

Even though the health infrastructure has been developed under the primary health care approach and the objective is to offer all the basic health services covered under the definition of primary health care, the government health system has *de facto* focussed only on a few selective interventions such as sterilisation in family planning and immunisation in child health. All other health care activities have been neglected. This has eroded the capacity of state to provide comprehensive health services even those classically defined as public health priorities, such as maternal and child health (especially maternal care during delivery), management of locally endemic diseases, and health promotional activities such as health education and nutrition. Also, many needs of the community are not recognised as public health priorities. Some examples are women's reproductive diseases, sexually transmitted infections, sexual problems, and violence against women.

Inadequate training at various levels

Training is the basis for human resource development. Several problems have emerged in the area of training over the past few years. Basic medical education has a heavy focus on urban curative care and is provided in tertiary care settings. This does not prepare doctors for their roles in the rural primary health care system. There is hardly any system of induction training for medical officers of the primary health centres when they join the government health system. Furthermore, the medical officers do not have any public health or management training even though they are supposed to manage the staff under them. The human aspect of care is missing in most training programmes. There is no training for health education, interpersonal communication, doctor-patient and doctor-staff interactions and counselling. The technically oriented training does not help to bridge the gap between the doctor, who is regarded as supreme, and the clients who are usually poor and illiterate.

At the lower level, the auxiliary nurse midewife's training is also mostly technical with a very limited component on social aspects of health, community involvement, mobilisation, health education etc. In recent years, even the technical training has deteriorated and become very theoretical with little emphasis on practical skills of conducting deliveries and other procedures. Our experience from an action research project in one state, and consultancy work in other states, showed that many auxiliary nurse midwives do not master basic skills such as taking blood pressure, testing urine for sugar and albumin, making sugar-salt solution for management of diarrhoea in children, and managing cases of acute respiratory infections.

The Independent Commission on Health in India observed that the standard of teaching in training schools for auxiliary nurse midwives was very low and that *"the main reasons for substandard patient and community care are: substandard training, especially in the staff nurse, midwife, and auxiliary nurse midwife training courses, the lack of a proper system of training; and absence of regular reorientation courses."* (VHAI, 1997). The male multi-purpose workers receive even less training. Many of them originally joined as small pox vaccinators, malaria workers, family planning workers etc. Hence their ability to carry out basic health and family planning work is at best limited.

Supervisory level lady health visitors, or female health supervisors and male health supervisors, are the weakest link in the system. Many of them have even less training than the workers they are meant to supervise. The quality of their training is poor, and their role is unclear. Their main job seems to be to compile the reports of the workers. There has been no systematic effort to improve their supervisory functions.

At the district and state level, key managerial positions are held by doctors and top posts are filled by officers of the Indian Administrative Service. There is no uniform system requiring these officers to have any public health qualification or management training. Management training in the primary health care system is weak (Mavalankar, 1998b), and programmes are run in a very bureaucratic and hierarchical fashion without the application of modern concepts of management or public health.

The poor quality of the training is the result of deterioration at the level of medical colleges and para-medical training institutions. Medical colleges increasingly focus on high-technology, private medicine rather than on community oriented primary care. Nursing and paramedical education deteriorated due to lack of resources, leadership and rapid expansion without attention to quality. The training infrastructure created by the Department of Family Welfare, including the regional health and family welfare training centres, state institutes of health, and the National Institute of Health and Family Welfare, is also plagued by lack of good trainers, and resources. Lastly, the link between the health system and the training institutions became weaker over time, and the training that was provided lost much of its relevance to the actual work.

There has been little in-service training in the primary health care system until very recently. Fortunately, of late, under the World Bank-assisted India Population Projects, a systematic effort was made to provide in-service training in many states. This effort, however, is far from adequate as it provides only two to three days training, once every two to three years, for each worker. The effectiveness of this effort is largely unknown.

A recent review of training programmes under the World Bank-assisted population, health and nutrition projects in India from 1972 to 1997, indicated that in a total of 22 projects, costing 3.2 billion dollars, only 7.6 percent of the project budget was spent on training. Even in projects specifically aimed at strengthening training, only

13 percent of funds were used for training. The review found that, "knowledge and skills related to some specific areas of service delivery ... were poor among the health workers and that there was a need to enhance training skills of most trainers at state and district level." (Ramaiah, 1998). In summary, it is clear that training has been a neglected area in the health sector.

Lack of availability and accountability of the staff

Given the deterioration of the work ethic in the public system over the past few decades, many of the lower level staff, such as the auxiliary nurse midwives and medical officers at the primary health centres do not stay at their place of posting. A recent study conducted by the Indian Council of Medical Research (ICMR) in 23 districts in 14 states, showed that only 5 percent of the auxiliary nurse-midwives and 57 percent of the medical officers stay at their place of posting (ICMR, 1997). Many of the staff prefer to, and are allowed to, stay in a nearby city or town from where they commute to their place of work. This means that the health services are not available 24 hours at the health centres as planned. In fact, our observations, and other studies, show that most staff spend only three to four hours at their place of work on a working day of eight hours (Mavalankar et al, 1998; Ghosh, 1994). Government services also have liberal holidays and leave provision for staff without provisions for covering leave period effectively. For example, the different kinds of leave due to staff, including Sundays and half Saturdays, add up to 42 percent of the days in a year.

At lower levels, such as community health centres, primary health centres and subcentres, there is no one to provide care when staff are on leave. To add to this, many workers do not go to their place of work regularly. There are also many other interruptions in the regular work such as meetings, sterilisation camps and special campaigns. A third level of problems is that at many places, posts are vacant due to lack of trained staff, or because of procedural delays in appointing staff. Thus, the primary health centre system largely provides out-patient services and even that quite unreliably.

The major reasons for these problems are a general lack of accountability in the public system, a lack of awareness among the clients and the political influence which protects poor performers.

Centralised planning and target-oriented performance appraisal

Central level planning has over the years, killed initiative at the state level to adapt, or augment health and family planning programmes to local needs. States lack public health expertise to develop new health programmes, and are not allowed to take direct assistance from foreign donors, or to collaborate with foreign partners in the health area without clearance from the central government.

Since 1966, the family planning programme has been target-oriented and time-bound. Given the weak supervision and managerial capacity, the target-oriented monitoring became a numbers' game. Under such a management system, no attention was paid to micro-level planning, skills development, supportive supervision, quality of services and ensuring supplies to meet programme needs. Providing primary health care and even critical services such as assistance during delivery became unimportant. For example, 130,000 auxiliary nurse midwives, who as the name suggests, are midwives, conduct only 13 percent of the deliveries in the country. Even now, about 65 percent of deliveries are conducted by traditional birth attendants and relatives (International Institute of Population Studies, 1995). Centralised planning and target-oriented monitoring lead to a deterioration of staff attitudes and values and has a negative effect on staff morale.

Lack of team work and referral system

The primary health care system has not done much to develop a team spirit and remains very hierarchical and bureaucratic. For example, an action research project in one state shows that in most meetings, the supervisors address subordinate staff not by their names, but by their designation and places of posting. The same thing is repeated at the monthly meetings of the primary health centre staff. There are many interpersonal problems between the staff at the primary health centre and staff of the district. At times, supervisors and subordinate staff do not talk to each other. All this gets reflected in the work performance of the primary health centre staff and their rapport with the community.

The referral system, which is the key to providing comprehensive health services and continuity of care, is either weak or non-existent. The primary health centres, the community health centres, and the district hospitals fall under different divisions of the health department, leading to a lack of functional coordination.

Rewards not linked to performance

In the health system, there are no concrete rewards except promotions and salary increments. All promotions and increments are linked to seniority in the system, vacancy and, at times, to caste and political connections. For many posts, promotions are few anyway. The current system of annual confidential reports does not reflect performance, as these reports are written as a routine procedure, indicating satisfactory performance except in very extreme cases. Postings and transfers are also not based on performance, but on the 'government's wish', for which there is a lot of scope for political and administrative contacts to be used. The staff who stay at their place of posting, and provide 24-hour service get the same salary as staff who are absent, or are available for only three to four hours a day. In such a system, many settle for the minimum acceptable level of performance. Further training is of little help, as staff do not see any personal benefit of the training.

Weak supervision at all levels

One of the weakest links in the primary health care system is supervision. Our studies and observations show that there is no effective supervision at the field level. The supervisors only monitor the work of their subordinates through the reports they submit of the numerical achievements of targets. Whatever little field supervision happens, is in the form of policing. The supervisor checks for the presence of staff and the completeness of records. There is no effort to supervise the service delivery process, the quality of work or client satisfaction. Supervision is also weak because there has been no training for supervision; there are no systems of supervision set in place and there is no review of the supervisor's role at any level. Supportive supervision and problem solving is entirely missing from the system.

Human resource related problems and performance of the health sector

The human resource problems discussed above have led to a situation where in spite of a large health infrastructure, the impact on health indicators has been modest. The birth rate and the infant mortality rate have declined gradually, while there has been no indication of any change in maternal mortality. On the other hand, HIV/AIDS is spreading rapidly in the country with estimates of one to four million people having been infected over the past ten years. Health needs of groups such as adolescents, post-partum women, and post- menopausal women are not addressed at all. Due to an over emphasis on sterilisation in family planning, the use of reversible methods has been very limited. Partly as a result of a gender bias in the family planning programme, almost all couple protection has been due to female methods with little contribution of male methods. Due to the general neglect of primary health care, many important health needs of women have not been addressed. For example, little attention has been paid to ante- and post-natal care, care during delivery, and management of reproductive tract infections and other gynaecological problems.

These problems have led to an unhealthy work environment at the primary health centre, and have frequently resulted in conflict, frustration and stress among staff. The target-oriented monitoring of the family planning programme has led to a decline of the quality of service and the unhealthy habit of over-reporting of performance.

Human Resource Management to Operationalise a Reproductive Health Approach

If reproductive health were another technical programme, such as control of acute respiratory infections or immunisation, one could have imagined a way to implement it through the primary health care system, using the same methods of training, supervision and monitoring used in earlier programmes. However, reproductive health is qualitatively and conceptually different from the previous vertical health programmes. Besides the addition of certain technical components, such as the treatment of reproductive tract infections and sexually transmitted infections, and adolescent reproductive health, the reproductive health approach requires a very different philosophy of work.

Rather than a vertical technical programme trying to eliminate a disease, efforts must be focussed on meeting clients' needs, and attention must be paid to issues of participation, gender, quality of care and comprehensive services. This is a paradigm shift that requires a major cultural and managerial change in the primary health care system. Such a change also has implications for human resource management. To radically change the system's perspective towards client-oriented ways of providing services, the training, supervision, performance appraisal and reward systems need to change so that there is the incentive and support for individuals to change their work behaviour, style of management and patterns of planning. In this section, the key implications of the reproductive health approach on training, supervision, monitoring and appraisal and reward systems in the primary health care structure will be discussed.

Implications for training

The new approach will need at least a week-long orientation for staff to understand the key features. The methodology for orientation programmes will also have to be different as it aims at changing the mind-set, and not only at providing information or knowledge. Considerable interactive work will be needed where the understanding, values and perspectives of staff are explored. For example, a basic difference in approach will be to provide a particular service because it benefits clients, rather than because the health department has ordained that it should be performed. Thus, the needs, demands, perceptions and satisfaction of clients will be of greater importance than government orders.

Before training programmes are designed, there has to be a needs assessment for training, and a task analysis to clarify what is expected of health functionaries at various levels. The training has to be task-oriented and practice-based. Skills training has to match the needs of the specific tasks and programme components. For example, medical officers and auxiliary nurse midwives may have to understand how to treat reproductive tract infections with real cases, so that they can learn examination skills, interpret signs and symptoms, treat and counsel, and refer and treat sexual partners. This may take up to five to six days given the level of understanding of most peripheral workers. Similarly, workers would have to relearn several other skills, such as conducting deliveries, managing acute respirary infections, and inserting intra-uterine devices.

Table 1 lists the new skills that need to be developed and refreshed or relearned. It is imperative that adequate time be devoted to training all levels of workers. The past training systems are not appropriate if the reproductive and child health programme is to be effectively implemented. At the same time, the basic training of the health workers would have to be reexamined and modified to include some of the concepts, approaches and skills related to reproductive health. A system of induction training with emphasis on reproductive health would be needed so that new staff have an understanding of the issues and problems before they start providing services.

TABLE 1: New Skills that Need to be Learned and Skills that Need to be Refreshed/Relearned by Doctors and Health Workers to Implement the Reproductive and Child Health Programme

New skills to be learned	Skills to be re-learned
Management of RTIs and STIs	Management of normal delivery
Management of gynaecological problems	Emergency obstetric care
Adolescent health, sexuality and gender education	Menstrual regulation, medical termination of pregnancy
Interpersonal communication and counselling	Sterilisation, IUD insertions, oral contraceptives
Neonatal care and care of low birth weight babies	Management of acute respiratory infections and diarrhoea
Use of partograph in management of labour	Information, education and communication

Training materials including case studies, exercises, examples, audio-visual materials etc. should be prepared before the training is started. Trainers' training and preparation of curriculum and training modules should be completed before training is imparted. Various types of training such as orientation, skills development, programme management, and information, education and communication, should be clearly defined and adequate time should be allotted to each type of training.

Performance appraisal and monitoring

For major changes in any programme direction, performance appraisal and monitoring become key tools. It is said that 'what gets done is what is monitored'; other things are neglected. Hence, for a reproductive health approach to be implemented, it is very important to develop appropriate monitoring indicators. The World Health Organization had already suggested global monitoring indicators for maternal health (WHO, 1994) and recently also for monitoring reproductive health (WHO, 1997). Satia and Subramanian (forthcoming), have also suggested indicators for monitoring the Indian family welfare programme. This will help shift the focus from target-oriented indicators to a broader set of indicators and will help improve access and service quality.

The new performance appraisal and monitoring system will require indicators for assessing the quality of the process of service delivery, for evaluating gender aspects, for capturing broader reproductive health concerns through the life cycle approach and for measuring the participation of the community in the service delivery. Indicators guide the performance of the system and hence, it is important to select those that are most appropriate and will lead to meaningful performance in the direction of the reproductive health approach. Also, it will be crucial to decide how the indicators will be used for monitoring. The monitoring process has to change from using the data and indicators to identify staff who under-perform for punishment, to identifying systems that lead to low performance, look for systemic causes, initiate problem solving and provide support. These kinds of changes will empower workers to use data that they collect, to ask for more resources and to help to improve performance, rather than falsify data to avoid punitive actions as happened earlier under the target-oriented family planning programme.

Implications for supervision and reward system

The reproductive health approach makes clients the focus of service delivery and the most peripheral worker is the 'hero or heroine' of the organisation as he or she serves the clients. The supervisors are there to support the grassroots level workers. This means that for implementing the reproductive health approach, the system of supervision has to change in style and content to be more supportive, and coaching in nature rather than policing. Supervisors must solve problems of the workers, facilitate their work and at the same time ensure that staff are accountable to the clients. Supervisors must treat their subordinates as internal clients and satisfy their justifiable and genuine needs so that they can perform better. The supervisor must also play the role of trainer, and reinforce the training provided by the training centres. Finally, the supervisor should demonstrate client-orientedness, concern for quality, gender issues and encourage decentralised decision making.

The reward system also has to be reworked so that employees who meet the needs of individuals and communities and provide high quality care leading to client satisfaction will get rewarded rather than those who fill up false reports to please their supervisors. This will require flexibility and initiative at the local level to adapt the services to meet the needs of the community.

Implications for accountability

The ICPD advocates reproductive health in the context of reproductive rights. A rights approach to health means that health care is a basic right of individuals. Such an approach imposes substantial accountability on the health care delivery system. Unfortunately, in the past, accountability of the system to deliver results was eroded for several reasons. To implement the reproductive and child health programme effectively, accountability has to be brought back. The programme has to be accountable to the community and the stated objectives. To bring accountability, an approach similar to the Citizen's Charter could be adopted. The health system would specify the services that citizens can expect, and systems would be set up to monitor compliance with the promises made to the community.

Human Resource Training

Even in the new reproductive and child health programme, training is not seen as part of a broader resource management or organisational development effort, but rather, as a stand alone activity. The resources devoted to training still remain small. Training efforts made so far have been scanty, ad hoc, inadequate and of poor quality. In particular, these efforts have not been linked to enabling factors such as supplies, reorganisation of work routines and supervision and monitoring. The overall reproductive and child health budget allocates 6 percent of the funds to training (Government of India, 1997), while for the World Bank-supported component, 11 percent of the funds are to be spent on training (World Bank, 1997).

Unfortunately, there is hardly any systematic external review of the training efforts of the government and hence the quality of the training and the impact are not really measured. Our observations indicate that the training programmes have a number of weaknesses: the skills component is weak; the training is very theoretical and not related to day-to-day realities; there is no follow-up by supervisors, and the quality of trainers is poor. These weaknesses have limited the usefulness of the training programmes. Unfortunately, there does not seem to be any qualitative change in training in the reproductive and child health programme and hence previous problems may be repeated.

After removing the contraceptive targets in 1996, the Government of India suggested major changes in planning and monitoring. However, these changes were so complicated, that in effect, little happened except that the pressure exerted for target achievement was reduced. There was no focus on quality or clients' needs in most states, and the proposed approach did not link rewards to performance, nor did it put in any problem solving process or better accountability mechanisms.

This indicates that training is still seen largely as an independent activity, and not as part of a process of human resource management. The result is that there is no effort to link training to other aspects of human resource management such as job specifications, monitoring and rewards, and consequently the effectiveness of the training intervention is reduced.

Challenges Ahead

Given the fact that four and a half years have passed since the ICPD, it is time to look back and see what has happened, and what has not, and then plan for the future. This review indicates that while there have been substantial policy changes in India in the area of family welfare, efforts made to reorient the programme have been ad hoc, and have focussed only on brief orientation type training. If the reproductive and child health programme is to become a reality, human resource management will have to be managed strategically and in an integrated manner. Here, we present a model which is adopted from Pareek and Rao (1992) and takes an integrated look at training and other key functions.

Figure 1: Integrated Model of Human Resource Management for Effective Implementation of the Reproductive and Child Health Programme

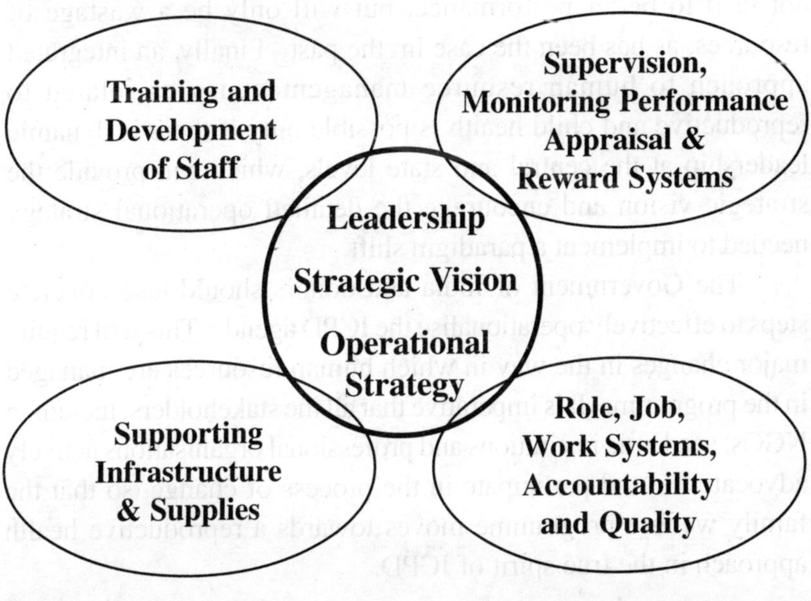

In order to be effective, the reproductive and child health programme needs to address all of the four major aspects of the above presented framework. Training must be seen as an integral and interlinked part of the package of interventions. It is important that training is linked to performance norms and measurement, and that it is reinforced by supportive supervision and problem solving. The performance indicators must monitor a broad range of services which the worker is expected to provide. The indicators must include quantitative and qualitative parameters, and be based on professional as well as community assessment. Workers who perform better on these indicators must be recognised and rewarded. Finally, the system should specify clear roles and tasks for all staff and staff should be accountable both to the community and to the programme managers. Systems for enforcing such accountability should be established, so that staff feel responsible and deliver the services they are expected to provide.

Quality assessment should be a part of the accountability and performance measurement system. Only such a comprehensive approach to human resource management in the context of reproductive and child health care will ensure programme success. Piecemeal ad hoc training, monitoring and supply interventions will not lead to better performance, but will only be a wastage of resources, as has been the case in the past. Finally, an integrated approach to human resource management issues related to reproductive and child health is possible only if there is dynamic leadership at the central and state levels, which can provide the strategic vision and encourage the detailed operational strategy needed to implement a paradigm shift.

The Government of India and donors should take concrete steps to effectively operationalise the ICPD agenda. This will require major changes in the way in which human resources are managed in the programme. It is imperative that all the stakeholders, including NGOs, academic institutions and professional organisations actively advocate for and participate in the process of change, so that the family welfare programme moves towards a reproductive health approach in the true spirit of ICPD.

References

The Futures Group International. 1998. Targets for Family Planning in India: An Analysis of Policy Change, Consequences, and Alternative Choices. The Policy Project, The Futures Group International, New Delhi, India.

Ghosh, B. 1994. Primary Health Care Time Management in Rural South India. *Journal of Health Management*, Vol. VIII, No. 2: 27-52.

Government of India. 1996 (a). In-service Training Under Family Welfare Programme: Guidelines for Developing In-service Training Plan at District Level. Department of Family Welfare, Ministry of Health, New Delhi, India.

Government of India. 1996 (b). Manual for Orientation of Auxiliary Nurse Midwives and Supervisors. Department of Health and Family Welfare, New Delhi, India.

Government of India. Undated (a). A Manual on Target Free Approach to Family Welfare. Department of Family Welfare, Ministry of Health and Family Welfare, New Delhi, India.

Government of India. Undated (b). Reproductive and Child Health Programme. Department of Family Welfare, Ministry of Health and Family Welfare, New Delhi, India.

Government of India. 1997 (a). Reproductive and Child Health Programme: Schemes for Implementation. Department of Family Welfare, Ministry of Health and Family Welfare, New Delhi, India.

Government of India. 1997(b). Training of Auxiliary Nurse Midwives (ANMs) for Building Effective Community Partnerships for Implementing the Reproductive and Child (RCH) Programme. Ministry of Health and Family Welfare in cooperation with United Nations Children's Fund, New Delhi, India.

Government of India. 1998. Manual for Community Needs Assessment Approach. Department of Family Welfare, Ministry of Health and Family Welfare, New Delhi, India.

Indian Council for Medical Research. 1997. A Baseline Survey of Reproductive Health Care Services in 23 Districts (14 States) of India. Indian Council of Medical Research, New Delhi, India.

International Institute for Population Studies. 1995. National Family Health Survey, India, (1992-93), 239. Mumbai, India.

Khan, M.E,. and Townsend, J.W. 1998. Has the Indian Family Welfare Programme Lost Momentum Under the Target-free Approach? Emerging Evidence. Paper prepared for a Workshop on the Target-free Approach. World Bank, New Delhi, April 2-3, 1998.

Mavalankar, D.V. 1998 (a). Management Constraints in Operationalisation of Reproductive Health Programme Interventions in PHC System in India. Indian Institute of Management, Ahmedabad, India. (Unpublished)

Mavalankar, D.V. 1998 (b). Need and Challenges of Management Education in Primary Health Care System in India. Working Paper No. 98-11-05. Indian Institute of Management, Ahmedabad, India.

Mavalankar, D.V. 1998 (c). Paradigm Shift In India's Family Planning Programme: A Review of Target Free Approach in Family Planning. Paper prepared for a volume being compiled for the ICPD +5 meeting at The Hague, Netherlands. International Council on Management of Population Programme, Malaysia.

Mavalankar, D.V., Sharma, B., and Sinha, H. 1998 . Qualitative Study of the Time Management and Work Schedule of Male Multipurpose Worker in Sanand Taluka of Ahmedabad District of Gujarat. Indian Institute of Management, Ahmedabad, India. (Unpublished).

National Institute of Health and Family Welfare. (Undated). Reproductive and Child Health Programme Trainers Modules for Management Training of Medical Officers (PHC). National Institute of Health and Family Welfare, New Delhi, India.

Pachauri, S. 1995. Defining a Reproductive Health Package For India: A Proposed Framework. South and East Asia Regional Working Paper No. 4. Population Council, New Delhi, India.

Pareek, U., and Rao, T.V. 1992. Concept and Boundaries of Human Resource Systems. In: Designing and Managing Human Resource Systems (2nd Ed.), 1-21. New Delhi: Oxford and IBH Publishing Company.

Ramaiah, S. 1998. Review of Training Programmes in Bank-financed Population, Health and Nutrition Projects in India (1972-1997). Paper presented at a Workshop supported by Operations Evaluation Division, April 2-3, 1998. World Bank, Washington D.C., USA.

Satia J., and Subramanian, S.S. (Forthcoming publication). Developing an Alternative System of Monitoring Indicators for the Family Welfare Programme. In: M. Koenig (ed.). Quality of Care in Indian Family Welfare Programme. New Delhi: Ford Foundation.

United Nations. 1995. Summary of the Programme of Action of the International Conference on Population and Development, 1994, 13. New York: United Nations.

Voluntary Health Association of India. 1997. Perspectives on Medical, Nursing and Paramedical Training and Education. In: Report of Independent Commission on Health In India, 24-34. Voluntary Health Association of India, New Delhi, India.

World Bank. 1995. India's Family Welfare Program: Toward a Reproductive and Child Health Approach. World Bank Report No. 14644-IN. World Bank, Washington D.C., USA.

World Bank. 1997. Project Appraisal Document (India): Reproductive and Child Health Project. World Bank Report No. 16393-IN. World Bank, Washington D.C., USA.

World Health Organization. 1994. Indicators for Monitoring Maternal Health Goals. WHO/FHE/MSM/94.1. Geneva: World Health Organization.

World Health Organization. 1997. Draft Report of the Interagency Technical Meeting on Reproductive Health Indicators for Global Monitoring. April 9-11, 1997. Geneva: World Health Organization.

8

Health Seeking Behaviour of Women and Costs Incurred: An Analysis of Prospective Data

Jagdish C. Bhatia
and John Cleland

Introduction

Reproductive health needs of women are now widely recognised. However, other aspects of women's health are still being neglected. A realistic formulation of policies and effective and efficient implementation of programmes require a better understanding of health care seeking behaviour-both in terms of utilisation of different sources of care and expenses on treatment of various illnesses. Resources available with governments to meet the ever growing health needs of the population, particularly those living in rural areas, are limited. In order to find additional resources, several cost recovery measures such as reducing subsidies and levying charges for services provided by public institutions have been suggested (de Ferranti, 1985).

Information on health care seeking behaviour and expenditure can be useful for assessing the feasibility and impact of such cost recovery efforts: how much can be recovered and from whom; what will be the impact on access to services, and ultimately, health? Some information on utilisation of public and private sources of care and direct household expenditure on health care is available from the developing countries. But this is largely aggregated at the household level, and is not separately available for women in the reproductive ages, a group which has hitherto remained neglected.

Information on household expenditure on health care in India is available from several small and large studies. In the late 1950s, the All India Institute of Hygiene and Public Health conducted a number of small studies in different parts of the country to collect data on private household expenditure on health care. The results indicated that per capita annual private medical expenditure in various states ranged between Rs 0.40 to Rs 7.20 (Seal 1961, 1962, 1963). Based on data from Narangwal studies in Punjab, Parker (1986) reported that per capita out-of-pocket expenditure on health care at 1970 prices was Rs 8.11 and 16.29 in 1968-69 and 1973-74, respectively. Thus, private expenditure on health care doubled in real terms in the five years between 1968 and 1973 – much of this was on the services of traditional and other non-allopathic practitioners who were readily available in the area.

There are some other smaller studies as well. Rao (1973) reported an expenditure of Rs 80 per family in the North Arcot district of Tamil Nadu and in a study conducted in a rural area of Bangalore district, Karnataka, Bhatia (1983) found that a household was spending Rs 39 per capita in a year on health care. A study of 82 poor rural families in South Kanara district of Karnataka and reported a yearly expenditure of Rs 270 per family, of which 60 percent was spent on private allopathic consultation and drugs.

More recently, studies to understand private health care expenditure have been conducted by the Foundation for Research in Community Health (FRCH). A pilot study conducted in Mumbai in 1984 revealed that middle class families with an annual income of Rs 10,000-25,000 incurred out-of-pocket expenditure of Rs 240 per capita (Rs 1,200 per family) excluding employer or insurance reimbursements. This amounted to approximately 7 percent of their annual income. Another sample from lower class, organised sector employees having an average annual income of Rs 7,000 per year spent Rs 176 per capita (Rs 880 per family) which works out to one-eighth of their average income (Duggal, 1986). Based on this experience, the FRCH conducted a major study on health care financing in Jalgaon district of Maharashtra in 1986. The results revealed an average per capita expenditure of Rs 183 per annum, of which Rs 154 was spent on doctor's fees, medicines, hospital costs and diagnostic tests; Rs 7 on transport, Rs 2 on rituals and Rs 7 on bribes, case paper charges and special diet (Duggal and Amin, 1989). The results of another study conducted in rural and urban areas of Madhya Pradesh in 1990-91 revealed a per capita monthly expenditure of Rs 24.93. The study found significant differentials in health care spending across economic classes ranging from Rs 10.68 for the lowest class to Rs 46.97 for the upper classes (George et al, 1994).

While most of the above studies were localised with small sample sizes, estimates of personal health care spending are also available from a few large national level studies. The National Sample Survey included three morbidity surveys, i.e; 17th round, 28th round and 42nd round of the survey. The 42nd round provides the latest information and data collected during this round pertains to the year 1986-87. The 28th round in 1973-74 estimated private health expenditure at Rs 14.05 per capita, which was three times over and above public sector expenditure in the same year (NSSO, 1982). The National Council of Applied Economic Research (NCAER) made an attempt in 1990 to provide macro-level household data on several aspects of health care. The sample consisted of more than 18,000 households spread over 21 states and union territories of India covering both rural and urban areas. According to this study, for the country as whole, the average household expenditure for treatment was Rs 142.60 per illness episode in urban areas and Rs 151.81 in rural areas (NCAER, 1992).

In 1993, the NCAER conducted a more detailed household survey of health care utilisation and expenditure, covering most of the states and union territories of India with a total sample of over 18,000. According to this survey, the per capita annual household expenditure on curative health care was about Rs 204, which was approximately 5 percent of the average household income. The average expenditure per illness episode was reported to be Rs 90 for rural areas and Rs 114 for urban areas (NCAER, 1995).

Most of the studies are based on single-visit interviews with a recall period of 15 days or one month except the FRCH study in Jalgaon district of Maharashtra which included three visits to the household in January, May and September to cover different seasons of the year. Neither do these studies provide a detailed breakdown of direct and indirect costs of treatment, nor the distribution of expenditure across different disease categories. None of the studies provides detailed statistical analysis of the relationship between health care expenditure and socio-economic characteristics. A review of the literature from developing countries has not revealed any longitudinal study on health care seeking behaviour and expenditure for women in the reproductive age group.

The main objectives of this paper are to analyse: (1) actions taken by adult women to alleviate symptoms of illnesses; (2) clinical practices of government and private medical practitioners; (3) detailed breakdown of expenses on government and private consultations for different disease categories; and, (4) the relationships between health expenditure and socio-economic characteristics of women.

Materials and Methods

A study was conducted in Karnataka which, according to the 1991 census, had a population of 44.8 million accounting for 5.3 percent of the total Indian population. The data used in this analysis were derived from a major research project, funded by the Ford Foundation, that was designed to investigate the pathways through which mother's education influences her child's survival. This study had several components: anthropologic studies; investigation of primary schools in three Indian states; a cross sectional survey, and a prospective study.

Indepth anthropologic research, carried out for more than a year, sought to identify possible linkages and develop instruments and methods for subsequent quantitative evaluation. During these investigations, the mother's health was found to be inextricably related to that of her child. It was decided, therefore, to collect detailed information in the cross sectional and prospective studies on different aspects of the mother's health. In the cross sectional study, a sample of 3,600 women (2,400 living in rural areas and 1,200 in towns) was selected. These women were asked questions about their gynaecological and obstetric morbidity and other matters (for details see Bhatia and Cleland, 1995a, 1995b and 1996). Given the objective of the main study, all women with children between 6 to 12 months (the most vulnerable age group) were included in the prospective study. In the original sample, 440 women met this criterion. All were married and younger than 35 years. They were interviewed at monthly intervals for one year. Information was sought on several aspects such as environmental sanitation and personal hygiene of the mother and the child, milestones and anthropometry of the child during the last one month, child rearing activities performed during the last 24 hours, immunisation status of the child, family planning, dietary pattern of the mother and the child during the last 24 hours, changes in the economic status and structure of the household during the last one month, and detailed sickness report of the mother and the child.

An analysis of health care seeking behaviour and expenditure incurred on illnesses reported by mothers is discussed in this chapter. For each reported illness, the woman was asked about the actions taken to alleviate the symptoms. In cases where a practitioner was consulted, information was sought about the type of practitioner, details of travel, consultation content and a detailed breakup of expenses. The data have been analysed using bivariate and multivariate statistical techniques.

Findings

Type of action by broad diagnostic categories

The symptoms reported by women were classified into 12 broad categories according to the International Classification of Diseases.

The results of our analysis indicated that out of 911 completed illness episodes, the symptoms were completely ignored and no action was taken in approximately one-sixth (15.9 percent) of the cases, (see Table 1). Self-medication was resorted to in about one-fourth (25.7 percent) of the episodes and in the remaining three-fifths (58.4 percent), a practitioner was consulted. The proportion of cases in which a practitioner was consulted was much higher for pregnancy/family planning (84.7 percent) and infective/parasitic diseases (71.0 percent). The latter category includes diarrhoea, unrelated fevers and other infective and parastic diseases. A large proportion (30.0 percent) of the genito-urinary problems and ill defined cases (24.6 percent) were completely ignored, and in a majority of nutritional deficiency and anaemia cases either no action was initiated or recourse was taken to self-medication. Resort to self-medication was reported to be quite high in episodes classified under the categories of nervous and sense organs (unrelated headache, inflamation of eye and ear etc), connective tissues

TABLE 1: Percent Distribution of Completed Illness Episodes According to Type of Action by Broad Diagnostic Category

Diagnostic Category	Action			
	No action	Self medication only	Practioner consulted	No. of episodes
Infective/Parasitic	4.7	24.3	71.0	169
Nutritional	20.0	32.0	48.0	25
Nervous/Sense organs	13.2	43.4	43.4	53
Circulatory/Respiratory	17.3	29.3	53.4	294
Digestive	16.7	22.2	61.1	54
Genito-urinary	30.0	15.8	54.2	120
Skin	13.0	26.1	60.9	23
Connective tissues	14.0	40.0	46.0	50
Injury/Poisoning	14.3	28.6	57.1	7
Pregnancy/Family Planning related	6.8	8.5	84.7	59
Ill-defined	24.6	21.1	54.4	57
Total	15.9	25.7	58.4	911

(unrelated bodyache, musculo-skeletal), ciculatory and respiratory (common cold, unrelated cough and other respiratory problems), accident/poisoning (superficial injuries, contusions etc).

Practitioner consultation and perceived seriousness of illness

A practitioner was consulted in approximately three-fourths (71.9 percent) of completed episodes that were perceived to be severe, and only one-half (49.7 percent) of illnesses that that were considered to be mild/moderate (see Table 2). These differentials in practitioner consultation and perceived seriousness of illness are statistically significant (Chi.square 38.49; p < .001). The relationship was further analysed with regard to the duration of completed episodes. Seventy two percent of completed episodes were of less than 15 days duration. A practitioner was consulted in a significantly higher number of severe cases as compared with illnesses of mild/moderate intensity, irrespective of the duration of illness. Thus, the decision to consult a practitioner is affected more by perceived severity of illness rather than its duration.

TABLE 2: Percentage of Completed Illness Episodes in which a Practitioner was Consulted by Perceived Severity and Duration

Severity	Duration		Total
	<15 days	>15 days	
Mild/moderate	49.9 (413)	49.4 (172)	49.7 (585)
Severe	69.6 (204)	77.8 (81)	71.9 (285)
Can't say	89.7 (39)	50.0 (2)	87.8 (41)
Total	58.4 (656)	58.4 (255)	58.4 (911)

Chi.Square=38.49 p < .001 (whether consulted vs. severity)
("can't say" excluded from the analysis) Note: Denominators are in parenthesis

Number of practitioner visits and perceived seriousness of illness

For each completed episode in which a practitioner was consulted, an average of 1.76 visits were made (see Table 3). The number of visits for moderate and severe cases were 1.55 and 2.19, respectively. These differences are statistically significant (Chi.square 13.23; $p < .001$). The number of visits for episodes of less than 15 days duration for moderate and severe cases were 1.52 and 1.84, respectively (Chi.square 5.32; $p=0.02$). Similarly, for episodes of more than 15 days the corresponding visits for moderate and severe cases were 1.51 and 2.97, respectively. This differential is also highly significant (Chi.square 7.95; $p < .01$). Thus, for all durations, the women made more visits to practitioners for episodes which they perceived to be severe than for those considered to be mild/moderate.

TABLE 3: For Completed Illness Episodes in which a Practitioner was Consulted, the Mean Number of Visits by Perceived Severity and Duration

Severity	Duration		All
	<15 days	>15 days	
Mild/moderate	1.52 (206)	1.61 (85)	1.55 (291)
Severe	1.84 (142)	2.97 (63)	2.19 (205)
Can't say	1.09 (35)	2.00 (1)	1.11 (36)
All	1.60 (383)	2.19 (149)	1.76 (532)
Chi.square	5.32	7.95	13.23
p-value	0.02	< .01	< .001

("can't say" excluded from the analysis)

Type of first consultation and perceived severity of illness

In the course of a single episode, patients may shift from one type of practitioner to another. For example, the patients might first consult a government practitioner and then, if they were not cured, a private practitioner or vice versa. It was, therefore, important to understand whether perceived seriousness of illness affected their choice of first consultation.

Table 4 shows, that in about 70 percent of the cases, first consultations were with private medical practitioners, and this proportion is more or less the same for moderate and severe cases. A further analysis does not change the picture. It, therefore, appears that choice of the first consultation with a private medical practitioner was not affected either by perceived severity or duration of illness.

Table 4: For Completed Illness Episodes in which a Practitioner was seen, the Percentage of First Consultations that were with a Private Practitioner, by Perceived Severity and Duration

Severity	Duration		All
	<15 days	>15 days	
Mild/moderate	70.4 (145)	65.9 (56)	69.1 (201)
Severe	76.1 (108)	61.9 (39)	71.7 (147)
Can't say	62.9 (22)	100.00 (1)	63.9 (23)
All	71.8 (275)	64.4 (96)	69.7 (371)
Chi-square q-value	1.36 0.24	0.25 0.62	0.40 0.53

("can't say" excluded from both analyses)

Travel characteristics of government and private consultations

A total of 745 consultations were made with practitioners (see Table 5). The average reported travel time, both for government and

TABLE 5: Percent Distribution of all Government and Private Consultations by Travel Characteristics.

Travel Characteristics	Type of Practice		Total	Chi.square and p-value
	Government	Private		
Travel time (min.)				13.41
<15	22.2	11.6	13.8	< .01
15-29	19.0	21.5	20.9	
30-59	35.4	45.3	43.2	
60+	23.4	21.6	22.0	
Mean	43.36	43.65	43.59	
Distance (km)				12.99367
<=2	59.5	48.4	50.7	< .01
2-5	15.8	12.8	13.4	
5-10	14.6	28.1	25.2	
10 +	10.1	5.50	5.20	
Mean	4.11	5.50	5.20	
Mode of travel				12.99367
Foot	53.2	39.0	42.0	< .01
Bus	34.2	46.7	44.0	
Other	10.1	12.8	12.2	
Don't Know/ Not applicable	2.5	1.5	1.7	
Number of escorts				17.33014
Nil	39.9	23.3	26.8	< .001
1 +	60.1	76.7	73.2	
Consultations	158	587	745	
Total visits	242	939	1181	

Note: The denominator is the total number of practitioner consultations for all episodes.

private practitioner consultations, was about 44 minutes. However, there are significant variations in the distribution by time. While in 22.2 percent of consultations with government practitioners, the travel time was less than 15 minutes, the proportion of private practitioner consultations for which travel time was less than 15 minutes was only 11.6 percent. Thus, more patients visited government facilities if they could be reached within 15 minutes.

With regard to distance travelled, three-fourths of consultations with government practitioners and three-fifths with private practitioners were within a distance of 5 kilometres. Visits of distances over 5 kilometres were most likely to involve private practitioners.

An analysis of information about the mode of travel showed that for consulting government practitioners, a higher proportion of patients walked, while a much greater proportion of those who travelled by bus consulted private practitioners. In approximately three-fourths of the consultations, the patients were accompanied by another person. Also, a higher proportion of patients were escorted while consulting a private practitioner.

Clinical practice of government and private practitioners

The patients who consulted a practitioner were asked details of their interactions with the practitioners. In all cases, the practitioners, both government and private, asked the patients the history of illness (see Table 6). However, a much higher proportion of private practitioners did a physical examination as compared to government practitioners. This difference is statistically highly significant (Chi.square 16.72; $p < 0.001$). In a very small percentage of consultations, the practitioners performed or ordered tests/ investigations. The practice of giving injections was predominant among both government and private practitioners and more than four-fifths of the patients were given injections by both types of practitioners. It is a practice among general physcians that they dispense as well as prescribe drugs. The cost of drugs dispensed is

TABLE 6: Comparison of Clinical Practice of Government versus Private Practitioners

	Type of Practice		Total	Chi. Square	p-value
	Govt. %	Private %	%	%	
History taken	100.0	99.8	99.8	0.27	0.60
Clinical examination done	69.8	86.0	82.9	16.72	< .001
Test done/ recommended	6.9	6.3	6.6	0.06	0.81
Injection given	82.8	84.7	83.4	0.25	0.62
Other drugs given	83.6	72.1	75.2	6.39	0.01
Drugs prescribed	44.0	77.0	70.7	47.37	< .001
Total number of completed episodes	116	430	532		
Total number of consultations	123	466	590		

Note : The denominator is the number of completed edisodes that involve 1+ consultation with a specified type of practitioner. The numerator is the number of consultations in which specified clinical steps taken at any visit to the specified type of practitioner.

usually included in the fees and patients are asked to buy drugs which are either expensive and/or are not available with the practitioners. The proportion of patients who were dispensed drugs was significantly higher for government as compared to private practitioners (Chi-square 6.39;p=0.01). While more than three-fourths of the patients who visited private practitioners were asked to buy medicines, the correponding proportion was less than half for government practitioners (Chi.square 47.37;p < .001).

Type of expenses incurred by patients

An overwhelming majority of the patients (92 percent) incurred some expenditure when consulting practitioners (see Table 7). The

TABLE 7: Mean Expenditure and Percentage of Government and Private Consultations that Incurred any Expenditure of Different Types (All Episodes)

Type of Expenditure	Government		Private		Government and Private	
	Mean exp. (Rs.)	% incurring	Mean exp. (Rs.)	% incurring	Mean exp. (Rs.)	% incurring
Consultation	20.52	45.6	35.76	91.3	32.53	81.6
Drugs	30.84	40.5	25.62	73.1	26.73	66.2
Travel	8.74	40.5	6.28	54.7	6.80	51.7
Other indirect	5.97	15.8	6.93	15.8	6.73	15.8
Total	66.06	73.4	74.60	97.1	72.79	92.1
Number of consultations	158		587		745	
No. of visits	242		939		1181	
Cost per visit	43.10		46.60		45.90	

percentages for government and private practitioners were 73 and 94, respectively. The average expenditure per consultation was Rs 66 ($2.1)[1] for those visiting government doctors and Rs 75 ($2.39) for those visiting private practitioners. The expenditure per visit was Rs 46 ($1.46), which was more or less the same for both types of practitioners. Of a total expenditure of Rs 73 ($2.96), 45 percent was spent on consultation fees (which in some cases also included costs of drugs dispensed), 37 percent on drugs purchased, 9 percent each on travel and other miscellaneous expenses such as special nutrition/food prescribed. A breakdown of expenditure by practitioner indicates that those visiting government doctors spent less on consultation fees, but more on drugs purchased from outside.

Expenditure by type of illness

The average cost of treating a completed illness episode was Rs 63 ($2.00). The cost was highest (Rs 104) for genito-urinary diseases which are of a long duration, and lowest (Rs 19) for illnesses related

1 Average exchange rate at the time of the study was 1 US$ = Rs 31.40.

to nervous/sense organs (see Table 8). The latter category usually included problems of minor nature such as unrelated headache, inflamation of eye, ear etc. The other diseases on which expenditure was higher than the average related to the digestive system (Rs 92) and diseases in the infective/parastic category such as diarrhoea, unrelated fever and other parastic infections (Rs 79).

TABLE 8: Expenditure per Completed Illness Episode by Broad Diagnostic Categories

Diagnostic Category	No. of episodes	% incurring any cost	Mean cost (Rs.)
Infective/parasitic	169	91.7	77.8
Nutritional	25	68.0	66.4
Nervous/Sense organ	53	79.2	19.3
Circulatory/Respiratory	294	74.8	41.6
Digestive	54	81.5	92.4
Genito-urinary	120	63.3	103.7
Skin	23	78.3	35.9
Connective tissues	50	70.0	56.8
Injury/poisoning	7	71.4	36.3
Pregnancy/Family Planning related	59	76.3	55.8
Ill-defined	57	66.7	82.0

Expenditure by disease category and type of action

Out of a sample of 421 women who remained with the study until the last round of enquiry, 379 (90 percent) reported at least one episode of illness during the year (see Table 9). A total expenditure of Rs 72,538 ($2310) was incurred which works out to an average annual expenditure of Rs 172 ($5.48) per woman. A further breakdown showed that 60 percent and 14 percent of this expenditure incurred on private and government practitioner consultations, respectively, and 25 percent on self-medication. One-fourth of the total expenditure was on treating genito-urinary diseases, and another 20 percent and 18 percent on diseases falling into the infective/parastic and circulatory/respiratory categories, respectively. Thus approximately two-thirds of the total expenditure was incurred on these three categories. If we add the expenditure incurred on problems related to pregnancy/family planning and genito-urinary diseases, it appears that women incurred one-third of total expenditure for treating diseases of the reproductive system.

TABLE 9: Mean Annual Expenditure per Woman on all Episodes and Percentage of Women Incurring Any Expenditure by Broad Diagnostic Categories and Type of Practice

Diagnostic Category	Private		Government		Self-medication		All costs	
	Mean	%	Mean	%	Mean	%	Mean	%
Infective/Parasitic	19.77	21.38	3.97	4.99	11.11	15.91	34.86	30.40
Nutritional	3.30	3.09	0.57	0.71	1.45	3.56	5.31	6.65
Nervous/Sense organ	3.85	5.46	4.34	1.67	1.42	5.49	9.61	10.45
Circulatory/ Respiratory	24.01	23.52	2.00	9.03	4.84	24.70	30.85	40.14
Digestive	8.35	7.84	0.27	1.19	4.57	6.41	13.19	12.11
Genito-urinary	26.55	17.10	5.26	6.89	11.12	10.45	42.93	24.22
Skin	2.65	3.80	0.93	1.19	0.30	1.19	3.87	4.99
Connective tissues	4.53	7.60	0.86	0.71	3.06	4.28	8.45	9.50
Injury/Poisoning	0.48	1.19	0.00	0.24	0.18	0.71	0.66	1.19
Pregnancy/Family Planning related	5.42	7.13	0.95	2.85	4.13	3.33	10.50	8.08
Ill-defined	5.10	6.41	5.65	2.85	1.33	4.99	12.08	9.98
Total	104.0	59.14	24.80	24.23	43.50	56.29	172.30	90.02
No. of Women	294		102		273		379	

Note : Total expenditure (sum) = Rs. 72,538
Mean per woman (all) = Rs. 72,538 / 421 = Rs. 172.3

Expenditure and socio-economic characteristics

The relationship between annual health expenditure and socio-economic characteritics of women is shown in Table 10. This table shows that average expenditure incurred by urban women was significantly higher than by rural women. Urban women spent much

Table10: Relationship between Annual Health Expenditure (All Episodes) and Socio-economic Characteristics of Women

Characteristic	No.of Women	Mean Expenditure in Rupees				Mean-duration (days)	Ratio of exp. by duration
		Govt.	Pvt.	Others	Total		
1	2	3	4	5	6	7	8
Location							
Urban	103	6.63	166.7	63.36	236.7	117.6	201.3
Rural	318	30.68	83.71	37.07	151.5	95.00	159.5
p-value		0.18	0.0032	0.11	0.04	0.10	
Caste							
High/Middle	254	27.67	115.3	52.16	195.1	84.42	231.1
Lower	115	26.95	62.22	17.68	106.8	123.8	86.3
Non Hindus	52	5.98	141.4	58.31	205.7	127.7	161.1
p-value		0.66	0.08	0.08	0.08	0.0032	
Education							
None	232	34.62	84.49	41.20	160.3	109.2	146.8
1-5 Years	59	17.85	132.0	68.86	218.7	107.3	203.8
6+Years	130	10.41	126.1	36.08	172.6	82.05	210.4
p-value		0.35	0.20	0.33	0.56	0.11	
Monthly Income							
<=500	58	37.93	72.17	27.14	137.2	130.8	104.9
500-100	159	25.30	84.70	63.83	173.8	114.6	151.7
1000-2000	109	11.17	129.7	28.18	169.1	80.56	209.9
2000+	95	31.56	126.3	37.03	194.9	81.32	239.7
p-value		0.71	0.28	0.15	0.83	0.0105	
Age of respondent							
<20	54	21.54	89.26	28.85	139.6	86.15	162.0
20-24	180	29.16	105.2	36.52	170.9	90.87	188.1
25+	187	21.53	107.1	54.44	183.1	114.0	160.6
p-value		0.89	0.89	0.36	0.75	0.12	
Household size							
<5	128	21.28	110.9	36.02	168.2	95.66	175.8
5-9	230	28.34	98.80	46.55	173.7	107.4	161.7
10+	63	18.97	109.0	47.56	175.5	85.48	205.3
p-value		0.88	0.89	0.78	0.99	0.39	
Women's autonomy Index							
<20	115	31.76	80.03	37.73	149.5	103.3	144.7
20-30	183	24.37	96.43	48.50	169.3	102.2	165.7
30	123	18.92	137.7	41.46	198.1	95.44	207.6
p-value		0.82	0.17	0.18	0.59	0.86	
Total	421	24.79	104.0	43.50	172.3	100.5	171.4

Note : Column 8 refers to mean expenditure per 100 days of sickness

more money on consulting private practitioners and on self-medication compared with their rural counterparts. Muslim women depended more on the private health care system and spent more money than lower caste Hindus. Educational differences in health care spending were not discernible except that with an increase in educational level, expenditure on government practitioners decreased. There was no clear trend of the relationship between health expenditure on the one hand, and monthly income, age of the respondent and family size, on the other. There was a direct relationship between health care spending and the score on women's autonomy. Women with a higher score on autonomy spent, on an average, more money on private consultations and less on government consultations.

In order to analyse the net effect of selected socio-economic variables on the duration of illness and total expenditure on health care, analysis of covariance was performed (see Table 11). The results indicate that except for the effect of rural/urban residence and religion/caste on reported duration of illness, no other variable included in the analysis had a significant relationship either with the duration of illness and/or the total expenditure on health care. The total variation explained in these two dependent variables by the independent variables included in the equation was marginal.

TABLE 11 : Multivariate Analysis of Correlates of Morbidity

	F- Ratio and Level of Significance	
Characteristcs	Duration of illness	Total expenditure
Rural/Urban residence	3.93*	3.63
Religion/Caste	3.21*	1.72
Income	1.44	0.51
Education	1.17	0.00
Age of respondent	1.30	0.06
Family size	0.18	0.29
Woman autonomy index	1.27	1.35
R-squared	.047	.025

* Significant at 5 % level.

Discussion

In this chapter, we have described the health care seeking behaviour of young adult women in terms of self-medication, utilisation of government and private sources and spending on health care. More detailed breakdowns are provided by perceived severity, duration of illness, diagnostic categories and socio-economic characteristics. The total cost of treatment is separately calculated for consultation fees, drugs purchased, travel and expenses on special foods etc. The cost per episode of illness and per visit are worked out for both government and private consultations. The results of earlier work on health expenditure in India are reviewed. However, since most earlier estimates are based on cross sectional studies conducted among the general population, and have different time periods and definitions, the comparisons have little applicability to the present study which is specifically aimed at women in the reproductive age group.

Our results indicated that in approximately one-sixth of illness episodes reported, no action was taken. This figure rises to 20 percent for episodes of reported nutritional deficiency and further to 30 percent for episodes of a genito-urinary nature. A large proportion of women take these symptoms as a part of their life and do not take them seriously. In our study, the women resorted to self-medication in more than one-fourth of the illness episodes. Self-medication is a world wide phenomenon and has been reported by several researchers (Abosede 1984; Krishnaswamy, Kumar and Radhaiah, 1985; Greenhalgh, 1987; Kloos et al, 1987; Coppo, Pisani and Keita, 1992). The results of a longitudinal morbidity study in Kenya indicated that women reported more disease episodes and self-medicated more than adult males (Oranga and Nordberg, 1995). In India and most other developing countries, all types of drugs, including scheduled drugs, can be purchased over the counter without a prescription.

In addition, patients continue to buy drugs which are prescribed earlier. The probable reasons for self-medication are inaccessibility of health facilities, non-availability of doctors, and time and financial constraints. It has been argued that self-medication reduces the burden on the medical practitioner and decreases the cost of treatment and that restrictions on access to drugs should be relaxed (Cargill, 1967; Zapka and Averil, 1976). In order to achieve the goal of Health for All, the World Health Organization also advocates self-care, self-responsibility and self-coping mechanisms. Medical professionals, however, have argued against such permissiveness and have recommended stringent measures to control over-the-counter sales and dispensing of dangerous drugs by unqualified medical practitioners. In spite of the prevalent legislation on drugs in different countries, lay diagnosis and treatment of illnesses persist all over the world. If self-medication is restricted to symptomatic treatment of diseases and is accompanied by health education, it would relieve many patients of pain and misery who otherwise would remain without any form of care or treatment.

The results of our study also showed that symptoms are ignored or self-medication is resorted to generally in illnesses which the women considered to be of minor nature. In most illnesses which are perceived to be severe, irrespective of their duration, a practitioner was consulted. An overwhelming majority (78.8 percent) of these consultations were with private practitioners and women travelled longer distances to consult these practitioners than to consult government practitioners. The results of this study are in conformity with other studies which have shown high dependence of health care seekers on private practitioners (Duggal and Amin, 1989; Vishwanathan and Rhode, 1990; Yesudian, 1990; NCAER, 1992 and 1995). It could not, however, be ascertained if these practitioners were qualified or unqualified.

Several studies in India have shown that unqualified or indigenious medicine practitoners practise allopathic system of medicine (Neumann, Bhatia and Murphy, 1967; Bhatia, 1975; Chuttani et al, 1973). Patients from rural areas or small towns are not able to make a distinction between qualified and unqualified practitioners. According to Government of India's estimates based on 1981 census data, out of a total of 236,000 qualified allopathic medical practitioners, 69 percent are in private practice. In addition,

90 percent of an estimated 450,000 non-allopathic, qualified and unqualified practitioners work as private practitioners (Government of India, 1984).

In our study, we found a very high level of use of injections both by government and private doctors. This is because patients expect and have faith in injections. Since the placebo effect of injections is very high, doctors consider it worth giving injections rather than losing a patient for ever. A woman who consulted a practitioner, on an average, incurred an expenditure of Rs 73 ($2.32). The average for those consulting private and government practitioners was to Rs 75 ($2.38) and Rs 66 ($2.10), respectively. A further breakdown indicated that each visit to a government practitioner cost Rs 43 ($1.37) while it was Rs 47 ($1.49) for private practitioners. Thus, the difference in expenditure on these two types of practitioners is only marginal. It is also interesting to note that approximately three-fourths of the patients using government doctors incurred some expenditure. In theory, government health institutions are supposed to provide free services. However, in practice the patients have to give bribes, buy medicines from the market and incur expenditure on travel etc. Further, government and private practice may not be easily distinguished. Many government doctors practise privately outside working hours and encourage patients to visit them at home or in their private clinics. If the expenses incurred on visiting government and private practitioners are more or less the same, the patients would obviously like to patronise private practitioners where perceived quality of care is higher and doctor-patient rapport and interactions are presumably better. The average total expenditure on health care for the entire sample is Rs 172 ($5.45), and there is no evidence of significant socio-enomic differentials in spending. It is not, however, indicative of their ability and willingness to pay for services.

The results of this study reinforce the findings of other studies about the dominance of the private sector in the provision of health care. Not much is known about the quality of services provided by private practitioners, although some evidence indicates that they prescribe unnecessarily because of their excessive interaction with pharmaceutical companies who try to influence the prescribing behaviour of practitioners through their strong marketing strategies (Greehalgh, 1987).

In order to improve the health status of the people, particularly women in the reproductive age group, we have to look at the government and private sectors in a more rational manner. While there is a need to improve the quality of care at government facilities and make them more affordable for weaker sections of society, there is also a need for regulatory and supporting policy interventions to promote a viable and efficient private sector.

References

Abosede, O.A. 1984. Self-Medication: An Important Aspect of Primary Health Care. *Social Science and Medicine*, 19,7: 699-703.

Bhatia, J. 1983. Assessment of Health Care Needs in Rural Karnataka. Indian Institute of Management, Bangalore, India.

Bhatia, J.C., and Cleland, J. 1995a. Self-reported Symptoms of Gynecological Morbidity and their Treatment in South India. *Studies in Family Planning,* 26,4: 203-216.

Bhatia, J.C., and Cleland, J. 1995b. Determinants of Maternal Care in a Region of South India. *Health Transition Review*, 5: 127-42.

Bhatia, J.C., and Cleland, J. 1996. Obstetric Morbidity in South India. *Social Science and Medicine* 43,10:1507-1516.

Bhatia, J.C., Dharamvir, Chuttani, C.S., and Timmappaya, A. 1975. Traditional Healers and Modern Medicine. *Social Science and Medicine,* 9(1): 15-21.

Cargill, D. 1967. Self Treatment as an Alternative to Rationing Medical Care. *Lancet*, 1,1377.

Chuttani, C.S., Bhatia, J.C., and Timmappaya, A. 1973. A Survey of Indigenous Medical Practitioners in Rural Areas of Five Different States of India. *Indian Journal of Medical Research*, 61(6): 962-967.

Coppo, P., Pisani, I., and Keita, A. 1992. Perceived Morbidity and Health Behaviour in a Dogon Community. *Social Science and Medicine*, 34,11: 1227-1235.

de Ferranti, D. 1985. Paying for Health Services in Developing Countries; An Review. Staff Working Paper No.721. World Bank, Washington D.C., USA.

Duggal, R. 1986. Health Expenditure in India. Foundation for Research in Community Health Newsletter, 1,1. Mumbai: Foundation for Research in Community Health.

Duggal, R., and Amin, S. 1989. Cost of Health Care: A Household Survey in an Indian District. Mumbai: Foundation for Research in Community Health.

George, A., Shah, I., and Nandraj, S. 1994. A Study of Household Health. Expenditure in Madhya Pradesh. Mumbai: Foundation for Research in Community Health.

Government of India. 1984. Hand Book of Health Statistics. Central Bureau of Health Intelligence, Ministry of Health and Family Welfare, New Delhi, India.

Greenhalgh, T. 1987. Drug Prescription and Self-medication in India: An Exploratory Survey. *Social Science and Medicine*, 25,3: 307-318.

Kloos, H., et al. 1987. Illness and Health Behaviour in Addis Ababa and Rural Central Ethiopia. *Social Science and Medicine*, 25,9: 1003-1019.

Krishnaswamy, K., Kumar, B.D., and Radhiaiah, G. 1985. A Drug Survey- Precepts and Practices. *European Journal of Clinical Pharmacology,* 29: 363-370.

National Council for Applied Economic Research. 1992. Household Survey of Medical Care. New Delhi: National Council of Applied Economic Research.

National Sample Survey. 1982. Report of the Third Round 1951-52. National Sample Survey Organisation, Government of India, New Delhi, India.

Neumann, A.K., Bhatia, J.C., Andrews, S., and Murphy, A.K.S. 1971. Role of Indigenous Medicine Practitioner in Two Areas of India: Report of a Study. *Social Science and Medicine*, 5137-149.

Oranga, and Nordberg, E. 1995. A Longitudinal Health Interview Survey in Rural Kenya: Potentials and Limitations for Local Planning. *East-African Medical Journal*, April 1995: 241-247.

Parker, R.L. 1986. Health Care Expenditures in a Rural Indian Community. *Social Science and Medicine*, 22,1: 23-27.

Rao, P.S.S., Rajamanickam, C., and James Fernandes, S. R. 1973. Personal Health Expenses Among Rural Communities of North Arcot District. *Indian Journal of Medical Research,* 61.

Seal, S.C. 1961,1962,1963. Reports of the General Survey in Madhya Pradesh, Bengal, Bihar, Rajasthan, Assam, Uttar Pradesh, Manipur, Delhi. All India Institute of Hygiene and Public Health. New Delhi: Directorate-General of Health Services.

Sundar, R. 1995. Household Survey of Health Care Utilisation and Expenditure. Working Paper No.53. New Delhi: National Council of Applied Economic Research.

Vishwanathan, H., and Rohde, J.E. 1990. Diarrhoea in Rural India: A Nationwide Study of Mothers and Practitioners. New Delhi: Vision Books.

Yesudian, C.A.K. 1990. A Study of Health Service Utilisation and Expenditure. Department of Health Services Studies, Tata Institute of Social Science, Mumbai, India.

Zapaka, J., and Averil. W. 1976. Self Care for Colds; A Cost-Effective Alternative to Upper Respiratory Infection Management. *American Journal of Public Health*, 68,9: 814-816.

PART TWO

Reaching Neglected Population Groups

1

Youth: A Resource for Today and Tomorrow

Sagri Singh

Introduction

Worldwide, youth[1] between the ages of 10-24 years make up about one third of the total population, with India accounting for approximately 17.7 percent (Population Reference Bureau, 1996). In India, the population of adolescents (10-19 years) is 21 percent with youth (10-24 years) contributing approximately a third of the total population (Alan Guttmacher Institute, 1998). So far, youth have remained largely invisible at the policy level where the focus has been on the problems generated by this age group including their contribution to the increase in future population growth (population momentum)[2], teenage pregnancy, addiction, illiteracy, and violence. Given the relative invisibility of the population and the sensitivity of certain issues such as sexuality, violence and reproductive health, the majority of innovative programmes that address youth health, literacy, and skills and vocational training needs is by the voluntary sector. Organisations have used a variety of approaches to address the needs of this group as well as to ensure

---

[1] In keeping with the WHO definition and for purposes of this paper, adolescents denote those between the ages of 10-19 years and youth between the ages of 10-24 years. For the most part, the paper will address the needs of adolescents with an extrapolation to the age 20-24 years.

[2] The population momentum is projected to account for over 61 percent of the total population growth between 1996 and 2101 (Visaria and Visaria, 1996).

that the information is based on the needs of the target group (Greene, 1997; Satia et al, 1995; Singh, 1998; Subramanian, 1998). For the most part, however, programmes for youth are in their nascent stage and have tended to focus on girls rather than boys and that too, on unmarried girls.

The International Conference on Population and Development (ICPD) in 1994 renewed the interest in youth and broke new ground in bringing global recognition of youth and their needs within the broader framework of rights, gender equity and equality. The ICPD Programme of Action (United Nations, 1994) recognises the contribution of youth and adolescents on two levels. The first takes a broader view highlighting the potential of youth as a future human resource and emphasises the importance of addressing them in their own right (that is, as an end rather than a means to an end) and in an integrated and holistic manner.

> To "*promote to the fullest extent the health, well-being and potential of all children, adolescents and youth as representing the world's future human resources, ... with due regard for their own creative capabilities, for social, family, community support, employment opportunities, participation in the political process and access to education, health, counselling, and high quality reproductive health services...*"
> (Chapter VI B "Gender Equality, Equity and Women's Empowerment").

At the second level, the document focuses specifically on the reproductive health and rights of youth. As stated in Chapter VII on Reproductive Rights and Reproductive Health:

> "*... to address adolescent sexual and reproductive health issues, including unwanted pregnancy, unsafe abortion and sexually transmitted diseases, including HIV/AIDS, through the promotion of responsible and healthy reproductive and sexual behaviour, specifically suitable for that age group;...*"
> (paragraph 7.44).

In this paper, an attempt is made to highlight the context in which youth (and adolescents) in India have been perceived vis a vis the government, the process of change underway post ICPD, and the opportunities and challenges that lie ahead in translating the rhetoric into reality.

The Context

Policy

Indian policy-makers have long recognised the potential of youth and made efforts to harness their potential and collective strength for social and economic development. However, the impetus has been paternalistic: To harness the energy of youth and channellise it into a positive force rather than to focus on identified needs and strategies. In 1985, the International Year of Youth, an independent Department of Youth Affairs and Sports was established within the Ministry of Human Resource Development. At the same time, parallel departments were set up at the state level. The National Youth Policy was formulated in 1986. It views youth (defined as 15-35 years) as:

> *"a vital and vibrant natural resource that has a right and an obligation to participate actively in national development... to create increasing opportunities for them (youth) to develop their personality and their functional capability and thus make them economically productive and socially useful"* (Government of India, Department of Youth and Sports Affairs 1985).

The policy instead of providing an enabling environment to understand and nurture youth, was based on what the state decided was best for youth.

Two recent documents, however, highlight the renewed commitment of the government to work with youth in a holistic manner. The first is the report of the Swaminathan Committee, comprising of a group of experts, convened in 1993 to draft a preliminary National Population Policy. The Committee clearly recognises the growing proportion of youth as a significant group albeit within the narrow framework of population control and population momentum. While it calls for *"every effort ... [should be] made to inculcate in youth the dynamics of population growth and the concept of responsible parenthood"* (Government of India, 1993), the document breaks away from traditional thinking to encourage *"school, college and university systems should have more vigorous population, family health and sex education modules as part of syllabi at various levels in order to crystallise the concept of responsible parenthood and safe sex."* Elsewhere in the document, there is a recognition that gender equity, empowerment and an integrated approach are crucial to the success of these activities.

The second, a draft Youth Policy (Government of India, 1997) acknowledges the lack of importance given to youth affairs both in budgetary terms and as an issue, and seeks to correct this oversight. This policy stipulates youth empowerment, gender justice, an inter-sectoral approach, and information and research networks as the four thrust areas of youth empowerment. Keeping in mind the principles of inter-sectoral linkages, partnerships and an integrated approach, consultations were set up on various youth related issues across the country to feed into the draft policy. As a document and philosophy, it is groundbreaking: it redefines the age group (earlier identified as 15-35 years and now 13-30 years) and attempts to address the varying needs of youth in an integrated manner.

Initiatives

A number of government schemes have emerged in an attempt to fill the information gaps of adolescents especially around the broad areas of health, education and employment and training opportunities. These initiatives have arisen at the national and state levels as well as through bilateral collaboration. At the national level, various departments are involved in these activities including the Departments of Youth Affairs and Sports, Women and Child Development and Education; Ministry of Health and Family Welfare; Ministry of Rural Development and Employment; and Ministry of Social Justice and Empowerment. A number of states have also undertaken various schemes to redress the gender disparity and provide opportunities through training and education to youth, especially girls. In addition, bilateral collaboration with other governments has led to innovative programmes at the state level focussed on education and the girl.

Social Development

Two major programmes of the Department of Youth Affairs and Sports are the National Service Scheme and the *Nehru Yuvak Kendras Sangathan*. The former targets university students with a focus on all-round personality development through community service including improving campuses, working on slum improvement projects, and education campaigns. A number of additional activities are held including awareness camps, sports competitions and issue based activities in order to expose the students and foster a healthy environment for their growth and development (Government of India, 1997).

The *Nehru Yuvak Kendras Sangathan* is an autonomous grassroots level organisation catering to the needs of out-of-school, rural youth between the ages of 15-35 years who are enrolled through village based youth clubs. There are approximately 500 functioning youth clubs across the country. The objective is to mainstream rural youth into becoming active participants and contributors toward national development. Programmes undertaken by the youth clubs include vocational training, training for self-employment, work camps, youth leadership and awareness campaigns, cultural and social programmes, national integration efforts, and health awareness camps (Government of India, 1997). Both programmes have been successful in reaching out to youth and linking them up with various types of activities. However, while the employment and education aspects of young people's lives are dealt with at some level, there continues to be a major gap in addressing the social roles of youth and issues related to their health and sexuality.

Health and Empowerment

Data indicate that while the legal age for marriage in India is18 years and 21 years for girls and boys respectively, approximately 12 percent of boys and about 38 percent of girls between the ages of 15-19 years are married. And that while half of all women are sexually active by the age of 18, approximately one in five are sexually active by 15 years (Jejeebhoy, 1996). Child bearing outside marriage, however, continues to be uncommon. In fact, low contraceptive use and high abortion rates among unmarried girls bear testimony to this fact. On the other hand, fertility among married adolescent girls is significant with close to 30 percent of girls experiencing a first birth by the time they turn 18 years (Alan Guttmacher Institute, 1998).

With the advent of the South Asia Association of Regional Cooperation (SAARC) Decade of the Girl Child (1991-2000), government efforts became more focussed especially on girls. Schemes launched include the Adolescent Girls Scheme within the existing Integrated Child Development Scheme (ICDS) that was initiated in 1991-92. While the ICDS focusses on the nutritional and health needs of mother and child, the *Balika Mandals* or girls' clubs attempt to address the overall needs of out-of-school girls between the ages of 11-18 years. The initiative is innovative in that it identifies out-of-school girls as a marginalised group and attempts to address their needs in an integrated manner through nutrition programmes, health awareness and education, and skill training under the guidance of the village *balwadi* (child care centre) worker. The goal is to enable the adolescent girl to learn a vocational skill, in this case how to run a child care centre, in the hope that she will take on this activity at a later stage (Department of Woman and Child, 1997-98). While this scheme operates in over 500 blocks, at present it has limited outreach (approximately 391,000 girls); the impact of the scheme has yet to be assessed.

Since the early 1980s, through its network of schools and colleges, the government has been implementing a programme of population and development and family life education in order to prepare young people to make personal and socially responsible choices. It was envisioned that this programme would form an integral part of the existing educational system and that society, teachers and parents would be an important part of the initiative (Sriram, 1998). However, its focus is limited to preparing youth to be responsible within the framework of population growth and its effect on development. Hence, the state has yet again assumed a patronising role in determining the 'problem' and what should be done about it. Youth are perceived as passive actors, to be encouraged to absorb the messages in the hope that these will translate into positive behaviour. These activities have not been successful in discussing youth problems and needs. Issues of sexuality, reproductive health, and choices and responsibilities have not been addressed by this programme (Mehta, 1998). In fact, micro-level studies indicate the existence of premarital sexual activity in both rural and urban areas and that it is on the rise (reportedly higher among boys) (Bang et al, 1989; ICRW, 1997). Sexually transmitted infections (STIs) including HIV are also prevalent in this population. Baseline surveys report the current annual incidence of STIs at 5 percent (approximately 40 million new infections), a significant percentage of which occurs among the youth population (Government of India, 1998; Alan Guttmacher Institute, 1998).

Given the vulnerability of youth and their potential as educators, the government has launched a number of HIV/AIDS prevention education programmes in universities and schools as well as through social marketing activities and media campaigns. Examples of such programmes include University Talks AIDS initiated in 1991 in 59 universities through the National Service Scheme. The aim is to identify the level of AIDS awareness among university students and to raise awareness through a series of activities. Similarly, education departments at the state level conduct AIDS prevention programmes in secondary schools. For example, the Maharashtra AIDS Cell of the Directorate of Health Services formulated and implemented an AIDS prevention programme in 1994. The programme is targetted at in-school, rural youth through a system of trained peer educators, nodal teachers and district tuberculosis officers (UNESCO, UNAIDS and UNICEF, 1998). Departments of Education and Health also collaborate (such as in the states of Madhya Pradesh, Maharashtra, and Kerala) to implement programmes of HIV/AIDS prevention in the school system (Andersson et al, 1996).

Other programmes have attempted to use a lifecycle approach to address issues of gender discrimination, social and economic empowerment of women, and training, employment and educational needs of youth. In the early 1990s, a number of states like Rajasthan, Haryana, Punjab, Tamil Nadu, and Karnataka initiated schemes to raise the status of the girl child. The schemes involve a lumpsum investment on the birth of a girl child[3] that is to be repaid to her when she reaches 18 or 20 years. In addition, scholarships for education and credit for income generation activities are also made available. Depending on the state, payment is made based on stipulated education, marriage and family planning criteria. For instance, in Haryana under the *Apni Beti Apna Dhan* Scheme, the girl is eligible for the invested amount (average of Rs 25,000, approximately US$ 600) when she reaches the age of 18 years provided she is unmarried.[4] The Prime Minister launched a national level scheme (*Balika Samriddhi Yojana*) along the same lines in 1997. The latter provides families with a girl child, living below the poverty line, with financial help of Rs 500 (approximately US$ 12). This money is paid to the mother on the birth of a girl child for their general nutrition and health needs.

---

[3] Only girls from families living below the poverty line, backward and scheduled classes are eligible.

[4] Documentation of Apni Beti Apna Dhan by Nandita Mathur on behalf of Population Council, draft.

Education and Employment

The Indian Constitution guarantees free education to all citizens up to the age of 14 years. However, literacy levels continue to be low, especially among girls. Data indicate that two out of three boys and two out of five adolescent girls are literate. In fact, gender disaggregated data clearly show that significantly fewer numbers of girls enroll in school and a higher number drop out after the primary level. Work force participation among adolescents also indicates the disproportionately high and invisible work burden shouldered by girls who take on domestic responsibilities as early as 5 years of age (Chaudhury, 1998; Government of India, 1998; Mehta, 1998; ICRW, 1997; Jejeebhoy, 1996).

In terms of primary education, the government has over the years poured energy and resources in trying to fulfil the terms of the Constitution. Efforts have been made to spawn a network of formal and informal education opportunities throughout the country, including literacy classes for school dropouts, distance education schemes, vocational training, and skill building. In addition, the Ministry of Social Justice and Empowerment has schemes that focus on increasing the level of education among tribal girls by setting up educational complexes and hostels, providing vocational training and disbursing scholarships to girls and financial incentives to parents to send their daughters to school. The Ministry of Rural Development and Employment under its Integrated Rural Development Programme (IRDP) has a sub-programme called Development of Women and Children in Rural Areas. Initiated in 1982, it aims to improve the overall socio-economic status of women through programmes of health, literacy, thrift and credit activities. Training of Youth for Self-Employment is another such programme under the IRDP that aims at providing basic technical and managerial skills to rural youth between the ages of 18 and 35 years from families living below the poverty line.

Two innovative schemes have been undertaken in collaboration with the Swedish and Dutch governments, *Lok Jumbish* and *Mahila Samakhya*. The objective of the former, initiated in 1992, is education for all through peoples' mobilisation and participation.

The programme, currently underway in Rajasthan, provides access to primary education to children up to 14 years, ensures quality education, creates structures to empower women, uses education as an instrument of equality, involves people in planning and managing the programme, and builds partnerships with local communities and the voluntary sector. Gender issues are addressed within the formal and non-formal educational systems in the state (Lok Jumbish Parishad, 1998).

The *Mahila Samakhya*[5] programme was initiated in 1989. This is a woman's empowerment programme that aims to create an enabling environment for women to acquire knowledge and information. It attempts to bring about changes in self perception and perception of society. The programme functions on the strength of its *Mahila Sanghas* or women's groups, the unit of organisation and mobilisation at the grassroots. Education of adults and children is the central concern of the *Sanghas*. It is this concern that gave birth to the *Mahila Shikshana Kendras* or non-formal educational centres for girls. There are 16 such centres spread across the states of Karnataka, Bihar, Andhra Pradesh, Gujarat and Uttar Pradesh that provide adolescent girls with a unique opportunity for residential learning, using a holistic approach that includes literacy, leadership, and life skills training.

Media and Social Debate

Indians are no strangers to the various health and social problems that youth face in growing up. The media too has picked up on these issues over the years with regular features appearing in newspapers and magazines. For example, in November 1978 the cover story in India Today, a newsmagazine, analysed the results of a survey conducted by the Social Research Unit of the Indian Market Research Bureau of 604 college students in Delhi, Calcutta, Chennai and Mumbai (Sanghvi, 1978).

---

[5] Documentation of Mahila Samakhya by Nandita Mathur on behalf of Population Council, draft.

The government owned All India Radio network broadcast two radio serials on adolescent issues by its Yuvavani or Youth Voice station. The first aired in 1988 was titled *Jeevan Saurabh* (Fragrance of Life) and was a 13-episode series that used a participatory message design process to address problems facing adolescents such as sexuality, intergenerational conflicts, career choices, and personality development (Bhasin and Singhal, 1998). The second serial *Dehleez* (Threshold) was broadcast in 1994. Because of the high demand it was extended from its initial 26 to 52 serials. It was translated in 10 regional languages and broadcast across the country (Anonymous, 1994). The success of both serials is attributed to their developing a sense of ownership in the target audience by encouraging letters and questions. The programme highlighted the emotional, social and psychological problems of youth. These radio programmes and follow-up activities addressed an important need of providing accurate information in a confidential manner to youth.

Comparing information from studies done in the previous decade and current research, it is interesting to note that the issues that adolescents face have not changed over the years. Youth continue to be perplexed with the physiological changes they undergo. They lack accurate and respectful information about their bodies and relationships. They have shared concerns regarding economic security and career issues. Youth continue to quote books, media and peers as their primary sources of information (Bhasin and Singhal, 1998; Watsa, 1993-94; Sanghvi, 1978).

The Process of Change

The impact of this conference will be measured by the strength of the specific commitments made here and the consequent actions to fulfill them, as part of a new global partnership among the world's countries and peoples, based on a sense of our shared but differentiated responsibility for each other and for our planetary home. (ICPD-POA, Preamble 1.15)

While India has a rich and varied history of working with youth, the tone is one of patron or parent as there continue to be lacunae in recognising and addressing youth in their own right. The discussions and ratification of the ICPD Programme of Action helped to address this issue as political representatives and activists grapple with adopting and implementing the broader framework. While ICPD redefined adolescents and youth in clear terms and their needs within a framework of rights and choices, the change has been slow in taking root. The ICPD advocated an integrated participatory approach for formulating and implementing strategies and utilising existing resources more efficiently. To this end, the various actors in India have been responsive in taking up the challenge. There is a paradigm shift from a demographic imperative to reproductive rights and health, within development.

Linkages: Reproductive Health, Population, Environment and Development

With growing globalisation and a shrinking world economy, resources and opportunities available to youth are few. The implications are enormous as the government and civil society get ready to shift toward a more humane paradigm that believes in the rights and dignity of human beings. The government and activists are realising the importance of working within the broader development paradigm if programmes are to be effective, especially in a resource poor country like India beset with inequities at all levels. For example, the current draft Youth Policy recognises these interlinkages and attempts to address the various facets that make up the life of youth, including health, education, training and employment, gender justice, sport, art and culture, and science and technology.

Special attention is paid to the environment and the need to protect and nurture it in order to avoid the ill effects of environmental degradation on future generations (Government of India, 1997). In order to have efficient use of scarce resources and sustainability of programmes, efforts will have to be made for initiatives to be truly integrative and collaborative. The government is collaborating with various partners – NGOs, donors, and others – to develop more efficient programmes on the ground. However, a more concerted effort and political commitment is needed to have true collaboration between the departments and ministries within the bureaucracy itself.

Cairo Ethos in Practice: Implementing Policy and Services

The process of government policy formulation has been heartening to witness. Two draft policies that have a direct impact on youth have been through open consultations with recommendations requested at each stage. The Youth Policy drafted in 1997 has undergone a series of consultations with experts, activists and others. Suggestions have been solicited and in some cases incorporated. Similarly, the draft National HIV/AIDS Prevention and Control Policy was circulated among political representatives, NGO, media, activists, academics, and others. Feedback was solicited through consultations. A document on the National Perspective on Youth is being prepared to highlight the ways in which youth issues need to be perceived and addressed. In addition, the Ninth Five Year Plan (1997-2000) clearly articulates the importance of adolescent health and the need to address it in a comprehensive manner (Government of India, 1998).

The government has been particularly receptive and proactive in attempting to translate the ICPD programme within the country. The government shifted its population policy to a Target Free Approach in 1996 and launched the Reproductive and Child Health Programme in 1997. In the new programme, the government recognises adolescent girls as a distinct group with specific needs and has charged a committee of experts to formulate a comprehensive package of services for girls. The government has also made some headway in involving NGOs in dialogue for possible future partnerships in implementing programmes at the field level. However, the implementation of the broad youth policy continues to be limited and services for youth elusive.

Rights: Rhetoric to Reality

While the ICPD Programme of Action stipulates the rights framework, a great deal remains to be done in furthering how the government and the civil society understand the meaning of rights and how it translates in everyday life. A first step has been the clear articulation of a rights approach in the draft Youth Policy. However, the rights discourse fades on the more contentious issue of sex education and health services for youth. NGOs, on the contrary, have been working on linking health and rights issues and have found it doubly challenging when working with youth. For example, Adithi[6], an NGO in Bihar, emphasises the rights framework in its work with marginalised populations and children of commercial sex workers. In addition, organisations working on violence, sexual abuse and incest such as Sakshi, Shakti Shalini and others use a rights angle in all their work.

The government and NGOs have been less successful in incorporating the rights framework in advocating for health, specifically that of women and adolescents. NGOs have been training political representatives, legislative members, other NGOs, and civil society members on the rights discourse and its centrality to other aspects of life. Efforts are now being made by donors and NGOs to initiate a discourse on human rights and women's rights. The objective is to better understand the issues, develop a common vocabulary and frame the arguments within a rights discussion. But these are early efforts and exploratory in nature.

Partnerships

While the ICPD document clearly states that partnerships are key to implementing the broad agenda, these partnerships vary in nature. The Asia and Pacific Regional Consultation on ICPD+5 determined that *"partnerhips should be defined as respecting, sharing and cooperating together in a systematic and sustained manner and facilitating the contribution of partners at all levels towards a common goal"* (Asia and Pacific Regional Consultation Report,

[6] Ongoing documentation of Adithi by the Population Council.

1998). Recent years have witnessed an emergence of partnerships between the government and the voluntary sector; within the voluntary sector; within departments/ministries of the government; and, between state and central governments. A recent initiative is the 'mother NGO' concept. Intermediary NGOs are identified to work with the government in implementing the Reproductive and Child Health programme including the adolescent girl scheme. These intermediaries provide funds and technical assistance to smaller NGOs. In addition, some intermediary NGOs, such as the Child in Need Institute (CINI) in West Bengal, are working with a donor and the state government to implement pilot programmes on adolescent health.

Partnerships between government departments and ministries are crucial. An example of such a partnership is seen in the HIV/AIDS sector where both at the national and state levels, departments of education and health collaborate to conduct HIV/AIDS prevention and family life education. All these activities are underway, but it needs to be said that only time will tell how true the partnerships are, and if they will hold out through the design, implementation, management and monitoring of the programmes. Especially important and difficult to achieve is cost sharing among various government departments.

Advocacy and Resources

The ICPD underscored the importance of advocacy as an important tool to advance the agenda. In a country where the concept of adolescence is relatively new, the government and NGOs are now talking about adolescence as a key phase in the lifecycle. There is discussion on the large numbers of youth in the country and the need for structured policies and programmes. Through a systematic advocacy programme, the draft Youth Policy and related policies have been critically reviewed by NGOs and researchers and recommendations provided. In addition, media advocacy through articles in newspapers and magazines have initiated public awareness and dialogue on the vulnerability of youth and the importance to address their needs in a confidential and respectful manner.

Ongoing research (ICRW, 1997) and documentation of existing innovative programmes (Population Council, ICOMP, UNESCO) are being conducted in an effort to better understand youth needs and experiences, and to design effective interventions. An example can be seen in a recent British Broadcasting Corporation World Service training conducted for electronic media producers in India. Four of the six programmes were independently conceptualised and developed for youth and their parents on sexual and reproductive health issues.[7] The producers are now in the process of disseminating their programmes. Through various meetings and conferences, networks of groups working on various aspects of adolescent/ youth issues have developed. For instance, the Population Council has convened a working group on adolescents that reviewed the two draft policies on youth and HIV/AIDS prevention, identified recommendations, and then met with representatives to discuss their implications.

While there is interest in adolescent and youth issues, the resources to act upon the identified priorities remain relatively slim. Few donors have adolescents as a priority group for funding and even when they have, little information has been available at the grassroots to identify activities that could be effectively implemented. The problem is further compounded by the lack of integration within the bureaucracy to operationalise programmes. Issues such as HIV/ AIDS and adolescent pregnancy continue to take precedence in both donor and government funding priorities. Services are implemented through vertical programmes. One of the key principles identified by Germain and Kyte (1995) to implement a reproductive health approach is to *"utilize resources we already have more efficiently; we do not have to wait for new money, new data, or new staff"*. Furthermore, policy implementation requires political will and concerted commitment on the part of its implementers.

---

[7] Information available from the Ford Foundaiton, New Delhi and BBC World Service Training in the U.K.

Opportunities and Challenges

Governments in collaboration with non-governmental organizations, are urged to meet the special needs of adolescents and to establish appropriate programmes to respond to those needs (ICPD-POA, paragraph 7.47).

There is ample opportunity for addressing the needs of youth as donors, NGOs and governments are beginning to perceive this as an important group. The government has a critical role in leading the way given the financial and human resources at its disposal, the existing infrastructure, and the mechanisms to implement programmes. It is time, therefore, to prioritise the needs, review existing research, activities and budgets, and reorganise and integrate programmes across the different ministries and departments so that the needs of youth are addressed through holistic, respectful and innovative programmes.

In the draft Youth Policy, the government has separated the *age of adolescence* (13 to 19 years) from *age of attainment of maturity* (20 to 30 years). The challenge now lies in prioritising competing interests, finding common ground or at least complementary activities to address diverse needs, and of equal importance, to avoid duplication of services. The government will also need to carefully formulate implementation plans to take into account the inherent gender bias that exists in the country. This bias works in two ways: (1) girls' lack of access to opportunities in the areas of health, employment and education as compared to boys and (2) the propensity for programmes to provide traditional opportunities that perpetuate the status quo and preserve the disparity rather than challenge it.

India is at the cutting edge in terms of formulating a policy that attempts to address youth in a holistic and integrated manner. A number of challenges, however, exist in implementing such a broad policy. Different departments of the government are responsible and accountable for various aspects of the programme; resources are widely dispersed with limited integration among departments;

and commitment to the issue remains scattered. Despite the innovative approach used to draft the youth policy through a process of consultations, for the most part, policies continue to be formulated based on criteria determined by experts and not by the target group. The result is that many vital issues and strategies are overlooked.

It has been observed that policies in India are more progressive than the communities they are formulated to serve or the service providers through whom they are implemented. Therefore, policies often end up being only partly implemented due to reluctance or perceived reluctance of the general public. In order to implement policies effectively, there is a need to prepare the civil society through systematic advocacy thereby fostering an enabling environment for programme implementation.

Mechanisms for advocacy exist as state-owned electronic media (*Doordarshan* and *Akash Vani* – television and radio, respectively) has wide outreach in both rural and urban areas. The government also has precedence is using media based messages for raising awareness. Country-wide advocacy campaigns have been conducted around population control and family planning. *Dehleez* and *Jeevan Saurabh* are but two examples of how youth interests have been successfully addressed through state-owned media. While advocacy is a key strategy for the government, the patronising attitude toward youth has led to the cancellation of more recent radio initiatives like *Balance Barabar*, a radio programme that addressed the health needs of youth. Therefore, the biggest challenge for political representatives today is to resolve the tension that exists between servicing youth needs and affirming cultural and traditional norms.

Most of the cutting edge initiatives underway in the country are situated in the voluntary sector. The government has in place wide outreach, existing infrastructure and resources that could be built upon. Upscaling small-scale programmes through the existing government infrastructure is critical. Some government-led innovative schemes such as *Lok Jumbish, Mahila Samakhya* and Gujarat Bicycle Scheme have a lot to offer in terms of their experiences and lessons that can be learnt. Shared learning to replicate successful innovations requires collaboration with different partners such as NGOs and other government departments. The challenge lies in conducting research, documentating experiences of NGOs and government initiatives and disseminating these to contribute to collective learning. The government should be open to innovate on its own or with NGO inputs. Likewise, a rigorous system of monitoring and evaluation needs to be put in place to determine progress and impact of programmes.

Putting youth at the centre and listening to their concerns and suggestions is the key to fostering ownership and success of programmes. Today, youth are articulate, ambitious, interested, and ready to stake their claim. Their concerns include gender discrimination and son preference; poor reproductive health; lack of decision making by girls and women; inadequate facilities; rampant illiteracy; unemployment; and pervasive gender violence that violates human dignity and rights (UNFPA and UNCDPA, 1998). It is essential, therefore, that youth are brought into the process as equal partners rather than token members because it is through them, and with them, that programmes will provide the required space to address the identified needs of this hitherto neglected population.

References

Alcala, M.J. 1995. Commitments to Sexual and Reproductive Health and Rights for All: Framework for Action. New York: Family Care International.

Andersson, A., Kumar, S., and Peterson, J.D. 1996. Promoting HIV/AIDS Preventive Education Within the Formal School System in India. Report of a Lesson Learned Seminar. New Delhi: Ministry of Education, Ministry of Human Resource Development, National AIDS Control Organisation and The Joint United Nations Programme for HIV/AIDS.

Annonymous. 1994. Insights into Adolescent Sexuality. "Dehleez" Emerges a Popular Programme on Yuvavani. *Focus on Population, Environment, Development,* 8(2): 5.

Bang, R.A., Bang, A.T., Baitule, M., Chaudhury, Y., Sarmukaddam, S., and Tale, O. 1989. High Prevalence of Gynaecological Diseases in Rural Indian Women. *Lancet,* I(8629): 85-88.

Bhasin, U., and Singhal, A. 1998. Participatory Approaches to Message Design: "Jeevan Saurabh," a Pioneering Radio Serial in India for Adolescents. *Media Asia,* 25(1): 12-18.

Chaudhury, R.H. 1998. Socioeconomic, Demographic and Reproductive Health Profiles of Adolescents in SAARC Countries. Paper prepared for United Nations Population Fund sponsored South Asia Conference on the Adolescent, July 21-23, New Delhi, India.

Commonwealth Youth Programme. Adolescent Reproductive and Sexual Health: A Situational Analysis. Chandigarh, India.

Department of International Economic and Social Affairs. 1986. The Situation of Youth in the 1980s and Prospects and Challenges for the Year 2000. New York: United Nations.

Germain, A., and Kyte, R. 1995. The Cairo Consensus: The Right Agenda for the Right Time. New York: The International Women's Health Coalition.

Government of India. Planning Commission. Ninth Five Year Plan, 1997-2002. Volume II. Draft.

Government of India, Ministry of Health and Family Welfare. 1998. India Country Paper. Theme Paper prepared for United Nations Population Fund sponsored South Asia Conference on the Adolescent, July 21-23 , New Delhi, India.

Government of India. 1997. Draft National Youth Policy. Department of Youth Affairs and Sports, Ministry of Human Resource Development. New Delhi, India.

Government of India. 1997. Annual Report. Department of Youth Affairs and Sports, Ministry of Human Resource Development. New Delhi, India.

Government of India. 1996-97. Annual Report. Department of Women and Child Development, Ministry of Human Resource Development. New Delhi, India.

Government of India. 1985. National Youth Policy. Department of Youth Affairs and Sports, Ministry of Human Resource Development. New Delhi, India.

Greene, M.E. 1997. Watering the Neighbour's Garden: Investing in Adolescent Girls in India. Working Paper 7, Population Council, South and East Asia Regional Office, New Delhi, India.

International Center for Research on Women. 1997. Adolescent Sexuality and Fertility in India – Preliminary Findings. Information Bulletin, January, Washington, D.C., U.S.A.

International Institute for Population Sciences. 1995. National Family Health Survey 1992-93: India. Summary Report. Mumbai, India.

Jejeebhoy, S.J. 1996. Adolescent Sexual and Reproductive Behavior – A Review of the Evidence from India. Working Paper No. 3., International Center for Research on Women, Washington, D.C., U.S.A.

Lok Jumbish Parishad. 1998. Lok Jumbish: Seventh Report. Jaipur, India.

Madhyam Communications. 1998. Youth Today: Desperately Seeking Direction. *Voices for Change*, 2(1).

Madhyam Communications. 1998. Young Today... What of Tomorrow? *Voices for Change*, 2(2).

Mavalankar, D., Bang, R., and Bang, A. 1998. Quality Reproductive Health Services in Rural India: The SEARCH Experience. Series on Upscaling Innovations in Reproductive Health in Asia, Vol. 2. Malaysia: International Council on Management of Population Programmes.

Mehta, S. 1998. Responsible Sexual and Reproductive Health Behaviour Among Adolescents. Theme Paper prepared for United Nations Population Fund sponsored South Asia Conference on the Adolescent, July 21-23, New Delhi, India.

Pathak, R, 1994. The New Generations. *India Today.* January 31: 73-87.

Sanghvi, V. 1978. The Cult of Virginity. *India Today,* November 1-15: 46-52.

Satia, J., Tahir, S., and Andersson, C. (eds.). 1995. Innovative Approaches to Population Programme Management: Youth Reproductive Health. Innovations 2. Malaysia: International Council on Management of Population Programmes.

Singh, S. 1998. Promoting Community Based Interventions for Adolescent Reproductive Health in India. Paper presented at the International Reproductive Health Meeting, Mumbai, India. (Submitted for publication)

Singh, S. 1997. Adolescent Reproductive and Sexual Health Needs in India. In Country Studies on Youth presented at the Workshop on Youth Across Asia, Kathmandu, Nepal, September 23-25. Asia and Near East Operations Research and Technical Assistance Project, Population Council, New Delhi, India.

Subramanian, S.S. 1998. Rural Women Take Reproductive Health Matters Into Their Own Hands: Rural Women's Social Education Centre. Series on Upscaling Innovations in Reproductive Health in Asia, Vol. 1. Malaysia: International Council on Management of Population Programmes.

Thapa, V.J., and Raval, S. An Early Awakening. *India Today*, September 21: 50-56.

The Alan Guttmacher Institute. 1998. Into a New World: Young Women's Sexual and Reproductive Lives. New York.

The Centre for Development and Population Activities and United Nations Population Fund. 1997. Youth Acting on Cairo and Beijing. New York, USA.

United Nations. 1994. Report of the International Conference on Population Development, Cairo, September 5-13.

United Nations Educational, Scientific and Cultural Organisation, The Joint United Nations Programme on HIV/AIDS, United Nations Children's Fund. 1998. Catch 'em Young: A Best Practice Case Study on School Based AIDS Preventive Education Programmes in Maharashtra, India. New Delhi: United Nations Educational, Scientific and Cultural Organisation.

Visaria, L., and Visaria, P. 1996. Prospective Population Growth and Policy Options for India, 1991-2101. Gujarat Insitute of Development Research, Ahmedabad, India, and Population Council, New York, USA.

Watsa, M.C. (ed.). 1993-94. Youth Sexuality: A Study of Knowledge, Attitudes, Beliefs and Practices among Urban Educated Indian Youth. Mumbai, India: Family Planning Association of India.

World Population Foundation. 1998. Draft Report of ICPD+ 5 NGO Forum, Consultation for Asia and Pacific Region, November 25-27.

2

Adolescent Reproductive Health: Experience of Community-Based Programmes

Masuma Mamdani

With assistance from:
Souhaila Abdulali, Sashwati Bannerji, Bishakha Datta, Renu Khanna, Sandhyarani Mohanty, Rukmini Rao, Sangeeta Subramanian Sokhi and Aleyamma Vijayanan.

This monograph is an outcome of a project funded by the Ford Foundation (New Delhi) to document the experiences of community-based programmes in addressing reproductive health needs of women in India.

Introduction

Adolescence[1] as a transitional period between childhood and adulthood is a relatively new concept in India. As a result, the relationship between the physical, social and psychological changes that are specific to adolescents, and their vulnerability to health problems, has remained largely unrecognised and unexplored. Thus, while there are about 190 million adolescent girls and boys between 10 and 19 years of age, accounting for about a fifth of India's population, their reproductive health needs remain ill-served (IIPS, 1995). Hardly any attention is given to their sexual health and development in the national programme. The problem is further exacerbated by the fact that Indian cultural values prohibit premarital sexual activity. Consequently, the needs of sexually active unmarried adolescents are rarely considered.

Adolescents represent a resource for the future whose potential can either be wasted or nurtured in a positive way. The information and means to protect themselves should be seen as a basic human right. But, in the absence of appropriate and effective programmes for sexuality and gender education, and in the absence of appropriate reproductive health services, adolescents continue to remain at risk.

Recognising this urgency, and despite great challenges, such as lack of political endorsement, and social, cultural and financial

---

[1] The World Health Organization defines the term "adolescence" as people between 10 and 19 years of age (WHO 1996, p4). The term is used rather loosely in this report and unless specified, often embraces both adolescents (married and unmarried) and unmarried men and women who are in their early adult years.

constraints, a number of community-based, private voluntary non- government organisations (NGOs) have begun to address the needs of adolescents. Most programmes have focused solely on health and educational activities aimed at unmarried adolescents, with the objective of inducing specific behavioural changes. Some have set their goals in terms of reaching out to adolescents with information and limited services. A few are challenging existing gender norms.

India is gradually coming to terms with a growing adolescent population, both in absolute terms and relative to other age groups. There appears to be an increasing recognition among policy makers of the need to address adolescents beyond the family planning framework. But, public sector programmes on the ground are relatively few and there remains a dearth of information.

This paper attempts to bridge the gap between the major issues facing adolescent girls in India today, and the extent to which NGOs have been able to address their reproductive health needs (see Appendix I for a brief summary). It is important to realise that most of these programmes are in their infancy and have not yet achieved significant community coverage. They have not operated for a sufficiently long period for any notable behavioural impact to be realised. Comprehensive evaluations are lacking. Nevertheless, given the limited available information, it is important to analyse their experiences, learn from their mistakes and highlight some of the essential components of a 'successful' adolescent programme. The next section provides an overview of reproductive health and risks in adolescent girls, and summarises some of the major obstacles confronting these girls in obtaining appropriate services. Section three reviews a cross-section of programme approaches across India and based on their experiences, delineates some of the crucial components involved in the delivery and acceptability of these programmes. The concluding section discusses the feasibility of expanding the coverage and range of adolescent programmes within the larger public health programmes.

Reproductive Health of Adolescent Girls in India

A number of recent publications have addressed the general issue of reproductive health and hazards among adolescents in developing countries (FHI, 1997; Goodburn and Ross, 1995; Harrison and Koblinsky, 1995; PRB, 1997; Senderowitz, 1995; The Alan Guttmacher Institute, 1997; United Nations, 1989; WHO, 1996). While there is a paucity of well-conducted studies on sexual activity of adolescents in India, the overall conclusions drawn from various sources of information are the same (Achhpal and Verma, 1987; Bhatia and Chandra, 1993; Gupta and Joshi, 1995; Jejeebhoy, 1996; Pathak and Ram, 1993; Sathe, 1987; Senanayake and Kleinmen, 1993; UNICEF, 1990). Their vulnerability caused by their young age, their ignorance on matters related to sexuality and reproductive health, their lack of factual knowledge on contraception and their inability or unwillingness to use family planning and health services, puts adolescents at a significant risk of experiencing negative consequences. As elaborated in the following sections, the stakes are particularly high for adolescent girls who are at risk of getting pregnant at an early age and once pregnant, for complications during pregnancy including unsafe abortions, for maternal death, as well as for poor infant outcomes. Sexually active adolescent girls are also at a higher risk for reproductive tract infections (RTIs), including sexually transmitted infections (STIs), with the risk of later infertility, or even death. Women are generally under-served in India; among them the most neglected are adolescent girls, and especially if they are unmarried, they are vulnerable, both biologically and socially.

Marriage patterns and fertility behaviour

For most women in India, sexual activity starts in adolescence and within marriage (UNICEF, 1990; IIPS, 1995). Early marriage was perpetuated in the past by tradition, beliefs about preservation of a girl's chastity, family honour and the need to reduce expenditure.

Present laws prohibit early marriages: the legal minimum age of marriage for girls is 18 years, and 21 for boys. Regardless, many girls continue to be married off at an early age and are expected to prove their fertility well before they attain full biological and emotional maturity.

Data from the 1992-93 National Family Health Survey provides some insight into marriage patterns and fertility behaviour of adolescent girls in India (see Table 1). There is some evidence of a modest increase in the average age for marriage; the Singulate Mean Age at Marriage (SMAM) for females has gone up by 4.1 years,

TABLE 1. Reproductive Health Profile of Adolescent Girls: Selected Indices

SELECTED INDICES	URBAN	RURAL	TOTAL
Percent aged: 10-14 years 15-19 years	 11.8 10.9	 11.9 10.6	 11.9 10.7
Singular Mean Age at Marriage (years)	21.5	19.3	20.0
Percent currently married: 10-14 years 15-19 years	 2.4 21.3	 7.0 44.7	 5.7 38.4
No. of births per 1000 (15-19 years)	75	131	116
Percent ever-married women (13-19 years) who are mothers pregnant with their first child	N/A* N/A	N/A N/A	46.0 11.7
Percent all women aged 13-19 years who are mothers or pregnant with their first child	N/A	N/A	17.0
Percent share of births occurring to women aged 15-19 years.	13.9	17.8	17.1

* *information not assessed*

Source: National Family Health Survey, 1992-1993 (IIPS, 1995)

from 15.9 years in 1961 to 20 years in 1992-93. In all, as many as 6 percent of 10-14 year olds and 38 percent of 15-19 year olds are currently married. Further, 58 percent of ever-married adolescent girls between the ages of 13 and 19 years have begun childbearing. This corresponds to 17 percent of all females aged 13-19 years. The situation appears to be particularly acute in rural India.

Stark variations in marriage patterns and fertility are evident (see Table 2) across the country (Aras, 1992; Bhattacharya and Joshi, 1995; Gupta and Khan, 1995; Roy and Nangia, 1995). For example, early marriages are much more common in the states of Bihar, Madhya Pradesh and Andhra Pradesh where more than 50 percent of adolescent girls between the ages of 15 and 19 years are currently married. In contrast, women in Kerala, Punjab and some other smaller states tend to marry much later: less than 15 percent of adolescent girls in the corresponding age group in these states are currently married. Teenage pregnancy is noted to be particularly high in Madhya Pradesh and Andhra Pradesh. Early marriages and childbearing in many of these states have often been associated with low levels of female literacy. For example, survey findings from the northern and central states indicate that only 25 percent of girls aged 10-14 years were enrolled in schools compared to 84 percent in Kerala (Bhattacharya and Joshi, 1995). While there is not much difference in the proportion of ever-married adolescents who have begun childbearing, between illiterate and literate adolescents with less than a middle school education, married adolescents who have completed high school are less likely to have begun childbearing (see Table 3).

There is growing evidence that sexual activity among unmarried adolescents is increasing, especially in the urban areas. In an excellent review of reproductive behaviour of adolescents in India, Jejeebhoy (1996) suggests that around 20 to 30 percent of all males and up to 10 percent of all females, mainly from the urban areas, are sexually active during adolescence before marriage. Given the sensitivities involved, few studies have considered the issue of sexual activity among unmarried adolescent girls, particularly in the rural areas. There are obvious difficulties entailed in obtaining accurate

TABLE 2. Reproductive Health Profile of Adolescent Girls: Selected States

STATE	Female 15-19 years currently married %	Births among (15-19 years) Urban No. by 1000	Births among (15-19 years) Rural No. by 1000	Ever-married women aged 13-19 years who are mothers or pregnant for the first time %	Women aged 13-19 years who are mothers or pregnant for the first time %	Singular mean age at marriage – SMAM (years)
North						
Haryana	44.1	75	166	62.9	20.7	18.4
Central						
Madhya Pradesh	61.9	92	173	54.9	26.5	17.4
Uttar Pradesh	39.6	62	128	49.4	14.1	18.6
East						
Bihar	50.3	89	127	48.2	18.6	18.0
Orissa	27.5	70	89	59.8	13.2	20.7
North East						
Assam	31.0	70	122	70.6	17.9	21.6
West						
Goa	3.1	19	11	67.6*	1.6	25.1
Maharashtra	36.2	88	183	68.1	19.9	19.3
South						
Andhra Pradesh	52.2	0.085	164	60.1	25.4	18.1
Kerala	13.4	0.033	147	59.2	5.9	22.1

* *Based on 25-49 unweighted cases*

Source: National Family Health Survey Data, 1992-1993 (IIPS, 1995)

TABLE 3. Percentage of ever-married women who have begun child-bearing by educational status, 1992-93

	Women 13-19 years:			
Educational status	who are mothers %	pregnant with first child %	who have begun childbearing %	number
Illiterate	48.1	10.2	58.3	6,359
Literate: Less than middle school complete	45.1	13.7	58.8	1,778
Middle school complete	39.3	15.6	54.9	787
High school complete	33.0	17.3	50.3	522

Source: National Family Health Survey, 1992-1993 (IIPS, 1995)

information. Except for a community-based study carried out among tribal women in rural Maharashtra (Bang et al, 1989), the bulk of the evidence is unrepresentative and comes mainly from two sources: indirectly, from reports of physicians, chemists or key informants of unmarried adolescents seeking assistance for abortion services or contraceptives (Abdulali, 1996; Bhende, 1994; Khanna, 1996) and, from hospital or clinic-based records of unmarried adolescents seeking abortions (Anonymous, 1978; Bhattacharya and Joshi, 1995; Chhabra, 1992; Purandre et al, 1978). Contrary to the findings of the Maharashtra study that suggests an exceptionally high level of premarital sexual[2] activity, available evidence indicates that although sexual activity among unmarried adolescent girls is not unusual and

[2] A cross-sectional study of gynaecological and sexual diseases in women was done in two villages. Of the 650 women studied, 92 (14 percent) were unmarried. Based solely on physical examination (criteria: the hymen was torn and the vagina easily admitted two fingers), the study concluded that 46.7 percent (43 out of the 92 girls examined) of the unmarried girls had had sexual intercourse.

appears to be increasing, it is limited – less than 10 percent (Jejeebhoy 1996). Nevertheless, reports of focus group discussions carried out with adolescents in several Indian cities suggest sexual activity among adolescents is occurring at increasingly younger ages (Anonymous, 1994). Further, results of an Indian Family Survey reveal that 13 percent of girls and 28 percent of boys approve of premarital sexual relations (Bhattacharya and Joshi, 1995). With the relaxation of social and cultural norms restricting sexual behaviour, and increased media and peer pressure to be sexually active, it is likely that premarital sexual activity will increase, particularly in the urban areas.

Reproductive risks

Wanted pregnancies

The consequences of early childbearing are acute (Aras, 1986; Aras et al, 1989, 1990; Jejeebhoy and Rama Rao, 1995; Kushwaha et al, 1993; Pachauri and Jamshedji, 1983; Pratinidhi et al, 1990). On a national level, adolescents account for a high proportion of maternal deaths in India. For example, as many as 45 percent of all maternal deaths in rural India occurred in women aged under 24 years (Registrar General, 1987; quoted in Jejeebhoy, 1995). Data from the NFHS 1992-93 (see Table 4) reveals that around 10 percent of all pregnancies in married adolescents aged 15-19 years result in a spontaneous abortion or still birth; the corresponding figure for 20-24 year-olds is 8 percent (see Table 4) (IIPS, 1995). Fragmentary data obtained mainly from hospital-based studies suggests the same. As is evident from results of selected studies (see Table 5), pregnant adolescents are at a much higher risk of dying compared to women over 20 years of age. Maternal mortality is around one-and-a-half to two times higher for adolescents than for older women. Complications of pregnancy, such as anaemia, spontaneous abortion and eclampsia are also significantly higher among adolescent mothers. The results also indicate that babies of adolescent mothers are more likely to have low weight, run a higher risk of being premature and have a higher perinatal mortality.

TABLE 4. Maternal Care: Selected Indices

SELECTED INDICES	URBAN (%)		RURAL (%)		TOTAL (%)	
Pregnancies in ever-married women resulting in:	15-19 years	20-24 years	15-19 years	20-24 years	15-19 years	20-24 years
induced abortion	3.3	2.2	1.4	0.9	1.7	1.2
spontaneous abortion	9.5	6.4	6.8	5.2	7.3	5.5
still birth	1.9	1.9	2.5	2.6	2.4	2.5
All births to women < 20 years not receiving any antenatal care*	NA	NA	NA		34.6	
All births to women < 20 years not given any iron-folic acid tablets	NA	NA	NA		48.2	

* *based on births in the four years prior to the survey i.e. for 35 percent of all births to women under 20 years, the mothers did not receive any antenatal care during pregnancy (antenatal care relates to pregnancy-related health care provided at a health facility or at home, by a doctor, a health worker, TBA (including hakims); 48 percent of all births to women under 20 years were to mothers who had not received any iron-folic acid tablets.*

Source: National Family Health Survey, 1992-1993 (IIPS, 1995)

The poor nutritional status of adolescent girls in India is well-documented (Gopalan, 1990; Kanani and Consul, 1990; Ramachandran, 1989). For example, results of a community-based study of 54 tribal (mainly illiterate) pregnant adolescents aged 13-19 years in Rajasthan revealed that 85 percent weighed less than 42 kg and 94 percent were anaemic (Sharma and Sharma, 1992). A South Indian study of 47 adolescent girls aged 13-18 years revealed poor growth in all age groups; 73.5 percent of the girls were classified to be anaemic (Jude et al, 1991). In yet another study carried out in 105 adolescent girls (10-18 years) living in the slums of Gujarat, 98 percent were anaemic (Kanani, 1994). Stunting, as a result of malnutrition, frequently means that girls have small or deformed pelvises, which may prevent normal delivery. Moderate

TABLE 5. Adolescent Pregnancies: Summary of Results from Selected Studies

Location	Methodology	Summary findings
Urban Uttar Pradesh (Swain et al, 1993)	Hospital-based, retrospective review of 2,051 deliveries occurring in 1988	Overall incidence of eclampsia was 22/1000 deliveries; eclampsia was more common in adolescent mothers than in older ones (5.2 % vs. 1.5-1.6 %, p<0.001); 43 out of 44 eclampsia cases had not received any antenatal care; eclampsia accounted for 13 (28.9%) of the 45 maternal deaths that occurred in 1988.
Rural Maharashtra (Hirve and Gantra, 1994)	Community-based, medical social workers followed-up a cohort of 1,922 pregnant women from 45 contiguous villages in Pune district at monthly intervals	29% of infants were low birth weight (LBW) infants; risk factors for LBW were: very low socio-economic status, mother's age < 20 year, first pregnancy, last pregnancy interval shorter than 6 months, non-pregnant weight < 40 kg. height less than 145 cm., haemoglobin less than 9 g/dl, third trimester bleeding, premature birth & low literacy levels.
Rural West Bengal (Mishra and Dawn, 1986)	Hospital-based, retrospective review of 10,920 pregnancies and labours occurring in 1978-82	2,730(25%) pregnancies were to women aged 12-19 years, complications of pregnancy (anaemia, spontaneous abortion, eclampsia and premature labour) were significantly higher among teenagers than in women over 20 years of age; corresponding to age groups 12-19, 20-30 and > 31, maternal mortality rate was 3.80, 2.55 and 1.07; perinatal mortality rate was 29%, 18% and 4%; incidence of premature infants was 20%, 16% and 11%.
Rural West Bengal (Parkasi, Sil and Dasgupta, 1985)	Hospital-based study of 5,117 single live births in 1976	Low birth weight babies were mostly pre-term, female, born to poor mothers, born to adolescent mothers, of birth order 1 or 4 and up, and delivered mostly in the monsoon season.

and severe anaemia, which often starts during adolescence, presents another serious risk; it is one of the most common contributing causes of maternal death and morbidity.

Iron-folic acid tablets distributed during the last trimester of pregnancy, primarily through antenatal care providers, has been the major intervention to prevent and treat anaemia caused by iron deficiency. But a micro-level evaluation by the Indian Council for Medical Research (ICMR) shows that this approach has had little effect on the prevalence of anaemia among pregnant women (1989). The reasons for this range from inadequate supplementation and low acceptance to the poor quality of tablets. Several studies have observed the poor compliance of oral iron supplementation, especially if women are unsupervised, and this may be influenced by both biological and cultural factors (MotherCare Project, 1993; Khanna, 1992).

Adolescence, malnutrition, anaemia and the extra nutritional demands exacerbate health risks during pregnancy. These risks may be further heightened due to the lack of antenatal care. The National Family Health Survey shows that 35 percent of pregnant women under 20 years did not receive any antenatal care (IIPS, 1995). Consequently, unlike in other countries, young women in India, particularly in the rural areas, experience slightly higher mortality rates than males;[3] largely as a result of a high maternal mortality attributable to their poor reproductive health. In all, 15 percent of all deaths of rural women aged 15-24 years are attributed to diseases of childbirth and pregnancy; the second largest cause of death following accidents and violence, which account for 34 percent of all deaths and which may often be associated with marriage or pregnancy (Ravindran, 1996).

There are many adolescents who have healthy pregnancies and healthy babies, and give birth without complications. But then, there are many who do not. Even when pregnancies among adolescents

[3] Age specific mortality rates in the 15-19 year age category is reported to be 2.2 per 1000 among males and 3.4 among females in the rural areas; and 1.3 and 1.7 respectively, in the urban areas (IIPS, 1995).

are planned, the health risks faced by these young mothers and their newborns are enormous, especially if they are malnourished.

Unwanted pregnancies

Overall, based on the available data on induced abortions, adolescent girls appear to suffer a disproportionate share of unwanted pregnancies. Estimates from the National Family Health Survey for married women reveal that induced abortion is somewhat more likely among adolescents aged 15-19 years than among 20-24 year olds: 1.7 percent and 1.2 percent of pregnancies, respectively (IIPS, 1995). Most of the available evidence comes from hospital based records. For example, adolescents accounted for 27 percent of the 2,755 abortions conducted in a rural hospital (Chhabra et al, 1988), and 30 percent of the 1,684 abortions conducted in an urban hospital (Solapurkar and Sangam, 1985), with a disproportionately large number of them being unmarried in both instances. Adolescents are also considerably more likely to delay seeking abortion services and undergo second trimester abortions which are not safe: 90, 81 and 66 percent of adolescent abortion seekers in Baroda (Bhatt, 1978), Mumbai (Purandare and Krishna, 1974) and Sevagram (Chhabra, 1992) respectively. Unmarried adolescents, in particular, are more inclined to delay seeking an abortion until late pregnancy mainly due to the lack of awareness as well as ignorance of services, and fear of social stigmatisation (Chowdhury and Mukherjee, 1979; UNICEF, 1990). For example, 45 percent of the 784 adolescents, who had undergone an abortion in an urban hospital, were unmarried; and compared to 25 percent of married adolescents, 58 percent of them were in their second trimester at that time (Aras et al, 1987). Health consequences of unsafe abortions are acute, ranging from complications such as a perforated uterus, cervical lacerations or haemorrhage in the short term to an increased risk of ectopic pregnancy, chronic pelvic infection and possible infertility in the long term. The problems are further exacerbated by the fact that existing health services are ill-equipped to address the needs of these young girls, including emergency and timely evacuations, post-abortion care, counselling and contraceptive services.

Sexually transmitted infections (STIs)

There are few studies of STIs (also referred to as sexually transmitted diseases or STDs) in adolescents. However, reports from STI clinics imply an increase in young people's attendance, mainly males, over the past few years (Watsa, 1993). The actual numbers may be an underestimate and are also difficult to interpret. An increasing trend could be a result of an actual increase in STI rates. It could also be due to several other factors, including a growing susceptible adolescent population, more adolescents resorting to STD clinics for treatment, and/or better reporting procedures. Notwithstanding this, these figures do indicate that STIs are not uncommon among adolescents. Early and unprotected sexual activity is likely to expose adolescents to an increased risk of contracting STIs, including HIV/AIDS. In general, female sex workers are reported to be an important source of STIs for the majority of adolescent and pre-adolescent boys seen at STD clinics (Bansal, 1992; Kanbargi and Kanbargi, 1996; Pandhi, Khanna and Sekhri, 1995).

Despite this frightening scenario, both unmarried and married adolescent girls continue to be vulnerable to early, and often, unprotected sexual activity. Adolescent girls are the least likely to seek assistance, especially if they are unmarried. Why is this the case?

Obstacles to Obtaining Appropriate and TImely Care

Ashish Gram Rachna Trust, Pachod, Aurangabad

"A case that nobody in the hospital has been able to forget is that of a 12-year-old girl who came in, wearing a child's frock, with a ballooning stomach. Her mother, who brought her in, complained that she was not starting to menstruate, which was a problem for the family as they wanted to marry her off as soon as she attained puberty. Examinations revealed that the girl was pregnant. The girl could not even understand the concept of pregnancy, let alone its cause. After much probing, she revealed that a male cousin had regularly been 'sticking something up her.' She didn't know or understand that this could cause pregnancy. According to Dr. Aruna Pattanayak, who has been a gynaecologist in the hospital for the last 15 years, cases of minor rape are common, which is why families want to get their daughters married off when they attain menarche. "We keep saying that the early age of marriage causes reproductive health problems, but if you want to postpone the age of marriage, can you also protect their daughters during this time?"

Gender norms

Social attitudes clearly favour cultural norms of premarital chastity in girls. Double standards exist. Reports from several community-based programmes reflect the different views: that boys having premarital sexual activity is accepted or even expected, but is unacceptable for 'respectable' girls. Contraception is seen as a woman's responsibility; but unmarried young women feel unable to seek contraception, or any other reproductive health service, for fear of being labeled 'sexually active' and therefore, promiscuous.

Boys and girls play different roles in Indian society. The dowry system is still a part of marriage. Females are widely considered to be a social and financial liability. Such gender norms lead to many abuses. Daughter neglect in terms of the biased allocation of food and health care is, arguably, one of the most common forms of discrimination in India, especially in the North (Das Gupta, 1987; Khan et al, 1988; Khanna, 1995; UNICEF, 1990). Girls are taken out of school at an early age,[4] usually soon after menarche. They are at risk of sexual violence, including rape or domestic violence. There is some evidence indicating that adolescent abortion seekers often become pregnant as a result of rape or non-consensual sexual activity (Mandal, 1982; Bhatt, 1978). For example, an estimated 25 percent of rape victims are young adolescents under 16 years of age (Ministry of Welfare, Department of Women and Child Development, 1990, quoted in Jejeebhoy, 1996). The involvement of young girls in sexual activities may also often be due to their inability to say no to older men because of a cultural tradition of respecting elders and men (Mavalankar, 1996).

Voices of Adolescent Girls: SUTRA, Himachal Pradesh

"They have no expectations from me except that I should get married, live in somebody else's house properly without disgracing them. I should do whatever my in-laws tell me to do and even if they beat me or insult me, I should listen to them. They tell me that I should learn to cook, cut grass and not argue. They tell my brothers to study even though they are not interested and don't go to school. I tell my mother to send me but she says who will do the work then?"

"I wish I could be born a boy in my next life. Girls have to do all the work and yet get all the curses that you don't do enough. My brothers do no work, once in a while, they plough the fields but otherwise they just enjoy themselves. They get up at 8 in the morning and go to sleep at 8 at night and I have to get up at 4 in the morning and go to sleep only at 10 at night. It's no use telling them to work with me: they say boys are not supposed to."

— *Source: Mahajan and van Zuijlen, 1994*

[4] 64 percent and 56 percent of girls between the ages of 10-14 years and 15-19 years respectively, are considered literate compared to 81-82 percent of boys in the same age interval; 54 percent of all males (15-19 years) have completed a middle school education compared to 35 percent of the girls aged 15-19 years (IIPS, 1995).

Ironically, it is often women who discriminate against their own sex (Thapa, 1995). Gender stereotypes are often so deeply ingrained that women see little contradiction in what they are saying or doing. For example, the Self-Employed Women's Association (SEWA), a long-standing community-based organisation in Gujarat, promotes social change both by transforming the conditions in which self-employed women live and work, and also by transforming women's self-perception, enabling them to transcend the psychological confines of poverty and the strictures of family and tradition. In a series of interviews with 32 SEWA members, Schuler et al (1995) noted that as a result of their increased roles in their families' economic support, SEWA members are able to increase their power and status within their households. But despite this, these women continue to be bound by tradition. While they reported that they treated their sons and daughters equally, and that they had high aspirations for their daughters, "it was obvious that girls often were being provided less education and made to work throughout much of their childhood".

Generally, even married adolescents have limited decision-making power in their sexual relationships. Preliminary findings from a study carried out in rural Maharashtra which involved in-depth interviews with married adolescent girls, their husbands and their mothers-in law show that where both adolescent girls and boys would have liked to have delayed their marriage and their first pregnancy, the decision was usually taken by the mother-in-law (ICRW, 1997).

The prevailing gender ideology, as reinforced by the media, parents, educators, religious leaders, family planning professionals, policy makers and politicians, profoundly affects the reproductive health and well-being of adolescents. It influences their views on sexuality, access to accurate information, and access to health services.

Insufficient information to seek timely care

It is clear that adolescents are often ignorant about the reproductive process and contraception and may not realise that their concerns need professional attention. For example, results of a hospital-based study show that 88 percent of the 100 unmarried mainly rural girls, who came seeking an abortion, did not know that sexual intercourse could lead to pregnancy or STIs, and 90 percent did not know about contraception (Chhabra, 1992). Results of another study, involving 85 adolescent girls and 125 adolescent boys residing in the slums of Mumbai found that only 16 percent of the girls and 54 percent of the boys reported that a woman could become pregnant after sexual intercourse; hardly 10 percent of the respondents had heard about STIs (Bhende, 1994). In addition, many adolescent girls may be totally unaware that they have contracted a STI either because they are asymptomatic or because they do not recognise the symptoms, there may also be denial on the part of these girls that they can contract STIs, contributing to the continued practice of high risk behaviour.

Seldom have studies considered the sexual vulnerability of newly married adolescents, who are equally ill-informed and, therefore, totally unprepared for sexual intercourse and its consequences. Overall, the fear of adult recrimination frequently prevents adolescents from asking questions or seeking help from their parents or adults. While a formal population education programme does exist and has been introduced in most universities, the curriculum covered rarely touches upon issues of sexuality and reproductive health; teachers often find the topic embarrassing and avoid it (Jejeebhoy, 1996). Thus, information on sexual matters tends to come either from peers, who may be equally uninformed, incorrectly informed and likely to be relatively inexperienced, or from the media which tends to represent either sexual and gender stereotypes or extremes (ICRW, 1997).

Inaccessibility of appropriate services

Adolescent health care in rural India is limited. As elsewhere, most public sector services target adult married women. They are not planned for adolescent use, especially if they are not married. Unmarried adolescents for example, often do not seek safe abortions for a number of reasons: fear that the services are not confidential;

inability to pay the required fees; the prerequisite of parental/ partner approval in some instances; or that health workers will react negatively and will be insensitive to their needs (FPAI and WHO, 1982; ICRW, 1997). For example, it was only after an intensive participatory training programme that was rooted in social realities, that auxiliary nurse midwives associated with the Briham Mumbai Municipal Corporation project were able to gain a better understanding of women's problems and their needs. For the first time, they were able to see issues such as poverty, premarital pregnancy and rape from the point of view of the slum women. Said one auxiliary nurse midwife: "Earlier, we used to see unmarried pregnant women as loose women." Another problem revolves around the very absence of appropriate and affordable facilities in the government health system. For example, reports from a community-based programme in rural Andhra Pradesh reveal that unmarried pregnant adolescents are often forced to resort to unsafe abortions; their mothers are usually quite supportive, but are simply unable to access cheap and safe abortions (Rao, written communication).

Contraceptive uptake is generally reported to be very poor among married adolescents (Bhattacharya and Joshi, 1995; Gupta and Joshi, 1995; Roy and Nangia, 1995). Nationally, only about 7 percent of married adolescent girls aged 15-19 are using contraception; as many as 30 percent report a desire to delay the next birth or limit childbearing, but are not using a contraceptive (IIPS, 1995). The family planning programme has, till recently, been dominated by demographic goals and targeted at married women. The focus has been on permanent methods aimed at older women. A consequence for adolescents being the non-availability of appropriate contraceptive methods, especially for spacing births, Female controlled barrier methods are unavailable. The condom is the only method available, but poorly promoted and, therefore, underutilised by both men and adolescent boys. In addition, few unmarried adolescents visit family planning clinics. The small minority who do seek help, do so when an unwanted conception outside of marriage occurs.

It is clear that marital status legitimises sexual activity and fertility and, therefore, the problems faced by married and unmarried adolescents are quite different. For instance, although Maternal Child Health and Family Planning (MCH/FP) services may not cater to adolescent needs (e.g. providing temporary contraceptive methods and a comfortable environment that is sensitive to their needs, etc.), they are, in theory at least, accessible to them, particularly after their first birth. Unmarried adolescents on the contrary, face other restrictions; perhaps legal, but also considerable cultural and social barriers. Thus, efforts to address problems associated with early sexual activity and childbearing within marriage will be relatively easier compared to those outside marriage. Sexual activity and fertility among unmarried adolescents has to be addressed within a very different context and with different challenges.

Addressing Adolescent Girls: Community-based Programmes

Adolescent reproductive health programmes on the ground are relatively few and recently implemented, mainly by NGOs. For the most part, their approach has depended on the stated needs, as identified by adolescents themselves, the feasibility of providing the required services and most importantly, the cultural and social norms of the target population to be served.

Two distinct models may be identified:

- Programmes that have focused solely on the provision of sexual information to unmarried adolescents.

- Programmes that are providing information and limited medical services; a few are even attempting to reach out to adolescents with literacy programmes and skill training activities.

Focus on sexual information

Most programmes are reaching out to adolescents on an informal basis, individually or collectively at *Mahila Mandals* (women's groups) via their community-based health workers; some are addressing adolescents in a more structured manner in a peer group environment, albeit in a village setting; and, a few are addressing adolescents in a peer group environment at residential camps away from the village setting. Many of these programmes aim to provide adolescents with sexual information with a view to change behaviour. Recognising that the reproductive health of adolescents is more than just a medical problem, and must be dealt with from more than just a medical perspective, a number of these programmes are incorporating a gender perspective into sex education. Some are addressing only girls. Others are reaching out to boys as well.

In the main, however, the design and implementation of some of these programmes – for example Baroda Citizens Council (BCC), Deepak Charitable Trust (DCT), Orissa Institute of Medical Research and Health (OMRAH), Krishan Nath Baba Memorial Charitable Trust & Health Centre (KNBMCT & HC) and Ashish Gram Rachna Trust – have been severely constrained by the existing cultural and social milieu. They have failed to incorporate a gender perspective. Their overall health programme has largely been limited to women, with a focus on provision of MCH services – a need-based entry point. Empowerment and sensitising the community to gender issues has not been a priority. Thus, to gain social acceptability, such programmes have been limited to providing basic sexual education sessions at the village level, often attended by mothers and daughters together. There are two obvious limitations to this approach. First, adolescent girls are not going to be at ease exploring issues pertaining to sexuality in such a setting. Therefore, they are unlikely to seek information on topics of concern to them. Second, the content of the sexual education sessions in itself has to be tailored to what is acceptable to the community at large. For example, 'family life education' projects have generally ignored sexuality and gender relations, promoting instead, norms of 'responsible parenthood' within marriage and abstinence outside it. Failure to challenge existing sex roles and attitudes toward male and female sexuality simply reinforces prevailing imbalances of power in gender relations. However, many of these programmes are in their early stages. They are functioning in an environment of strong social and cultural sensitivities. Their very ability to provide adolescents with information on sexuality and reproductive health, no matter how basic, should thus be viewed as an achievement.

It is clear that programmes which have been working towards women's empowerment on a broader level have been much more successful in their attempts at reaching out to adolescents. A notable example is the Society for Rural Education and Development (SRED) that works primarily with landless labourers and small farmers in rural Tamil Nadu. SRED does not run an adolescent reproductive health programme as such, but its clinic is open to men, women and adolescents. SRED's main focus is on providing safe, legal and confidential abortion services to adolescents. It is unique in its approach. Not only does the organisation facilitate and meet all the costs of an abortion if the girl elects to have one, but it also lends support to the unmarried adolescent mother to carry her baby to term if she chooses to do so. SRED tries to ensure that the mother and baby are accepted in the family and the community at large. It is worth noting that the impetus for starting SRED was the rape of an 11-year-old girl, and sexual violence remains a very important point of focus for the group. The suicide rate among young girls is reported to be high; illegal dangerous abortions are also reported to be very common; and SRED believes a lot of this is due to sexual exploitation. Thus, abortion is viewed to be a political issue and is the main focus of its women's clinic.

Another exceptional example in this regard is the Society for Social Uplift Through Rural Action (SUTRA) in Himachal Pradesh. It is one of the few programmes that has been systematically working towards challenging existing gender norms. Its *Yuvti Shivir* (young girl's camp) project – five-day residential 'awareness generation' camps for young unmarried women – provides opportunities and space to adolescent women to come together to discuss and understand the situation of women from a feminist perspective. This is a laudable achievement, given the immense social constraints on these girls, many of whom are often not allowed to step out of their home environment upon reaching puberty. As elsewhere in India, and perhaps even more, women at SUTRA live within a strong patriarchichal framework. Their lives are ruled by the concept of *izzat* (honour). How then did SUTRA succeed in getting these girls to attend such residential camps?

To begin with, these camps were initiated in direct response to demands placed by the *Mahila Mandals* (Mahajan and van Zuijlen, 1994). SUTRA's work pivots around the *Mahila Mandals*. Women are given a political understanding of their health. They are mobilised to break the culture of shame and silence surrounding their bodies. These women have been effective in agitating against liquor, in mobilising credit and development schemes, in using the legal system to secure justice, and in generating awareness on health, including reproductive health. The objective of the SUTRA camps was not only to provide access to maximum information, but also to give the women an opportunity to come together and spend time away from home, to enable them to reflect on their personal problems and situations from a wider social perspective. Hence, most mothers who had themselves attended SUTRA's awareness generation camps earlier believed that this could be a valuable experience for their daughters too. SUTRA also uses the strategy of *Sahyoginis* (village-based activists) to convince family members of the usefulness of allowing their daughters to attend these camps; and to accompany the participants to and from their home areas to SUTRA's headquarters. These *Sahyoginis* also play an important role in organising, attending and actively supporting the follow-up programme – *Yuvti Sangathans* – at the village level. In addition, SUTRA also tries to raise awareness about the gender stereotypes propagated in textbooks used in the government primary schools through its widely disseminated newsletter *Yuva Sathin*.

How effective has SUTRA been in its objective of empowering adolescent girls? "After working for 10 years, girls are now talking about incest. We consider this an indicator of success," says SUTRA's director.

The importance of providing sexual and gender education to adolescents is unquestionable. Such information helps adolescents understand how their bodies work and what the consequences of their actions are likely to be. It dispels myths and corrects inaccuracies. It can enhance their self esteem and clarify their values. It stresses the need for safe and responsible sexual behaviour. But, in the absence of accessible services, this knowledge does not always translate into action. For example, SUTRA's initial attempts at providing MCH services were unsuccessful, mainly due to lack of professional medical staff. SUTRA subsequently made a conscious decision to empower and mobilise the community to demand services from the government. This, of course, will take time to materialise and meanwhile, there remains a conspicuous absence of appropriate services.

On the whole, a number of these programmes are service-based. They do not offer reproductive health services that are tailored to adolescent needs. Nevertheless, these services are available to adolescents, and there is the occasional adolescent who does seek assistance, in particular for menstrual problems, white discharge and abortions. But, many in need do not. For example, although community health workers at OMRAH do encourage girls in need of a gynaecological examination and treatment to attend the clinic, few follow up on their recommendation. Two obvious factors deterring the girls from utilising these services are: their inability to meet the required 50 percent of the costs of any laboratory tests conducted; and, the prerequisite of parental permission. Given the prevailing gender ideology, confidentiality, especially in relation to use of services, is very important to adolescents. This is well illustrated by the experience of Ashish Gram Rachna Trust. When it became evident that many unmarried pregnant women were getting illegal abortions, the Trust used traditional birth attendants, with whom it had developed an ongoing relationship for the past 30 or so years, to ensure that these women were brought to the hospital in the first trimester where they could avail of legal, safe and confidential abortions. These traditional birth attendants are both trusted and respected by the community and have over the years developed a strong rapport with the girls in the villages. They have reportedly succeeded in identifying and referring many girls who have missed their first period. As a result, there are fewer cases of complicated septic abortions coming to the hospital.

Focus on information and services

Although the provision of health services to adolescents is increasingly being recognised as an essential addition to educational programmes, few groups have been able to go beyond and into actual service provision. In addition to the social and cultural constraints, there are the obvious restrictions imposed by scarce resources. Some programmes – Action India, Deccan Development Society and Sarada Valley Development Society (SVDS) – have begun to promote the philosophy of 'self-help'.[5]

Some of the most effective adolescent reproductive health programmes appear to be those that include more than information and services. They have incorporated a skill training component: Prerana's 'Better life programme for young women and adolescents' in New Delhi; Society for Education Action and Research in Community Health's (SEARCH) 'Youth Life Education and Personality Development Programme' for adolescent girls and boys from the tribal population in rural Maharashtra; and in particular, Rural Women's Social Education Centre's (RUWSEC) wide range of programmes for married and unmarried adolescent girls and boys in rural Tamil Nadu – for factory workers, school going adolescents, drop-outs (Subramanian, 1996). RUWSEC, in fact, is one of the few programmes that is also attempting to work with newly married adolescent couples (see Box).

---

[5] A number of programmes are working for alternatives in women's health based on the self-help methodology and plant-based medicines which are easily accessed and perhaps also more affordable. Their prime objective is to empower women to take greater control over their bodies and health, and train local women to recognise and treat common gynaecological problems.

Literacy programme for girls at RUWSEC

In response to its findings that about 60-80 percent of the girls in the 11-18 years age group were effectively illiterate, RUWSEC initiated the *Magalir Chudar Kalvi* scheme in December 1990. It is an education and empowerment programme for girls in this age group, with a focus on literacy training, and overall personality and assertiveness development. The programme also includes workshops on sexuality and gender education and is held three times a year. The success of this programme is reflected by the level of literacy skills gained by nearly all these girls: 22 of these girls now function as literacy teachers in their respective villages. Many of these girls are already married. RUWSEC has now initiated a contact-programme and is planning future workshops in order to respond to their changing needs — marriage and sexuality within marriage, gender relations within marriage, and assertiveness within the joint family context. Realising that these girls now have very different expectations of their marriage from that of their husbands, which often resulting in conflict in their marriages, RUWSEC also hopes to work with the husbands of these girls.

— Source: Subramanian, 1996

The focus of RUWSEC and SEARCH, and Prerana to some extent, is to help youth to enhance communication and negotiation skills; to enable girls to negotiate safe sex or say no to sex with confidence; and change risky behaviours. These linkages are essential to provide access to reproductive health services, help youth to translate knowledge into action. In the absence of any follow-up data, however, it is not clear how effective these programmes have been in their objective of addressing adolescent reproductive health needs. To date, Prerana has focused mainly on skill-training activities, perhaps a demand-based entry. The community has responded positively to the programme, essentially because some of these adolescent girls are now in a position to supplement the household income. RUWSEC's success may be judged by the success of its literacy programme; or, by the increasing demand for its adolescent girls' camps. The organisation has also had a very positive response from adolescent boys and young men. This is reflected in the increasing number of men who are beginning to approach their clinic for STI treatment and also in the steady increase in the demand for condoms.

There is also some anecdotal evidence that may well reflect the efficacy of SEARCH's programme. For example, one girl succeeded in getting the menstrual taboos against her mother lifted in the home after attending a camp. The other anecdote is of an adolescent girl who was about to get married. Inspired by the camp, she wrote an anti-dowry play, performed by a group of seven girls in the village. The play explores the marriages of two daughters; one bold, the other meek. It contained characters such as a demanding mother-in-law, a father crushed by a dowry demand for Rs. 50,000, a television set, and a motorbike. The climatic scenes are the burning of the meek daughter-in-law and the rebellion of the bolder one, who is about to walk out of her marital home - but her supportive husband actually persuades his mother to apologise to her for ill-treatment! After the performance, adolescent boys in the village were asked if they would take dowry on getting married. They all said no. However, it remains to be seen if this public posture would actually hold in their private lives.

Overall, in the absence of any data, it is impossible to ascertain the effectiveness of any of these programmes. For example, it would be of use to learn what proportion of all adolescents are covered? What proportion of adolescents are not allowed to attend and for what reasons? What indicators are used to assess change in behaviour? This is even though, judging by the heavy demand for such services by adolescents themselves – at SEARCH, RUWSEC, Ashish Gram Rachna Trust, SVDS, BCC, and others – it is obvious that all of these programmes are meeting unmet needs.

All the innovations started on a small scale and were improved upon, before broadening their base. The success of many of the programmes discussed above can be attributed to formulating strategies which matched their environment and paying attention to implementation details. Several issues, thus, need to be addressed when designing an adolescent reproductive health programme: what should the sexual educational curriculum include? Who should be involved in programme planning and implementation? And, where, how and to whom should the services be offered? The following section summarises some of the major lessons learnt from these programmes.

Lessons Learnt

A needs assessment of the target population: participatory design and evaluation

- Programmes need to be aware that adolescents are not a homogeneous group and their needs will vary accordingly.

- In order to ensure that their specific needs are being met, it is important to listen to adolescents and attempt to understand how they perceive their own needs, and where possible, involve them in designing programmes. This will also enhance their commitment.

Adolescent needs will vary according to their age, sex, marital status, whether they are in school or not, urban or rural, and others. The decision on who to address and the actual content of the sexual education module will obviously depend on several of the above factors, the objectives of the programme, available resources and the cultural setting. For example, due to socio-cultural constraints, BCC made a conscious decision to start their adolescent programme by informally reaching out to older girls – over 15 years of age through income-generating activities (sewing classes). It was hoped that via these older girls, some of the information would permeate to younger siblings. Also, it was only after a year's interaction with these girls through informal weekly meetings and group discussions on health, nutrition, personal hygiene, reproductive health, and family planning, did it successfully hold a two-day residential camp away from the village setting.

Ashish Gram Rachna Trust's decision to target girls between 9 and 15 years of age was based on the realisation that young girls still get married at 14-16 years, and are typically taken out of school shortly before this. They have no access to vital health information that they need at this stage. Thus, the programme's main objective has been to provide them with basic information via its traditional birth attendants.

Likewise, RUWSEC's decision to address class 8 students in its school health programme was based on the fact that a large number of girls dropped out of school after this age. RUWSEC's sexual education programme was drawn up in a participatory way, taking into consideration the target population. The curriculum used in RUWSEC's school health programme was based on information seeking questions posed by the students themselves. Topics covered included: our bodies, friendship, relationships with parents and teachers, status of women, how to approach boys (or girls), married life, bad habits (drinking, smoking), and future life plans. Separate sessions are now held for boys and girls. Of the seven topics, six are common to both girls and boys; the content of one is different. The topics for girls also include menstruation, pregnancy, whom to approach in case of problems, exercises and activities to build self confidence. The same seven topics are repeated with the non-school going group of girls at the village level. Also, topics taught at the adolescent check-up camps included white discharge, prolapse, anaemia – all complaints that girls had initially reported. The pre-adolescent camps cover some very basic health issues – first aid, vitamin A deficiency, water stagnation, need to clean ground wells, how to prevent disease, how to take care of siblings, etc. And, as a way of evaluating the effectiveness of the school health programme, RUWSEC compared the responses to 10 questions posed to them in the first session with their answers in the last session.

SEARCH's decision to initiate sexual educational sessions and to address the issue of STIs in its residential camps was based on various factors: the high prevalence of STIs amongst the general tribal population that it works with; the fact that a few adolescents had been diagnosed as HIV positive; and because premarital sex appeared to be quite common amongst adolescent girls. In a manner somewhat similar to RUWSEC, one month after each camp at SEARCH, a meeting is held in villages from where more than 15 participants had attended the camp. Participants are then asked to evaluate their experience, and rank sessions in order of utility; these inputs are used to modify the programme. This follow-up meeting is also used to test how much information participants still retain. Specific health problems are tackled at subsequent monthly meetings.

Involvement of boys (and men)

- To be successful, adolescent programmes must address the severe imbalances in power between adolescent boys and girls, and promote safe and responsible sexual behaviour in adolescent boys as well.

With the exception of Centre for Health, Education, Training and Nutrition Awareness (CHETNA) which works with adolescents in an urban setting, all the other programmes, which happen to be rural-based, have found it necessary to address adolescent girls and boys separately. Some programmes like BCC, OMRAH and Ashish Gram Rachna Trust, for example, have not involved adolescent boys because to date, their health programmes have largely been limited to women. BCC tried but was unable in its initial attempts as it did not have male health workers and cultural considerations preclude female staff from discussing sexual issues with boys/ men.

Appropriate and acceptable approaches

- Sex education is noted to be most effective when it is interactive and participatory, and held in a supportive environment.

- Incorporating sexual education into a broader health education package is more acceptable and works well in a culture where sexual education for unmarried adolescents, girls in particular, continues to be taboo.

Various means have been effectively used to disseminate information — film songs, role plays, skits, slides, flash cards, posters, booklets, informal group discussions and individual counselling. Counselling, based on a relationship of confidentiality, trust and ongoing dialogue, is essential to provide the support that young people need in exploring issues of sexuality. For example, in the absence of any data, it is difficult to ascertain to what extent adolescents are making use of RUWSEC's and SEARCH's 'women-centred' health services. There are, of course, reports of adolescents seeking assistance on an ad hoc basis. But, in as much as both these programmes found it necessary to reach out to adolescents separately, and judging by the increasing demand for their camps, it is clear that adolescent needs can be addressed much more effectively when provided in the context of broader services designed specifically for them. An important contributory factor to SEARCH's or SUTRA's success is that their camps are residential and held in a supportive environment at the organisation's campus. SEARCH's initial attempts to hold such camps in village settings had failed. Adolescents were not at ease. Passing villagers observing youngsters viewing slides of STIs, or hearing them discussing sexual issues, complained of young minds being polluted by dirty talk. Even now, girls recommend these camps to their friends in an indirect manner, by saying they will get 'good information' there. They do not as yet, openly admit to attending sexual education sessions.

While there is no standard formula of reaching out to adolescent boys, it is interesting to note the strategy used by some of the programmes. SEARCH, for example, did it by involving the right people – two young men who had been trained at a prestigious body building institute and who commanded respect from the adolescent boys they were to lead; and by including strategic activities such as sports. In a similar manner, DCT is beginning to target adolescent boys by sponsoring cricket matches between villages where they also hold meetings. Instead of hiring their own 'men', RUWSEC implemented a very brilliant and innovative programme of supporting independent men's organisations to carry out their agenda on gender sensitisation and responsible and safe sexual behaviour with adolescent boys and men in the villages. RUWSEC also adopted the strategy of running a youth recreation centre to reach out to boys; and through schools.

All programmes have adopted the strategy of incorporating sexual education into a broader health education package; as noted earlier, some have combined this with a number of other strategic activities such as sports, skill-training and income-generating activities. This combination of fun and learning, imparting skills and information seems to have worked well. Adolescents find the sessions enjoyable. They are comfortable attending them.

It is important to create social acceptability and the look of it can result in some difficulties as witnessed by the experience of Chinmaya Tapovan Trust in Himachal Pradesh, when it first started its adolescent girls' groups. "The minute we started talking about menstrual cycle and conception, there was a sudden drop in attendance," says Dr. Metre of the Trust. "Mothers would say 'What kind of things are you teaching them?' Other girls started referring to members as 'dirty girls.' And the girls themselves were shy of talking about these things. The fault was not theirs but ours. Our training was at fault." The Trust is now redesigning its programme. "Maybe we'll drag mothers into the group and make them talk about issues like menstruation," says Dr. Metre. The number of groups has been reduced from 145 to 90, and safe topics like knitting and pickle-making are to be integrated into the meeting. "It's easy for a girl to go back and say she learnt about *gobi ka achar* (cauliflower pickle)," says Dr. Metre, "rather than that she learnt about menstrual hygiene."

Training of providers

- Providers need to be trained and sensitised to the special and different needs of adolescent boys and girls, and to the dynamics between young boys and girls. They also need to be sensitive to how gender norms in a given society affect adolescents' decision-making about reproductive health behaviour and how these norms affect access to health services.

It is essential for providers to view reproductive health not only in terms of services but also in terms of attitudes and quality of care. Their views concerning gender norms will most certainly affect the services they provide. Provider training must include topics such as understanding sexuality, body changes during adolescence, feelings, and relationships. Very often the physical aspects are talked about but not the last two.

Few programmes have invested in developing training programmes for providers of adolescent reproductive health programmes. At RUWSEC for example, a five-person team, all of whom have reportedly received some form of formal training on how to work with adolescents, (e.g. adolescent psychology), supervises all on-going work with adolescents. In addition, community-based workers (including traditional birth attendants) have been pivotal to providing information to adolescent girls. However, they have not received specific training with regard to working with adolescents per se. Further, the fact that none of these programmes have systematically evaluated the quality of counselling is an issue that needs to be addressed.

Community support

- Community involvement is essential to sustain any gains made and to provide support.

SEARCH and RUWSEC made a conscious attempt to work together with community leaders, religious groups, teachers and parents, and sought their support in order to overcome any opposition that may be based on fear and mistrust. DCT and OMRAH enlisted the support of mothers and held sexual educational sessions for mothers and adolescents together. Prerana held sensitisation workshops for parents and for community leaders not only to gain acceptability for their programme, but also to ensure a conducive environment for the adolescents at home. The male and female health workers of Social Action for Rural and Tribal Inhabitants of India (SARTHI) are planning to hold separate gender sensitisation meetings with mothers and fathers in an effort to pave the way for their adolescent girls' programmes.

Most of the documented innovations conducted surveys in their communities and shared their findings. In an attempt to raise awareness vis-a-vis women's health, SEARCH also shared the findings of its study on gynaecological morbidity in women through an innovative community education drive – a women's awakening and health fair in 11 villages, which were attended by about 30,000 people. This was an intensive, 12-hour educational and cultural programme, developed by local artists and the SEARCH team and arranged by village groups. Through the use of a picture exhibition, a team of women from each village helped explain the findings of the gynaecological study and other issues of women's lives and social life. There were slide shows for men and women on various reproductive health and related social issues; songs on women's lives; a play entitled 'When the husbands get pregnant' which attracted huge crowds. The result: a demand by males for a study on STIs and women and youth requesting more information on women's health issues. This led to a series of three-day camps for women and youth, and the formation of women's and youth groups in many villages; and an emerging movement against men's alcoholism.

Above all, it is clear that a shared commitment from the community and a conducive environment is necessary for such programmes to be effectively implemented. It is also important to note that SEARCH's health education activities for adolescents followed a gradual progression – from lectures and slide presentations on sexuality and sex education to adolescents in nearby schools, followed by a similar programme for teachers to organising residential camps for adolescent girls and boys.

Sustainability

- Continued advocacy is important to sustain programmes aimed at unmarried adolescents.

- In order to assess the impact of the specific interventions implemented and make optimal use of scarce resources, it is important for programmes to implement a simple mechanism for ongoing monitoring and evaluation.

- While adolescent health needs can be addressed much more effectively when provided in the context of broader services designed for adolescents only, the potential for cost recovery is low.

As always, prior to recommending the implementation of an intervention, one needs to consider its sustainability. On one level, one must assess the extent of community commitment. There is still hesitation on the part of parents, community leaders and teachers to allow unmarried adolescents to be exposed to sex education. Continued advocacy is important to enhance social acceptability of such programmes. Programmes that have been working towards women's empowerment on a broader level have found it much easier to reach out to adolescents – SUTRA, RUWSEC, SEARCH, and SRED. SUTRA's experience clearly shows that in most instances, where the mother herself was an active *Mahila Mandal* member and had attended camps held by it, the daughter met with little resistance when seeking permission to attend adolescent girls' camps. Some of these programmes have also been able to go beyond the provision of sexual and gender education, to providing services in an 'adolescent friendly' environment. In the long run, in order for such programmes to gain acceptability in the community at large, and dispel fears that information on sex education encourages or increases sexual activity, it will be important for them to demonstrate that their interventions are having a measurable impact towards safe and responsible sexual behaviour and may well lead to: safer pregnancies in younger women; or, a reduction in STI cases, premarital pregnancies, illegal abortions, and other essential negative outcomes. To this end, it is important for these programmes to establish a mechanism for ongoing monitoring and evaluation.

On another level, is the issue of costs of adolescent programmes. These are difficult to estimate for they are components of broader or larger programmes with which they share facilities and resources. Nonetheless, it is evident that many programmes are constrained by their limited resources and are unable to meet the increasing demand by adolescents for information and services. Some groups like RUWSEC, SEARCH, SUTRA, and Ashish Gram Rachna Trust, are adopting the strategy of training 'peer educators' to sustain sexual education programmes, once established. Though SEARCH and RUWSEC have been able to provide separate services to adolescent, these have been on a small scale and mainly focused on RTIs and abortions. Also, due to a paucity of funds, both programmes have been forced to restrict the number of girls it can reach out to. It is clear that where programmes may be able to sustain educational interventions in the long run, the feasibility of providing continued and separate services for adolescents is questionable. The potential for cost recovery is low.

Expanding Coverage and Range of Adolescent Programmes

Adolescents make up a large and growing proportion of India's population. They are gradually being recognised as a high risk group: girls, particularly for their poor nutritional status, their early initiation into motherhood, and their poor reproductive health outcomes; and both sexes, for their lack of factual knowledge regarding issues pertaining to sexuality and contraception, and for their high risk behaviour. There appears to be an increasing recognition among policy makers for the need to address adolescents beyond the traditional family planning framework; to respond to their reproductive health needs in ways which are sensitive to the socio-cultural constraints adolescents, and unmarried girls in particular, face in obtaining services and expressing their health needs.

To date, NGOs have been at the forefront for providing services to adolescents, albeit mainly limited to provision of sexual information. Further, most have targeted unmarried adolescents. In general, there are very few programmes that have considered the needs of newly married adolescent couples. On a larger scale, 'Sex Education, Counselling, Research and Training/Therapy' (SECRT) centres run by the Family Planning Association of India, is one such organisation which provides counselling services for young couples about to be married and also for married couples (Manorama, 1990; Sathe, 1992). These centres also provide a range of confidential and free medical services, but only to married adolescents. In addition, though SECRT holds seminars and workshops in rural areas, the centres themselves are urban-based – Mumbai, Bangalore, Lucknow, Chennai, New Delhi, Rajkot and Pune.

There is no doubt that NGOs are able to manage small-scale projects, but these projects are only reaching a limited number of adolescents, leaving the majority without access to either information or services. The challenge now is to bring sexual education and appropriate services to the larger audience of unreached adolescents. Such efforts will require resources, both financial and manpower, and commitment at the national level. It is, therefore, crucial to sensitise policy makers and generate their commitment for a national policy that helps establish a comprehensive supportive environment for adolescents.

An assessment of NGO activities highlights the following:

- the need to incorporate sexual education sessions into a broader health education package in the school curriculum and provide adolescents with factual information on anatomy and physiology;

- to respond more sensitively, and in less judgmental ways to the special needs of unmarried adolescent girls and boys; and,

- to provide appropriate counselling services to newly-married adolescents.

Several other programme recommendations stand out clearly from the literature review:

- to acknowledge the role of literacy in postponing early marriage and early pregnancy among adolescent girls and, therefore, promote girls' access to and participation in educational opportunities;

- to address the nutritional needs of adolescent girls and to use existing programmes to improve their iron status;

- to promote suitable contraceptive methods to delay age at first pregnancy and to increase intervals between births for adolescents; and,

- to make sure that adolescent mothers receive appropriate antenatal care.

Governments and decision-makers are key to determining the degree of information and assistance accessible to young people. The government, for example, can implement policies that could encourage girls to stay longer in school by ensuring their safety there, establishing schools closer to home, increasing the proportion of female teachers, making school hours more flexible, or by offering an alternative to formal education and teaching adolescents income-earning skills. The government can also take some immediate steps towards incorporating gender perspectives in education, services and training. The government can propagate healthier social practices via the media, promote positive role models, educate the community about the risks of early childbearing, the importance of providing sexual education sessions to adolescents, the need for young women to be healthy and discourage gender differences in food intake, with particular attention to the senior women of the family who are often the key decision makers.

The introduction of a sex education component into the government school curriculum will not only cover a majority of children, but will also create a conducive climate for NGOs to reach out to working children. Further, parents will perhaps be able to accept sex education more readily when it is a part of school activities. It is here where the government can positively collaborate with and learn from the NGO experience. For example, to gain acceptability within the community at large, sex education may need to be introduced into the school curriculum in phases and possibly be incorporated into a broader curriculum on health education rather being in its own area of study. Various model materials will need to be developed for specific target groups. Teachers will also need to undergo an intensive training programme so that they are able to and are comfortable with providing such sessions to adolescents.

The government also needs to look into appropriate and feasible strategies towards improving the iron status of adolescents. Clearly, providers themselves will need to be convinced of the importance of taking such supplementation before they can relay these to adolescents. Steps will also need to be taken towards ensuring an adequate supply of good quality iron-folic acid tablets. Educational campaigns aimed at mothers, mother-in-laws and adolescents, emphasising the importance of a diet which includes available foods rich in iron, and foods that enhance iron absorption will be equally important. In addition, there are other factors such as malnutrition, malaria, bacterial infections, blood loss from abortion, delivery or extremely heavy menstruation, intestinal parasites such as hookworm, and inhibitors in food taken with the tablets (e.g. coffee, tea) which may interact with and reduce the adolescents' uptake of iron, and which will need to be taken into consideration. All in all, the prevention and control of anaemia calls for a much more comprehensive approach than the present practice of distributing iron and folic acid tablets during the last trimester of pregnancy.

Several questions remain unanswered and these need to be addressed. For example, in light of scarce resources, and with India in the process of structural adjustment and of introducing 'user fees', what priority should be given to providing separate services tailored to adolescent needs? The NGO experience has shown that the potential for cost recovery is low. Charging adolescents for services, no matter how nominal, will often deter adolescents, especially unmarried ones, from using the necessary services.

It is clear that for any long-term strategy to be effective, it will have to depend on the public health system in rural India. To this end, there is need for qualitative studies on how existing health and information services can be structured to respond to adolescent needs, taking into consideration the social, cultural, and economic constraints that adolescents in India face. For example, service provision can be integrated through the auxiliary nurse midwives. BMC's sexual education programme may be in its very early stages, but it does demonstrate that given appropriate gender-sensitive training and support, the midwives can effectively reach out to women and adolescent girls; they can provide family life education and life options information to adolescents; and perhaps, also offer appropriate family planning and reproductive health services for adolescents. The example of Ashish Gram Rachna Trust well demonstrates the potential of training traditional birth attendants to reach out to adolescents and ensure that those in need seek timely assistance. It is also clear that if existing services are to cater to adolescents then health care providers, lay workers, paramedical and specialist staff will need to be sensitive to their needs. This means including the subject of adolescent sexuality into their training curriculum; physical, gender and psychological aspects. In one small study for example, interviews with members of the medical profession revealed that a small but significant number, considered the general attitude of health workers doctors, nurses, teachers, etc. to be opposed to the provision of contraceptive counselling for adolescents (FPAI and WHO, 1985). Few doctors really reflect on the emotional needs of adolescents. Many have not had the relevant training or time to devote to drawing out problems of shy and reticent adolescents, especially those seeking abortion services.

Perhaps, the main question that remains unanswered and needs to be addressed is that, knowing the risks of STIs, including HIV, and the consequences of unwanted pregnancy for unmarried adolescents, to what extent can programmes support the healthy development of adolescent sexuality? There may be a shroud of secrecy surrounding premarital sexual activity in rural India, but this is an open secret. Girls are coerced quite often, but they are also consenting partners at times. Notwithstanding this, all these girls pay a heavy price for becoming pregnant outside marriage.

The adolescent period is a time in which individuals explore and develop their sexuality. It is the start of behaviours that may become life-time habits that can result in diseases many years later. As future adults and parents, it is imperative for health planners to consider their health and development a priority, and address it in a holistic manner: from a physical, psychological and social perspective. Investing in adolescent health is essential for the national economy and general well being.

References

Achhpal, B., and Verma, A. 1987. Towards Better Families: An Integrated Approach to Family Life Education and Family Welfare. Monograph No.12, 106. Department of Human Development and Family Studies, Maharaja Sayajirao University, Baroda, India.

Anonymous. 1994. Insights into Adolescent Sexuality. "Dehleez" Emerges a Popular Programme on Yuvavani. *Focus on Population, Environment, Development,* 8(2): 5.

Anonymous. 1978. Kerala: Legal Abortions Increased 15X, 1972-76. *International Family Planning Perspectives and Digest,* 4(1): 31-32.

Aras, R.Y. 1992. Towards Child Health: Through Mother's Health and Education. *Indian Journal of Maternal and Child Health*, 3(2): 52-53.

Aras, R. 1986. Teenage Pregnancy: An Epidemiological Perspective. *Journal of Family Welfare,* 32(3): 65-74.

Aras, R.Y., Pai, N.P., Baliga, A., Jain, S.G., and Naimuddin. 1989. Pregnancy at Teenage – Risk Factor for Lower Birth Weight. *Indian Pediatrics,* 26(8): 823-825.

Aras, R.Y., Pai, N.P., and Jain, S.G. 1987. Termination of Pregnancy in Adolescents. *Journal of Postgraduate Medicine*, 33(3): 120-4

Aras, R.Y., Pai, N.P., and Purandare, A. 1990. Perinatal Mortality – A Retrospective Hospital Study. *Journal of Obstetrics and Gynaecology,* 40(3): 365-369.

Bang, R., Bang, A., Baitule, M., Chaudhury, Y., Sarmukaddam, S., and Tale, O. 1989. High Prevalence of Gynaecological Diseases in Rural Indian Women. *Lancet,* I(8629): 85-88.

Bansal, R.K. 1992. Sexual Behaviour and Substance Use Patterns Amongst Adolescent Truck Cleaners and Risk of HIV/AIDS. *Indian Journal of Maternal and Child Health,* 3(4): 108-110.

Bhatia, B.D., and Chandra, R. 1993. Adolescent Mother-An Unprepared Child. *Indian Journal of Maternal and Child Health,* 4(3): 67-70.

Bhatt, R.V. 1978. An Indian Study of the Psychosocial Behaviour of Pregnant Teenage Women. *Journal of Reproductive Medicine,* 21(4): 275-278.

Bhattacharya, M., and Joshi, P.L. 1995. Teenage Pregnancies: Present Trends and Future Prospects. In: R.B. Gupta, and S. Joshi (eds.). Workshop on Strategy Formulation to Reduce Teenage Fertility in Uttar Pradesh, India. Uttar Pradesh Academy of Administration, Nainital, India. Final Report.

Bhende, A. 1994. A Study of Sexuality of Adolescent Girls and Boys in Underprivileged Groups in Bombay. *The Indian Journal of Social Work,* LV(4): 557-572.

Capoor, I., and Mehta, S. 1995. Talking about Love and Sex in Adolescent Health Fairs in India. *Reproductive Health Matters,* 5: 22-27.

Chhabra, S. 1992. A Step Towards Helping Mothers with Unwanted Pregnancies. *Indian Journal of Maternal and Child Health,* 3(2): 41-42.

Chhabra, S., Gupte, N., Mehta, A., and Shende, A. 1988. Medical Termination of Pregnancy and Concurrent Contraceptive Adoption in Rural India. *Studies in Family Planning,* 19(4): 244-247.

Chowdhury, N.N., and Mukherjee, K. 1979. Sociological Implications of Pregnancy in Unmarried Teenagers. *Journal of Obstetrics and Gynecology of India,* 29(2): 308-312.

Das Gupta, M. 1987. Selective Discrimination against Female Children in Rural Punjab, India. *Population and Development Review,* 13(1): 77-100.

Family Planning Association of India and World Health Organization. 1985. Adolescent and the Medical Profession. Unpublished Report.

Family Planning Association of India and World Health Organization. 1982. The Adolescent and Availability of Family Planning Services. FPAI-WHO Survey. Unpublished Report.

Family Health International. 1997. Adolescent Reproductive Health. *Network,* 17(3): 9-31.

Germain, A., Holmes, K.K., Piot, P., and Wasserheit, J.N. 1992. Reproductive Tract Infections: Global Impact and Priorities for Women's Reproductive Health. New York: Plenum Press.

Goodburn and Ross. 1995. A Picture of Health. A Review and Annotated Bibliography of the Health of Young People in Developing Countries. WHO/FHE/ADH/95.14. Geneva: World Health Organization.

Gopalan, C. 1990. Women and Nutrition in Developing Countries: Practical Considerations. In: H.M. Wallace, and K. Giri (eds.). Health Care of Women and Children in Developing Countries, 252-63. Oakland, California: Third Party Publishing.

Gupta, R.B., and Joshi, S. (eds.). 1995. Workshop on Strategy Formulation to Reduce Teenage Fertility in Uttar Pradesh, India. Uttar Pradesh Academy of Administration, Nainital, India. Final Report.

Gupta, R.B., and Khan, M.E. 1995. Teenage Fertility in U.P.: Some Results from Baseline Survey in Uttar Pradesh. In: R.B. Gupta, and S. Joshi (eds.). Workshop on Strategy Formulation to Reduce Teenage Fertility in Uttar Pradesh, India. Uttar Pradesh Academy of Administration, Nainital, India. Final Report.

Harrison, A., and Koblinsky, M. (eds.). 1995. Young Adults - Is Age a Risk Factor? *MotherCare Matters,* 5(2/3): 1-2.

Hirve, S.S., and Ganatra, B.R. 1994. Determinants of Low Birth Weight: A Community Based Prospective Cohort Study. *Indian Pediatrics,* 31(10): 1221-1225.

Indian Council of Medical Research. 1989. Evaluation of the National Nutritional Anaemia Prophylaxis Programme – an ICMR Task Force Study. Indian Council of Medical Research, New Delhi, India.

International Centre for Research on Women. 1997. Adolescent Sexuality and Fertility in India – Preliminary Findings. Information Bulletin. International Centre for Research on Women, Washington, D.C., USA.

International Institute for Population Sciences. 1995. National Family Health Survey, 1992-93. Mumbai, India.

Jejeebhoy, S.J. 1996. Adolescent Sexual and Reproductive Behaviour: A Review of Evidence from India. ICRW Working Paper No. 3. International Centre for Research for Women, Washington, D.C., USA.

Jejeebhoy, S.J., and Rama Rao, S. 1996. Unsafe Motherhood: A Review of Reproductive Health. In: M. Das Gupta, L. Chen, and T.N. Krishnan (eds.). Women's Health in India. Risks and Vulnerability, 122-152. Oxford: Oxford University Press.

Jude, P.M., Chandrakala, S., Jayalakshmi, S. et al. 1991. Status of Adolescent Girls in a Rural South Indian Population. *Indian Journal of Maternal and Child Health,* 2(2): 60-63.

Kanani, S. 1994. Combating Anaemia in Adolescent Girls: A Report from India. *Indian Journal of Maternal and Child Health,* 13(1): 1-3

Kanani, S., and Consul, P. 1990. Nutrition Health Profile and Intervention Strategies for Underprivileged Adolescent Girls in India: A Selected Review. *Indian Journal of Maternal and Child Health,* 1(4): 129-133.

Kanbargi, R., and Kanbargi, S. 1996. Sexually Transmitted Diseases in Bangalore City: Some Findings from an Exploratory Study. *Journal of Family Welfare,* 42 (1): 30-37.

Khan, M.E., Anker, R., Ghosh, Dastidar, S.K., and Bairathi, S. 1988. Inequalities Between Men and Women in Nutrition and Family Welfare Services: An In-depth Inquiry in an Indian Village. *Social Action*, 1998: 38.

Khanna, R. 1992. Taking Charge: Women's Health as Empowerment. The SARTHI Experience. SAHAJ/ SARTHI Godhar West, India.

Khanna, S.K. 1995. Gender Discrimination, Maternal Health, and Pregnancy Outcomes in North India. Ann Arbor, Michigan: UMI Dissertation Services [3], xi. 303 p. (UMI No. 9619044)

Kushwaha, K.P., Rai, A.K., Rathi, A.K., Singh, Y.D., and Sirohi, R. 1993. Pregnancies in Adolescents: Fetal, Neonatal and Maternal Outcome. *Indian Pediatrics,* 30(4): 501-5.

Mahajan, A., and van Zuijlen, M. 1994. Emerging Challenges, Society for Social Uplift Through Rural Action, Jagjit Nagar, India.

Mamdani, M., and Sen, G., 1996. SEWA's Health Project: An Evaluation Report. Unpublished.

Mandal, K.T. 1982. Problem of Unmarried Mothers: A Study of Sociopsychological Aspects of 100 Women Seeking MTP. *Journal of the Indian Medical Association,* 79(5-6): 81-86.

Manorama, H.S. 1990. India: Sex Education Counseling Research Training Therapy / Family Life and Marriage Counseling Centres. *Planned Parenthood in Europe,* 19(3): 15.

Mavalankar, D.V. 1996. Quality Reproductive Health Services in Rural India: The SEARCH Experience. Malaysia: International Council on Management of Population Programs.

Mishra, S., and Dawn, C.S. 1986. Retrospective Study of Teenage Pregnancy and Labour During 5 Years Period from January 1978 to December 1982 at Durgapur Subdivisional Hospital. *Indian Medical Journal,* 80(9): 150-152.

MotherCare Project. 1993. Anaemia and Pregnancy. *MotherCare Matters,* 3(1/2).

Pachauri, S., and Jamshedji, A. 1983. Risks of Teenage Pregnancy. *Journal of Obstetrics and Gynaecology,* 33(3): 477-482.

Pandhi, R.K., Khanna, N., and Sekhri, R. 1995. Sexually Transmitted Diseases in Children. *Indian Pediatrics,* 32(1): 27-30.

Pakrasi, K., Sil, S., and Dasgupta, P. 1985. Body Weight at Birth and Incidence of Low-Weight Babies in Calcutta (India). *Anthropologie*, 23(1): 81-94.

Pathak, K.B., and Ram, F. 1993. Adolescent Motherhood: Problems and Consequences. *The Journal of Family Welfare,* 39(1): 17-23.

Population Reference Bureau, 1996. The World's Youth. Chart. Washington, D.C., USA.

Pratinidhi, A., Shrotri, A., and Shah, U. 1990. Risk of Teenage Pregnancy in a Rural Community of India. *Indian Journal of Maternal and Child Health,* 1(4):134-138.

Purandare, V.N., Chaudhary, R.F., Raote, V.B., and Krishna, U.R. 1979. A Study of Psychosocial Factors of Out-of-wedlock Pregnancies. *Journal of Obstetrics and Gynaecology of India,* 29(2): 303-307.

Purandare, V.N., and Krishna, U.R. 1974. Pregnancy and Abortion in Adolescence. Paper Presented at a World Health Organization Meeting on Pregnancy and Abortion in Adolescence, Geneva, June 24-28. Geneva: World Health Organization.

Ramachandran, P. 1989. Nutrition in Pregnancy. In: C. Gopalan, and S. Kaur, (eds.). Women and Nutrition in India. New Delhi: Nutrition Foundation of India.

Roy and Nangia. 1995. Teenage Fertility Behaviour in Uttar Pradesh: An Empirical Investigation of Levels, Trends and Differentials. In: R.B. Gupta, and S. Joshi (eds.). Workshop on Strategy Formulation to Reduce Teenage Fertility in Uttar Pradesh, India. Uttar Pradesh Academy of Administration, Nainital, India. Final Report.

Sathe, A.G. 1992. Issues and Problems in Introducing Family Life Education for Boys and Girls of Secondary Schools. *Journal of Family Welfare,* 38(1): 56-67.

Sathe, A.G. 1987. The Adolescent in India: A Status Report. *Journal of Family Welfare,* 34(1): 11-19.

Schuler, S., Hashemi, S., and Pandit, H. 1995. Beyond Credit: SEWA's Approach to Women's Empowerment and Influence on Women's Reproductive Lives in Urban India. Self-Employed Women's Association, Ahmedabad, India. Unpublished Report.

Senanayake, P., and Kleinman, R.L. (eds.). 1993. Family Planning. Meeting Challenges: Promoting Choices. The Proceedings of the IPPF Family Planning Congress, New Delhi, October 1992. Carnforth, England: Parthenon Publishing Group.

Senderowitz, J. 1995. Adolescent Health: Reassessing the Passage to Adulthood. World Bank Discussion Paper No. 272. Washington, D.C. USA.: The World Bank.

Sharma, V., and Sharma, A. 1992. Health Profile of Pregnant Adolescents Among Selected Tribal Populations in Rajasthan, India. *Journal of Adolescent Health,* 13(8): 696-699.

Solapurkar, M.L., and Sangam, R.N. 1985. Has the MTP Act in India Proved Beneficial? *Journal of Family Welfare,* 31(3): 46-52.

Subramanian, S.S. 1996. Quality Reproductive Health Services in Rural India: The RUWSEC Experience. Malaysia: International Council on Management of Population Programmes.

Sundari Ravindran, T.K. 1996. From Rhetoric to Action, *Seminar,* 447, (November): 43-49.

Swain, S., Ojha, K.N., Prakash, A., and Bhatia, B.D. 1993. Maternal and Perinatal Mortality due to Eclampsia. *Indian Pediatrics*, 30(6): 771-773.

Thapa, P. (Undated). Disappearing Women: A Paradox of Social Compulsions and Individual Choice. In: The Girl Child and Adolescent Women. IPPF Discussion Paper 3: 12-15.

The Alan Guttmacher Institute. 1997. Risks and Realities of Early Childbearing Worldwide: Issues in Brief. The Alan Guttmacher Institute, New York, USA.

United Nations. 1989. Adolescent Reproductive Behaviour. Volume II. Evidence from Developing Countries. New York: United Nations.

United Nations Childrens Fund. 1990. Children and Women in India. A Situation Analysis. New Delhi: United Nations Childrens Fund .

Watsa, M.C. 1993. Unmet Needs in Family Planning: Youth (an Indian Viewpoint). In: P. Senanayake, and R.L. Kleinman (eds.). Family Planning. Meeting Challenges: Promoting Choices. The Proceedings of the IPPF Family Planning Congress, New Delhi, October 1992. Carnforth, England: Parthenon Publishing Group,

World Health Organization. 1996. Adolescent Health – Investing in the Future. *Safe Motherhood,* 22 (3).

Appendix

COMMUNITY-BASED PROGRAMMES ADDRESSING WOMEN'S REPRODUCTIVE HEALTH NEEDS IN INDIA

This project started in December 1994. Its prime objective was to document community-based programmes addressing women's reproductive health needs in India. The project consisted of four phases.

Phase One: As a starting point, around 300 organisations (non-governmental, academic institutions, women's groups, donors) were contacted. The objective was to identify a diverse range of reproductive health care programmes being implemented throughout the country.

Phase Two: A screening questionnaire sent to each of the organisations (mainly non-governmental identified in phase one), provided the initial information on the specific reproductive health needs being addressed. The return rate was around 80 percent. Every attempt was made to follow up on those NGOs that failed to respond.

Phase Three: Based on information obtained during phase two, field visits were made to 70 NGOs. The selection criteria were as follows: the programme had been established for at least five years; and, it should be somewhat innovative in its approach (other than the conventional maternal child care and family planning programmes). Another objective was to get a spread of groups across most, if not all, of the states across the country. Information from these preliminary visits has been compiled and published as a monograph entitled 'Community-based Programmes addressing Women's Reproductive Health needs in India: A Documentation' (Mamdani M (ed.), 1998). These documentations provide a 'snap shot' of reproductive health interventions being implemented by some of the community-based organisations within India.

Phase Four: Repeat visits were made to 33 of the programmes screened in the third phase. The objective was to get specific information on one or more of the following reproductive health interventions being implemented: reproductive tract infections; family planning (including spacing methods, infertility, abortion); safe motherhood; adolescent reproductive health; and, male involvement. Some issues of interest were: how these interventions are being implemented at the community level; the operational factors involved; the major obstacles met; and, where possible, get a notion of the incremental costs involved in implementing the specific intervention(s) of interest. About 4-7 days were spent with each of these programmes.

Apart from trying to get a geographic spread of programmes, a number of factors dictated the choice of groups selected. One obvious criterion was that the programme's approach was perceived as having been quite 'successful.' Another was to get a mix of 'models' (i.e., addressing the needs of a poor urban versus rural population, and clinic-based versus community-based programmes). The final choice also depended on the possibility of conducting another follow-up visit to that programme. Often programmes had several important items on their agenda and thus failed to accommodate our visit. Or, for example, due to unexpectedly bad cyclones in Andhra Pradesh, we failed to follow up on a number of programmes.

Major limitations:

1. We were unsuccessful in obtaining quantitative data of good quality, mainly because of a poor information system; a problem inherent in most programmes. A few programmes do have a systematic data collection procedure, but much of this information remains unanalysed.

2. It was not possible to get any valid information on the incremental costs involved in implementing a specific intervention. These are difficult to estimate for they are components of broader or larger programmes with which they share facilities and resources.

Information obtained from phase three and four has been used towards writing the following three issue-based monographs:

1. Community-based Management of Reproductive Tract Infections in Women in India: Lessons from the Field.

2. A Decade of Safe Motherhood: Initiatives in India.

3. New Priorities: Adolescent Reproductive Health in India.

3

Men as Supportive Partners in Reproductive Health: NGOs Pave the Way

Saraswati Raju

The author would like to thank Dr. Stina Almroth for her editorial insight and immense help in giving this paper its final shape.

Introduction

The Programme of Action globally endorsed at the International Conference on Population and Development (ICPD) propagated reproductive health as a human rights issue. Individuals are not the means to achieve demographic targets, as has largely been the approach the world over. Instead, they have the right to attain their personal goals within the broader sphere of reproductive health. Given this perspective, gender relations and human sexuality become closely interdependent and the role envisaged for men as supportive partners to women in their joint agenda for positive health outcomes, particularly those relating to reproduction, becomes crucial.

A review of demographic literature reveals that the role identified for men in the entire spectrum of reproductive health has been limited. The absence of men from this area is embedded in the societal roles of men and women, including how children are socialised into gender relations in their formative years. A reproductive health framework that advocates shared responsibilities and gender equity, therefore, requires taking a life-cycle approach, whereby adolescents become as significant a group as men or women in terms of their reproductive and sexual health needs. Thus, supportive partnership is not a techno-medical issue, but has to be situated within a socio-cultural milieu, particularly within a framework of gender relations. Although not explicitly stated, the agenda really is about social change towards a more gender egalitarian society.

This chapter attempts to take stock of post-ICPD activities in India as they relate to male partnerships in reproductive and sexual health. A brief historical account of how women's roles have been articulated in various policy documents provides a backdrop.

The Backdrop

The Constitution of India adopted in 1950 was most progressive. It not only granted equality to women and imposed a fundamental duty on every citizen to refrain from practices derogatory to the dignity of women, but also empowered the State to adopt measures of affirmative action in favour of women. However, the concept of gender equity was never examined by a nation state that essentially saw women as mothers and keepers of the family (Kumar, 1993). This perhaps explains why the Hindu Code Bill, that proposed equal inheritance for women, prohibition of polygamy and liberal divorce and custody rights as ways to concretise gender equity, was not accepted.

Despite an expressed concern to link family planning with the wider development process, efforts to monitor population growth in India have continued to place the responsibility of family planning on women. Various plan proposals for the apparent well being of women turned out to be mere means to the end of attaining demographic targets (Government of India, 1978; Raju and Kumar, 1992).

The 1990s witnessed feminist scholarship and activism that highlighted the inadequacies of the techno-medical approach to population control. This drew attention to the unequal negotiating positions between men and women, and the consequences for reproductive behaviour whereby women were assigned disproportionate responsibilities without any decisive powers. This, together with a supportive international environment helped change the vocabulary of the Indian planners. Women are now increasingly viewed as equal partners in the development process. The Swaminathan Committee that looked at population issues in India in 1993, for example, advocated a holistic approach to health in general, and gender equity in particular. It argued for inculcating a culture of joint responsibility in all matters relating to the family through various steps, including the removal of gender bias (Government of India, 1993).

While this was a refreshing change from earlier planning statements, there still remained a clear undercurrent through the report, of women being viewed as primarily responsible for reproductive health and men as an ad hoc constituency. Men's involvement in reproductive health remained essentially confined to contraception. The problem seems to lie in the interpretation of the word 'gender'. Gender is often used to mean only women rather than the socially constructed roles for men and women that require changing idioms for both. Thus, one looks in vain, in the Swaminathan Committee Report for effective ways to operationalise the concept of joint responsibility of men and women.

More recently, while implementing the reproductive and child health programme, the government declared that:

> *It is a legitimate right of the citizens to be able to experience sound reproductive and child health and therefore, the reproductive and child health programme will seek to provide relevant services for assuring reproductive and child health to all citizens ... [this is because] it is now well established that parents keep the family size small, if they are assured about the health and longevity of the children and there is no better assurance of good health and longevity of the children than health care for mothers and for young children* (Government of India, 1997:3).

It is evident that women's identity as citizens (supposedly a gender-neutral term) in the public discourse is not the same as in the private sphere of domesticity where the primary construct is that of motherhood. Health care for mothers is, in fact, aimed at children's health. The father remains conspicuous by his absence, even though his sexual behaviour and neglect of his own reproductive health may have a strong bearing on the mother's health.

Although issues concerning maternal health and development find mention of men, no particular role is envisaged for them in terms of child survival, health and development. In reproductive health, men's roles are typically limited to fertility regulation and contraceptive use (Kaza, 1998). Khan et al, in a policy review of men's involvement in reproductive health remarked:

> *Despite . . . top programme managers [being] aware of the need of pursuing a broader approach to reproductive health issues and the importance of involving men, their main concern is at present limited to strengthening delivery systems, with limited initiatives for involving men . . . in introducing no scalpel vasectomy and promoting the use of condom.*
> (Khan et al, 1998).

In sum, efforts to translate gender equity in terms of empowering women, and enhancing men's partnership in reproductive health are limited and narrowly defined. Yet, the appropriation of the ICPD language is a significant first step.

Non-governmental Organisations Pave the Way

While government efforts have not moved beyond planning, NGOs through their community-based programmes have found ways to approach reproductive health from a broader perspective that includes not only women, but also men (see Annexure 1). It is difficult to state conclusively whether it was the ICPD that propelled their interest in working with men or whether it was something they were likely to have done anyway. An examination of NGO

TABLE 1: Content Analysis of Various Programme Documents.

Name of the document	Year	Content with respect to male involvement
Action Plan for Revamping the Family Welfare Programme	1992	• No mention of gender disparity • No mention of male involvement.
Draft National Population Policy	1994	• Suggests a holistic approach to family welfare programme. • Issues of gender inequality brought up prominently • Male involvement is discussed in a gender framework.
Manual of Target Free Approach in Family Welfare Programme	1996	• No reference to gender issues • No reference to male involvement • Forms designed to collect data by sex.
Manual of Community Needs Assessment Approach	1998	
Reproductive and Child Health Programme-Schemes for Implementation	1997	• Gender issues not mentioned • Male involvement not mentioned • Counselling on sexuality and gender
Reproductive and Child Health Programme-Progress Report up to March 31, 1998	1998	• No reference to gender • No reference to male involvement.
Population, Family Welfare and Health: Chapter in Approach Paper to Ninth Five Year Plan 1997-2002	1998	Two-line reference to: • Promoting male participation in planned parenthood • Increasing vasectomy
Survey Instruments for RCH Baseline Survey	1998	• No questions on husband-wife communications • No question on gender issues • Questions to male members on STD and AIDS awareness

Adapted from: Khan, M.E., Gupta, R.B., and Haider, N. 1998. Involving Men in Reproductive Health: Policy and Programme Perspectives. Paper presented at the Workshop – Men as Supportive Partners in Reproductive and Sexual Health, Kathmandu, Nepal. June 1998. Population Council, New Delhi, India.

reports from different parts of the country preparatory to the ICPD, indicates that the latter is the more plausible proposition (Khanna et al, 1998).

While the efforts of NGOs to reach out to men have sprung largely out of their own programme activities, they clearly were able to do more because donor support was available after the ICPD. As most NGO initiatives are still in their infancy, it is important that donors keep alive their interest in supporting research and interventions that focus on men's partnerships in reproductive health. Government funding is yet to be earmarked for these initiatives.

Involving men for women's sake

In the overwhelming majority of cases, it is clear that the initiatives to include men were motivated by a concern about women's reproductive health which showed little improvement without men's support and active involvement. None of the NGOs focussed initially or exclusively on men. Men's inclusion was part of an evolutionary process, a consequence of ground realities within the context of women's health. For example, a number of NGOs found that sexually transmitted infections (STIs) could not be treated by simply providing physical access to women-friendly health care services. For women, a more crucial question was that of social access, which invariably included what men in their families had to say. As high as 50 percent of the women in a tribal area of Gujarat who had STI symptoms and had agreed to get themselves examined and treated, backed out because the male members did not allow them to attend the camp (Khanna et al, 1998).

In the course of their intervention, Community Aid Sponsorship Programme in alliance with Foster Parents Plan International (CASP-PLAN) realised that many women with STIs attending their gynaecology clinic were not showing satisfactory improvement. A closer probe made it clear that these women required 'partner compliance', which was lacking. The women in their project areas often insisted that their husbands should also be contacted and sensitised to the fact that their behaviour has a bearing on the reproductive health of their women partners. A common refrain was,: *"Aap hame to samjha dete ho, per hamare admi ko kaun samjayega"* [you make us understand everything, but who is going to make our men understand?] (Pal, 1998). Data collected by the Rural Women's Social Education Centre (RUWSEC) on reproductive health problems showed that a significant proportion of reproductive tract infections (RTIs) among women were a direct result of men's promiscuity (Subramanian, 1998).

In order to solve the practical problem of getting pregnant women to antenatal care clinics, the Deepak Charitable Trust started the *Pati Sampark* (literally 'contact the husband') programme, which contributed to an increase in women's attendance. Also, in the project area where husbands were contacted, women had a more in-depth understanding of antenatal services compared to women whose husbands had not been included in the programme. Although the exact role of husbands is not conclusive, qualitative research shows that the husbands in the project area held a more positive view of their potential roles to assist their wives during pregnancy (Dev, 1998).

Society for Education, Welfare and Action-Rural

An important learning has been that health and well being should be approached in a holistic manner, whereby the family is seen as a unit and a comprehensive package of health services is delivered according to the specific needs of the respective member of the family, whether it is the management of a minor or major illness, the care of a pregnant mother or child, the needs of adolescent youth or newly married couples, other married couples and elderly members of the family. The underlying fabric of socio-cultural traditions and the economic milieu has to be kept in mind while introducing any strategy. And lastly, but most importantly, 'man' is always there and cannot be bypassed in the overall interests of the society and towards building a true partnership with women counterparts.

SEWA–Rural Research Team, 1998

In an attempt to increase hospital referrals for high risk pregnant women, the Society for Education Welfare and Action (SEWA-Rural) sent postcards to the male members of the families of such women. They found that hospital referrals did increase and that there was a tangible increase in the level of awareness among family members. About 65 percent responded to suggestions for appropriate care as outlined in the postcards (SEWA-Rural Research Team, 1998).

Involving men for their own sake

As discussed, even when NGOs provided services especially for men, their concern remained women. In most cases, these services were for treatment of STIs and were provided within the existing health care facilities for women. CASP-PLAN, for example, used their existing antenatal clinics, extending clinic hours on week days and adding Sundays. Moreover, from having started out as an 'STD Clinic,' the clinic was later called the 'Male Clinic.' Similarly, at RUWSEC, when men approached male health workers for STI treatment, they were referred to the reproductive health clinic where a male doctor was available on specific days of the week. While RUWSEC has plans to expand services to bring in more male clients, their main aim remains treating partners of their women clients. (Subramanian, 1998).

In some cases, men became curious when they learnt that the women were being made aware of their bodies, sexual functioning, safe sexual behaviour and so on. The men also demanded such services.

In one case, an NGO that provides family planning services, Parivar Seva Sanstha (PSS), undertook community research and found a high unmet demand for male reproductive health services. As a result, PSS started a separate 'Male Only Clinic' in Chennai. Focus group discussions and in-depth interviews with potential clients indicated that it was important that the name of the clinic conveyed no stigmatising image or value judgement. The clinic was named, *Purush*, which simply meant 'men' (Sharma and Arora, 1998).

Concerned about preventing sexually transmitted infections including HIV/AIDS, the Bhoruka Public Welfare Trust established an intervention programme for the mobile population of truckers at strategic halt points. Drop-in-centres cum clinics were set up at the India-Nepal and India-Bangladesh borders as well as in Andhra Pradesh. These drop-in centres resembled resting places rather than medical clinics. Since the basic purpose was HIV/AIDS prevention, services included treatment of STIs, condom distribution, HIV testing, information, education, and counselling. As the services gained popularity among the truckers, they began bringing their families with them for general health care. Being a community-based organisation, the Trust felt that it should respond to this demand. Services were diversified from treatment of STIs to general health care (Majumdar, 1998).

Strategies for reaching out to men

Almost without exception, NGOs not only cater to the community but also draw upon the community's human resources for their work. A commonly adopted strategy is to train peer educators, paid or unpaid. Carefully selected peer educators often act as role models. From exclusively male or female teams of peer educators, some NGOs began to form mixed teams of both males and females. These teams were able to approach families in a more integrated way. This mixed team approach also had the benefit of team members learning from each other and dealing with their own shortcomings (Gupta and Joshi, 1998).

A common observation was that male workers intuitively possessed far less information than their female counterparts. Training and discussions with male workers brought forth a range of concerns and apprehensions regarding sexuality, pregnancy, abortion, and infertility. A number of NGOs firmly believe that to be effective, workers have to come to grips with their own ignorance and be able to deal with their own sexuality.

A particular strategy adopted by some NGOs, has been to train so called 'inner groups' who are then encouraged to pass on messages to the 'outer groups'. In one case, the inner group consisted of husbands who were attending health education camps with their wives. These men would then pass on their learning to their peers, the outer group. (Barua, 1998).

Another strategy has been to work with young husbands and wives as teams. *Swaasthya*, for example, is experimenting with activities to improve husband-wife communication. SEWA-Rural organises special programmes for newly-weds as a way to reach young couples with reproductive health information at a relatively early stage. Their way of approaching this target group is unique. They begin by contacting the young man well before he is married and thereby build rapport. Given the role other family members can play in a newly-wed couple's life, the in-laws are also brought into the picture from the very start. The future wife, who usually resides elsewhere, cannot be reached at this stage.

After marriage, the couples are brought out of their homes for a one-day *Nav Dampati Mela* (gatherings for newly-weds). Each couple is presented with a token gift, including condoms and oral contraceptives. Interestingly, the man gets the oral contraceptives and the woman the condoms. If the couples express an interest to learn more about fertility regulation, the health workers counsel them. As a follow-up activity, the newly-wed couples are encouraged to form their own small support groups. The coming together of young couples in public spaces, often for the first time, seemed to instill in them a sense of camaraderie, provided opportunities to unwind and help develop a sense of togetherness.

The observation that children were a point of converging interest in many settings, led some NGOs to take advantage of this as entry points to reach out to men. For example Social Action for Rural and Tribal Inhabitants of India (SARTHI), found that men took an interest in growth monitoring sessions for children. This NGO began providing information to men on child care during these sessions. Similar experiences are cited by the Centre for Health

Education, Training and Nutrition Awareness (CHETNA), CASP-PLAN, and the Family Planning Association of India (FPAI).

Concluding Comments and Future Challenges

In the absence of systematic base-line and post-intervention data, it is difficult to ascertain to what extent NGO interventions have helped. We do not know the proportion of men in different regions who do not avail the different types of services NGOs have to offer. Most importantly, how much of an attitudinal change is there and does it translate into real action? One NGO, that collected both quantitative and qualitative pre- and post-intervention data was able to demonstrate a positive impact of its efforts in improving the health seeking behaviour of pregnant women when husbands were contacted, compared to when they were not (Dev, 1998).

It is important to recognise that the NGOs themselves are not operating independent of the context and prevailing gender ideology. In traditional and conservative settings, it is especially difficult for NGOs to initiate discussions around gender justice while addressing men, lest it becomes a 'battle of the sexes'. In order to circumvent this hurdle, they must use the existing social construct of gender roles, at least to begin with. Consequently, they use existing spaces to propagate altered male behaviour in a gender-sensitive manner. For example, the Society for Integrated Development of Himalayas (SIDH) found that, in the process of sensitising male youth about the unequal position of women vis-a-vis men, any attempt to talk about women's issues made men defensive. They built immediate alliances among themselves to face the threat to their patriarchal hold. After much trial and error, SIDH developed ways to negotiate interpersonal relations within the existing context.

Understandably, NGOs have not been able to touch the underlying patriarchal base. The dilemma NGOs face is that they have to work at the grassroots level with the community and cannot always go against region-specific social and cultural norms. While NGOs have not really been able to engineer much social change, their very efforts to bring men in as supportive partners within the orbit of reproductive health has meant questioning the prevailing constructs of stereotype gender roles. NGOs are aware of this and often get frustrated because of their inability to raise questions of gender injustice. The message that comes across is that, as of now, programmes that operate without questioning the existing paradigm of gender constructs beyond a certain limit are more successful.

NGO experiences have been able to shed some light on issues debated in academic circles. For example, they clearly question the tendency to posit men as a generic category and to persist with stereotypes of men as 'uncaring and unconcerned'. To see men as an undifferentiated category negates the whole range of male behaviour and yet, it makes a big difference in terms of interventions. There are men who are supportive and caring. There are also men who want to be supportive and caring, but either do not know what to do or how to do what they are supposed to do. This may be because they are entrapped in the social construct of their contrived roles as sex partners, husbands and fathers, and fear being ridiculed as *ḅiala* (effeminate) or *joru ka gulam* (slave of the wife).

Social Action for Rural and Tribal Inhabitants of India

Our current understanding of empowerment has expanded. We believe that power has to be defined not in terms of 'power over others', but in terms of self reliance and inner strength, the ability to determine choices and exercise control over one's own life. This holds true for women as well as men. Just as women need to liberate themselves from patriarchal strongholds, men need to be liberated too from the patriarchal construct of masculinity.

Source: Khanna et al, 1998.

A hotly debated issue has been whether involving men might mean encroaching upon women's domain and their limited rights to privacy and control over their bodies. RUWSEC found that working with men helped them understand the dynamics of gender relations better. More importantly, bringing in men did not result in any 'dilution in the existing focus on empowerment of women'. Instead, men became more aware and more willing to seek help for their reproductive and sexual problems. In addition, the feedback from men's programmes helped RUWSEC improve their future activities for women (Subramanian, 1998).

Before any conclusive statement is made regarding the appropriation of women's domain, we need to understand how exactly men are being brought in. It can be convincingly argued that domain identification is itself an outcome of age-old social conditioning about responsibilities that are socially constructed as 'typically female' or 'typically male'. On the contrary, if men participate because of a demand from women, we can actually start talking about a shift in the social construct that is spearheaded by the women themselves.

However limited their efforts may have been, NGOs have been in the forefront in terms of addressing men as a constituency. And yet, their reach in terms of population and geographical spread remains restricted. The challenge now is to use these rich NGO experiences and upscale their efforts. The goal is to move the agenda of male involvement upfront as a part of the process of translating the rhetoric to action.

While most NGO initiatives so far have been concrete activities of involving men in practical matters related to reproductive health, the ultimate goal is about changing an unequal gender equation. It is about social change within the wider realm of gender equity. Freeing men from gender stereotypes will not only open up new spaces for men, but will also help women expand their capabilities. How to do this remains a major future challenge.

Such efforts will require financial and human resources of a magnitude that can only be provided by the State. NGOs can provide learning experiences that can be replicated, but the actual implementation and upscaling of proposed interventions still depends on political will and support. For example, bringing in men requires a variety of institutional support systems to be in place. To name a few, when it comes to reaching out to men for reproductive health services, clinic timings are crucial and there is a need to provide more flexible time schedules. To promote joint responsibilities in parenthood, men may be asked to accompany their wives for ante and postnatal check-ups, delivery, etc. This may require the provision of 'parental leave'.

What is disturbing, however, is the tendency of the State to expect the NGO sector to shoulder responsibilities of this nature. Policy documents mention delegating tasks to NGOs that the government system, *"is not in a position to even attempt"* (Government of India, 1997). Even if this candid submission is to be interpreted as a genuine confession of inadequacy on the part of the government and a desire to involve the NGO sector as a partner, there is a real danger in such a proposition. What is really being said is that any efforts to change attitudes, to erode the patriarchal bases of structures and to spearhead social change are not the State's responsibility. Time and again, it has been demonstrated that efforts, however sincere, cannot be sustained unless there is an institutional framework to support them and only the government has the legitimacy and power to do that. Joint efforts drawing from each other's strengths is a clear requirement.

These are not impossible dreams. To its credit, the government has moved away from a top-down approach. There is an openness and a willingness to build partnerships and alliances with multiple stakeholders. Teething problems and tensions are characteristics of all transitions. Joint efforts by the government, NGOs and the civil society should make a difference. However, such efforts must be sustained to move the agenda forward.

References

Barua, A. 1998. Young Husbands' Involvement in Reproductive Health in Rural Maharashtra. Paper presented at the Workshop on Men as Supportive Partners in Reproductive and Sexual Health, Kathmandu, Nepal, June 1998. Population Council, New Delhi, India.

Dev, A. 1998. Involvment of Husbands' in the Antenatal Care Evaluation of Deepak Charitable Trust' Outreach Programme, Paper presented at the Workshop on Men as Supportive Partners in Reproductive and Sexual Health, Kathmandu, Nepal, June 1998. Population Council, New Delhi, India.

Government of India. 1993. National Population Policy. Mimeo. Department of Family Welfare, Ministry of Health and Family Welfare, New Delhi, India.

Government of India. 1997. Reproductive and Child Health Programme – Schemes for Implementation. Department of Family Welfare, Ministry of Health and Family Welfare, New Delhi, India.

Government of India. Undated. Draft Statement on National Population Policy. Mimeo. Department of Family Welfare, Ministry of Health and Family Welfare, New Delhi, India.

Gupta, P.K., and Joshi, A. 1998. Leadership and Gender Sensitisation. Paper presented at the Workshop on Men as Supportive Partners in Reproductive and Sexual Health, Kathmandu, Nepal, June 1998. Population Council, New Delhi, India.

Kaza, R.C.M. 1998. Vasectomy Revisited. Paper presented at the Workshop on Men as Supportive Partners in Reproductive and Sexual Health, Kathmandu, Nepal, June 1998. Population Council, New Delhi, India.

Khan, M.E., Gupta, R.B., and Haider, N. 1998. Involving Men in Reproductive Health: Policy and Programme Perspectives. Paper presented at the Workshop on Men as Supportive Partners in Reproductive and Sexual Health, Kathmandu, Nepal, June 1998. Population Council, New Delhi, India.

Khanna, R., Patel, H., Pagi, B., and Singh, N. 1998. Men's Involvement in Women's Health. Paper presented at the Workshop on Men as Supportive Partners in Reproductive and Sexual Health, Kathmandu, Nepal, June 1998. Population Council, New Delhi, India.

Kumar, R. 1993. *The History of Doing*, New Delhi: Kali for Women.

Majumdar, A. 1998. Halting AIDS on the Highway. Paper presented at the Workshop on Men as Supportive Partners in Reproductive and Sexual Health, Kathmandu, Nepal, June 1998. Population Council, New Delhi, India.

Pal, P. 1998. Working with Men to Improve Reproductive Health in a Delhi Slum. Paper presented at the Workshop on Men as Supportive Partners in Reproductive and Sexual Health, Kathmandu, Nepal, June 1998. Population Council, New Delhi, India.

Raju, S., Kumar, S. 1992. Who Rock the Cradle? Women, Fertility Control and Technology in India. *Indian Journal of Public Administration*, 3: 323-332.

Society for Education, Welfare and Action-Rural Research Team. 1998. Enhancing Roles and Responsibilities of Men in Women's Health. Paper presented at the Workshop on Men as Supportive Partners in Reproductive and Sexual Health, Kathmandu, Nepal, June 1998. Population Council, New Delhi, India.

Sharma, M., and Arora, P. 1998. Purush: Male Only Clinic. Paper presented at the Workshop on Men as Supportive Partners in Reproductive and Sexual Health, Kathmandu, Nepal, June 1998. Population Council, New Delhi, India.

Subramanian, S. S. 1998. Rural Women Take Reproductive Health Matters Into Their Own Hands. Rural Women's Social Education Centre. Series on Upscaling Innovations in Reproductive Health in Asia, No.1. Malaysia: International Council on Management of Population Programmes.

Women's Health Training Research Advocacy Centre Team. 1998. Men's Roles and Responsibilities for Women's Health. Paper presented at the Workshop on Men as Supportive Partners in Reproductive and Sexual Health, Kathmandu, Nepal, June 1998. Population Council, New Delhi, India.

Annexure 1. Community-based Intervention and Research Activities on Men*

NGO	Population	Coverage	Approach	Activities	Strategic Intervention
ARCH	Married and unmarried rural tribal and non-tribal population in the age-group 15-37 years	Five villages in Gujarat	• Purposive sample • In-depth interviews	• Research	• To be planned following the research findings
CASP PLAN	Husbands of women in reproductive age-group	Urban slum, Delhi covering approximately 12,000 households	• Pre-intervention base line survey • Ethnographic study	• Research • Family Planning • Maternal Care • STD/HIV/AIDS Awareness	• Workshops • Healthy couple programme • Male clinic
CHETNA	Men and women	Gujarat and as a training centre, much wider catchment area	• Gender as a framework	• Training of health providers • Development of IEC material	• Developing gender-sensitive action plan during training • Creating body awareness
CINI	Married men in the age group 25-45 years	One village	• Situation analysis	• Intensive focus group discussion	• Cadre of peer group educators • Opening up of men's drop-in centres (proposed)
DCT	107 husbands contacted between Sep. 1996-Sep. 1997	20 villages Nandesari Baroda district	• Contacting husbands through outreach workers (men and women) and trained mid-wives	• Research on existing knowledge and intervention • Awareness creation about anternatal care • Identification of high risk pregnancies for husband's	• The *Pati Sampark* (literally meeting husbands) programmes. Evaluation of reproductive health in *Pati Sampark* group

Annexure 1. Community-based Intervention and Research Activities on Men*

NGO	Population	Coverage	Approach	Activities	Strategic Intervention
DCT			• Formal visits with men and informal visits with women	acceptance and support for their wives needs for antenatal care and for safe child-birth	vis-a-vis non-*Pati-Sampark* groups.
FPAI	Men, women and adolescents	2,400 slum and non-slum households	• Community participation conceived at three levels : 1. Involvement 2. Partnership 3. Action	• Group meeting • Face to face interaction	• Wife -to- wife network to reach mobile husbands • Referral services
IIPS	Local practitioners married and unmarried men	Slum in Mumbai	• Structured interview • In-depth face to face • Interview, free-listing • Pile sorting and rating	• Research	• Not applicable
KEM	Married and unmarried rural adolescents between the age group of 14-22 years	Research sample drawn from 2 villages in Pune district	• Meeting with village elders, school teachers • Meeting with youth leaders • Meeting with *panchayat* members	• Focus group discussions • Research • Quantitative • Qualitative	• Intervention is being designed
PSS	Married and unmarried men in the age group 18 to 45	Urban clients in Chennai	• Needs assessment based on extensive field survey	• Clinical services • Counselling	• Male only Clinic

Annexure 1. **Community-based Intervention and Research Activities on Men***

NGO	Population	Coverage	Approach	Activities	Strategic Intervention
SARTHI	Women, men, newly wed couples	150 villages in tribal *taluka* Gujarat area	• Training of health workers • Community awareness through intensive workshops and follow-up.	• Research • Management of STDs and RTIs. • Training village youth as health workers • Community work with men • Holding couple *melas*	• *Vansh velo talim* (family awareness education training) • *Savaali Ram ni Peti* or Mr Question Box • Different strategy for different age-groups of men
SEWA -Rural	• 60,000 people covered through various activities • Newly-wed couples	125 couples in batches in six *Melas*. 50 such Melas held so far Tribal region of Bharuch district in Gujarat	• Sensitising the newly weds through rapport building • Providing sex information to newly weds, basic health checks, family life education	• Safe motherhood initiative	• All doctors' team • Use of local calendar and events as reminders of expected date of delivery • Three sets of post cards to keep track of -Care of pregnant mother -Care of pre-term/low-birth child at home • Monitoring child growth up to 2 years • Reaching out to men and other family members to fix responsibilities • Infertility

Annexure 1. Community-based Intervention and Research Activities on Men*

NGO	Population	Coverage	Approach	Activities	Strategic Intervention
SIDH	Unmarried youth (boys and girls) from villages between the age group of 12-20 years	40 villages in Uttar Pradesh	• Training of the core group • Four-day intensive training in residential camps for boys and girls and follow-up by one-day refresher course.	• Developing training modules	• Extensive background research that went into preparing the training module
SWACH	Married and unmarried men	Rural Haryana	• Behavioural research (proposed)	• KAP study • Body mapping	• Use of popular providers (proposed) • Capacity building among popular providers
WHOTRAC	Men	Conceptualisation of male involvement	• Participatory and interactive based survey • Verbatim individual responses • Integration and documentation	• Research	• Not applicable

* Note : 1. All these NGOs are engaged in multi-faceted, multi purpose projects and activities. This table is not by any means exhaustive. Its focus is on activities that relate to men and boys.

2. Based on documentation for the workshop on Men as Supportive Partners in Reproductive and Sexual Health at Kathmandu, Nepal, June 1998.

4

Forging New Partnerships: Towards Empowerment

Swapna Mukhopadhyay
and
Jyotsna Sivaramayya

Introduction

If there was one overriding feature of the International Conference on Population and Development (ICPD), 1994, that demarcated it from earlier conferences of its kind, it was the strong need to recognise the essential interlinkages between the various dimensions of sustainable development. The recognition that population, poverty, patterns of production and consumption and the environment are so closely interconnected that none of them can be considered in isolation[1], provides the backdrop against which the goals, objectives and Programme of Action of the ICPD are to be viewed.

In India, the most important fallout of the ICPD has been that the reproductive health approach has replaced the narrower family planning programme as the major plank of population policy. An essential corollary of the reproductive health approach is women's empowerment, which is also cited as one of the principles that the ICPD is committed to: "*Advancing gender equality and equity and the empowerment of women, and the elimination of all kinds of violence against women, and ensuring women's ability to control their own fertility, are cornerstones of population and development – related programmes.*"[2]

---

[1] Para 1.5, Chapter I, Preamble, POA of ICPD.

[2] Principle 4, Chapter II, POA of the 1994 ICPD.

It is important to underscore the point that while women's empowerment is seen as an end in itself, and that it is one of the basic premises on which the entire ICPD edifice stands, it is also an inalienable instrument of perceived change; an essential ingredient of the strategies that are needed to make the vision of ICPD a reality. For, if fifty percent of the population continues to be disempowered and lack autonomy, no development worth its name can be sustained for long.

The Programme of Action also recommends partnerships between different agencies, especially between official and non-governmental organisations (NGOs):

"The increased level of interest manifested by non-governmental organizations, first in the context of the United Nations Conference on Environment and Development and the World Conference on Human Rights, and now in these deliberations, reflects an important, and in many places rapid change in the relationship between governments and a variety of non- governmental institutions. In nearly all countries, new partnerships are emerging between government, business, non-governmental organizations and community groups, which will have a direct and positive bearing on the implementation of the present Programme of Action."[3]

The need to forge partnerships with NGOs and other social actors derives directly from the condition of isolation and powerlessness of individual women. Change in gender relations which subordinate women and legitimises such subordination through unequal control over assets, ideas and ideology, can be brought about, and sustained, only when large numbers of women can be mobilised to question patriarchal norms, beliefs, attitudes and behavioural patterns. Such change can, of course, be initiated, as it often is, by some external actor or group of actors operating as a catalyst. The history of the women's movement in India, and elsewhere, is replete with instances where poor, dispossessed women have come together to question oppression, fight social evils and

[3] Para 1.14, Preamble.

confront state power demanding access to resources. Often the role of the catalyst has been played by groups of activists or an NGO. The point to emphasise is that without the strength of an organisation and/or the support of partnering agents, it is difficult for the process of empowering the powerless to start off. However, there are instances, that once started and given the right environment, it can sustain itself.

Towards Women's Empowerment

Empowerment is more about a continuous process than about a final outcome. It manifests itself in changed attitudes, leading to questioning of the norms of female subjugation, and in assertive and more autonomous behaviour reflecting an altered state of knowledge and consciousness.

It would, therefore, be a fruitless endeavour to try to measure the impact the ICPD may have made on the fruition of such a complex process in the context of half a billion women in India coming from widely divergent socio-economic backgrounds. All one could posit is that by putting women's empowerment centre stage, the thrust of the ICPD would have contributed to the ongoing process of restoring a balance in gender relations. The most concrete manner in which the ICPD has been instrumental in feeding into the process has been its contribution to the replacement of the old family planning programme with its sole emphasis on fertility control, by a broader and more inclusive reproductive health approach. The latter, among other things, makes a distinction between wanted and unwanted pregnancies and seeks to facilitate control of only the latter through informed choice by the couple. It also aims to meet other reproductive health needs of women, thereby, addressing the issues of women's dignity and human rights violations in contrast to the top-down policies of the past, which were often coercive.

A similar statement can be made about the impact of the ICPD in the area of forging partnerships in the development field, especially in the area of health and family welfare. NGOs, primarily the welfare-oriented ones, have had a long history of social action in India. The need for forging alliances with NGOs has also been recognised in official thinking for some time now. The efficacy of such partnerships was outlined in an official document for the first time in the Sixth Plan (1979-84). In view of their perceived flexibility, greater community outreach and more intimate knowledge of local conditions, it was felt that NGOs would be more effective in the delivery of official poverty alleviation and rural development programmes. Many such programmes carried out by NGOs have been funded by the government for some years now.

The Reproductive and Child Health programme has taken this trend one step forward. By involving NGO representatives at all stages of the design and implementation, by putting in place the concept of 'mother NGOs' and by placing the latter in strategic positions for training smaller NGOs in different regions of the country, the concept of NGO partnership has been built into the design of the programme itself.

The Reproductive and Child Health programme also involves the concept of community needs assessment. The involvement of community members and groups is thus foreseen though not clearly laid out in the programme design. There is some experience in India, built up over the last couple of decades, of government agencies working with community groups, especially women's groups. Some large government programmes, like the Development of Women and Children in Rural Areas which is based on the concept of providing production credit to groups of women, are designed on the principle of coordination between community groups and official agencies. Much experience has been built up over the years within the women's movement itself in organising grassroots women for advancing the cause of empowerment and channelling their demands for resources and services towards existing official programmes. Thus, several models of partnerships between government agencies and community groups have emerged in the country in recent years.

The ICPD also happened to take place at a time when another significant development was taking place in the area of women's political empowerment. This was the passing of the 73rd and 74th Amendments to the Constitution of India, whereby one-third of all seats in three-tier elected local government bodies (*panchayats*) in the country were reserved for women. By the time the Reproductive and Child Health programme went on stream, over 800,000 women, many of them from impoverished and socially depressed backgrounds, had been chosen as people's representatives in thousands of villages across the country. This opened up enormous possibilities for advancing the ICPD agenda.

In 1996, the Institute of Social Studies Trust, New Delhi, launched a project designed to build on this synergy. The presence of a large number of women representatives in local government bodies provided an opportunity to focus on issues pertaining to women's health, choice and rights in reproductive matters as entry points to achieve the goal of women's empowerment. The *panchayats* provided the forum, legitimised by a country-wide constitutional mandate, and a local NGO in each selected location was expected to play the role of the catalyst within the structure, thereby strengthening the partnership angle.

In three years, the project has demonstrated how the ICPD vision regarding women's empowerment both as a means and as an end can be advanced by relocating it within the context of the new opportunities unleashed by the presence of nearly a million of women in positions of power in local governance structures. It also demonstrated the strategic role of the catalyst, the local NGO in this case, in bringing the vision closer to reality. The distance to be covered and the nature of the obstacles to be tackled have clearly been functions of the ground conditions. By locating itself in three very divergent local contexts in three different states, the project demonstrated the crucial role of the agent as well as the environment in determining the nature and degree of success achieved under different circumstances. The experience gained under this project succinctly outlines what has been achieved and what has not. It also suggests what can be achieved under reasonable restructuring of ground realities and what cannot.

Reproductive Health Through Panchayats

The project was launched in three states of the country, that is, Himachal Pradesh, West Bengal and Karnataka. The choice of these states was guided primarily by the status and development of *panchayats* in these states on the one hand and by the situation of women on the other. In addition, the project sites were situated in varying geographical and socio-economic contexts.

Status of panchayats

Panchayats are institutions of local governance which have existed in some form or the other in India since ages. These village bodies with judicial and police powers looked after the overall administration of the village (ISST, 1994). The present concept of a three-tier *panchayat* structure from the district to village level is based on the same principle of decentralised administration and community participation. Even though it has been recognised that rural development programmes would not be successful without peoples' participation, an institutionalised village agency for representing the people, elected *panchayats* were not made mandatory until the recent Constitutional amendments were passed. It was left to individual states of India to make provisions for the establishment of *panchayats*. There has always been resistance from members of state legislative bodies and the bureaucracy to devolution of power to the grassroots. Therefore, the involvement of *panchayats* in community affairs and their level of development varies from state to state. This is also seen in the three states where the study was carried out.

In West Bengal, *panchayats* have been functioning very successfully; the only state to have had regular *panchayat* elections for the last 20 years. The most notable aspect has been the political will of the state government facilitating the devolution of power and resources to the *panchayats* since 1985-86. As per the devolution policy, planning committees were formed at the block and district levels comprising heads of the *panchayats* and government functionaries. These committees were given budgetary provisions and the power to formulate district and block level plans.

In Himachal Pradesh, the Panchayati Raj Act of 1968 provided for the representation of women and scheduled (untouchable) caste members in case they were not elected. The act also conferred about 27 administrative duties on *gram* (village) *panchayats* but did not provide adequate funds. Therefore, it was just not possible for a *gram panchayat* to perform even the basic duties. The real powers were vested with the state bureaucracy and not with the panchayats. In fact, the *panchayat* chiefs had to seek permission of the district officials in most matters severely undermining their independence (ISST, 1994). In Karnataka, the development of *panchayats* has seen many highs and lows. The Karnataka Act of 1983 was a landmark in that the state government divested itself of substantial powers and duties in favour of the panchayats. It entrusted to the district level *panchayat* the responsibility of planning for the district. But change of state government in 1990 resulted in an erosion of the powers of the *panchayats*. It is only with the passing of the 73rd Amendment, the *panchayats* were reviewed in 1993.

Women in panchayats

The successful devolution of powers to panchayats in a bid to increase community participation in planning, however, does not translate into women's empowerment in the community. An examination of the indicators used to measure women's status shows no correspondence to increased community participation. Himachal Pradesh for instance, has not had a *panchayat* system representing grassroots democracy before the 73rd Amendment. It is also low in terms of standard development indicators. In spite of this, the status of women as measured by conventional indicators is remarkable. More than 50 percent of the women there are literate as compared to the country average of 39 percent. Similarly, the sex ratio (females per 1,000 males) and the participation of women in officially recognised economic activity is also much higher than the national average. But, West Bengal, despite a high degree of decentralisation because of the Left Front government, the position of women has not improved to the same extent. The sex ratio and female labour force participation are much lower than the country average.

Empowering the community for us has meant empowering women who constitute nearly one half of society. The project has endeavored to activate the *panchayats* by making them take cognisance of the health needs of women, and the community. This has given women, especially those from the marginalised sections of society, the opportunity to interact with the rest of the community. Reproductive health is a very natural focal point for women's empowerment as it is a mirror to the overall life situation of women. Our experience is that the reasons for the lack of political participation and the reasons for not utilising health care have common elements e.g. lack of time, poverty, low self confidence and strong cultural taboos.

NGO involvement

The design of the project is also built on the experience that women cannot make a difference in their private and public life without a support structure. The cultural ethos in India celebrates meekness and submissiveness in women. It is this, that has prevented women's empowerment in domestic as well as public life. Restrictions in the domestic sphere have also restricted their participation in public life. Even those women who are not hampered by restrictions from the family face resistance from men in the *panchayats*.

As a result, women do not often participate in the discussions. In addition, as they have been elected for the first time, they are not aware of their rights and responsibilities; of the procedures that are to be followed; and, the jurisdiction of the panchayats. Therefore, empowerment of women can only be achieved if they are provided with a support structure to fight these restrictions. In this context, the ICPD statement regarding the involvement of NGOs is of great significance. It recognises the contributions that NGOs have made in all sectors of development and *"the support their activities engender from the community as a whole."* The project design was based on the active involvement of grassroots NGOs, who have been working in the areas for some years and have established a rapport with the community. In addition, there is a strong taboo associated with the discussion of reproductive health in India. More often than not, women will not speak about their reproductive health problems unless they are confident that the information will not be misused. Therefore, the necessity to involve NGOs with credibility in the community. The other kind of support that NGOs have provided has been in the form of training programmes for *panchayat* members, especially women. These programmes provide guidance to members as to their responsibilities and powers, and the procedures for utilising them.

Reproductive health survey

An important outcome of the ICPD in India has been to bring issues of reproductive health to the centre stage for the first time. In terms of government policy, it has resulted in a paradigm shift from maternal health to reproductive health. As the emphasis had so far been on maternal health, government policies before this had failed to take into account many other aspects of reproductive health. The most serious omission being the failure to address the incidence of reproductive tract infections (RTIs) and sexually transmitted diseases (STDs).

The Reproductive Health Through Panchayats project was initiated by conducting a household questionnaire survey. As no database existed on the incidence of reproductive morbidity in the country, this baseline survey helped us to understand the nature of health problems affecting women. The survey covered four *panchayats* comprising 3,445 households in West Bengal; two *panchayats* comprising 2,004 households in Karnataka; and, four *panchayats* consisting of 1,052 households in Himachal Pradesh.

Though the emphasis was on the reproductive health of women, the survey recorded the general health status of all individuals in the *panchayats*. The reproductive health status was recorded on the basis of symptomatic self-reporting. The questionnaire was administered to all females aged 12 and above. This enabled us to address the health problems of adolescents as well as post-menopausal women whose problems do not get recorded as they do not fall in the conventional 15-49 years reproductive age category. Many ailments afflicting older women are a consequence of their life styles and reproductive health problems they had in their reproductive years. Reproductive health problems of adolescents must also be addressed to reduce their burden of ill health in later years.

Our survey revealed that in spite of the differences in the location of the project areas, the most commonly reported reproductive health symptoms show little variance. These symptoms include tiredness/ paleness, backache, vaginal discharge, giddiness, and abdominal pain. The range of reported reproductive health symptoms from different study locations is summarised in Table 1.

TABLE 1: Most Commonly Reported Reproductive Health Symptoms*

Symptoms	Himachal Pradesh	Karnataka	West Bengal
Vaginal Discharge	63 - 36	85 - 29	52 - 41
Tiredness / Paleness	67 - 52	90 - 76	68 - 41
Backache	72 - 50	92 - 50	30 - 21
Abdominal Pain	58 - 40	82 - 48	49 - 30
Giddiness	41 - 33	84 - 47	70 - 48

* Percentage of women reporting symptoms.

The survey provided us with a means for initiating a discussion on reproductive health in the community. During our work, we found that reproductive morbidity was not a priority for the people.

The reason for this is partly cultural. There are strong taboos associated with discussing reproductive health. Women do not speak openly about their problems for fear of being accused of infidelity and being sent back to their natal homes. In addition, many women view these problems as 'natural', that all women have to bear. The process of women's empowerment has to first tackle the problem that women do not feel the need for help or are not able to articulate their health needs. In our experience, women would not speak in front of their mothers-in-law or male members, including their husbands. In some places, men were hostile and suspicious. There is the need to empower women both in their private lives as well as public lives before they can feel confident to take up these issues in the *panchayats*. NGOs have initiated discussion on reproductive health through the formation of *mahila mandals* (women's groups) and awareness groups. At some places, NGOs had established and had supported *mahila mandals* for many years and at other places, they were established as part of this project. These groups have had a special role to play in the community wherever the *panchayat* structure has been weak.

Community needs assessment

The Government of India's family welfare programme has moved from a contraceptive target-oriented approach to a community needs assessment approach. The former was based on achieving a definite number of contraceptive acceptor targets set by higher authorities, resulting in a coercive programme. The community needs assessment approach, on the other hand, is about providing contraceptive services in accordance to the community's needs, symbolising a reversal of the top-down approach. Under the new approach, the auxiliary nurse midwife assesses the needs of the community and determines targets in consultation with the *panchayat* or the health committee of the *panchayat*, the *anganwadi* workers, traditional birth attendants, women's health committees and families.

As the new approach builds on the old family welfare programme, it still incorporates some of the earlier drawbacks. Even now, the emphasis is on increasing contraceptive use and child survival without adequate importance to women's health and reproductive morbidity. This problem is compounded by the fact that there is no database in the country on the incidence of RTIs and STDs. Some independent studies on the prevalence of RTIs and STDs have found that 70-90 percent of rural women have one or more such infections (Bang et al, 1989). Fertility, pregnancy and child survival are adversely affected by these infections. RTIs may, therefore, lower contraceptive demand; and, if the symptoms of RTIs are seen as side-effects, it may lead to rejection of contraceptives (Pachauri, 1995).

Varied estimates of the incidence of RTIs make it imperative to develop a methodology for their detection. Under the community needs assessment approach, the auxiliary nurse midwife and male multi purpose worker have been instructed to refer people suffering from RTIs and STIs to primary health centres and hospitals. If women do not speak openly about reproductive health problems, there is no process delineated for recording the incidence of RTIs and STIs. This approach also does not address the most important issue of raising awareness and empowering women to seek reproductive health care.

Millions of women in India go through their lives silently suffering from RTIs without ever seeking treatment. There is, therefore, a need to create a database on the prevalence of these infections and to make the community as well as the health workers sensitive to these issues. Through surveys and participatory rural appraisal, our project generated a cost-effective method of collecting health status information, based on self-reporting of symptoms by women particularly those associated with reproductive health. One of the criticisms about self-reporting for reproductive health morbidity has been that it is unable to capture the full extent of its incidence (Bulut et al, 1995). But clinical and laboratory examinations are very time-consuming and expensive. The advantage of self-reporting is that it provides estimates of the community's perceived needs for reproductive health care.

Involving panchayats

The results of the survey on the general and reproductive health status have been utilised as talking points for health in the community and the *panchayats*. An important component of the project was disseminating information: people can take cognisance of an issue only when they are made aware of the existing situation. Our experience of working with *panchayats* has been that health is not considered a priority area. Most *panchayats* are more concerned about other issues, such as building roads or digging wells which are more 'visible' benefits. This does not mean that these issues are not important. They do have a bearing on the health status and health-seeking behaviour of the community.

Making health an important issue requires a sustained effort on the part of the people and the *panchayats*. *Panchayats* have been involved in government health programmes such as immunisation. But, *panchayats* have only been implementers and not initiators of these programmes. An important factor deciding the involvement of *panchayats* in community health is the extent to which they are functional and active. Wherever members are articulate, (not necessarily about reproductive health), *panchayats* have started discussions on reproductive health issues much faster than in areas where *panchayats* have very little role to play in community life. In the former case, it means the decentralisation process is becoming functional.

In West Bengal, where *panchayats* have been functioning for 20 years there is a perceptible difference in the level of decentralisation. All the three tiers of the *panchayats* are actively involved in the management of village issues.

In comparison, in Himachal Pradesh, they have started functioning only since the passage of the 73rd Amendment. As a result, the upper tiers of the *panchayats* are inactive. However, village *panchayats* have taken up issues concerning the villagers. In Himachal Pradesh, in the areas where the project is currently going on, due to the role of the NGO, people have started to demand action from the *panchayats* regarding health matters. In one instance, the auxiliary nurse midwife, who is the government health functionary in maximum contact with the people, was neither attending the health sub-centre regularly nor visiting the villages. Through the *panchayat*, the villagers persuaded her to write on a public notice board the days on which she would be available at the health centre and the days she would visit the village. In another instance, the doctor at a primary health centre was transferred because a complaint was filed against him by the *panchayat*.

In Karnataka, *panchayats* at the district levels are the only ones which are functioning. As the block and village level *panchayats* are inactive, people's involvement in *panchayats* is minimal. Though the people are enthusiastic, they do not have a forum to address their demands.

Our experience is that where there is government support, reproductive health issues receive attention. In West Bengal, for instance, the state government has given a directive to form health committees at the sub-centre level (a sub-centre serves a population of 5,000). The *panchayat* member of this area is a member of this committee and nominates other members. As a result of this support by the government, a discussion has been generated where no interest in health existed.

Whither Now: Some Reflections for the Future

What emerged from our experience corroborates what one has learnt from many grassroots initiatives in women's health in recent years: issues related to health and sanitation, especially women's health, are very low down in priority and unless reproductive health problems become really serious, they are kept under the wraps, from a sense of shame and the fear of desertion on charges of infidelity.

The flip side of this is that organisations and partnerships can help; that catalysts are important; and, that structures and institutions are necessary for sustaining the results of efforts at breaking down age-old barriers. There is also evidence of the essential interconnectedness of issues. Women's health cannot be dealt with in isolation. It is deeply embedded in the health status of the community. It is also integrally linked with livelihood issues and women's status. The interconnectedness of issues, the need for integrated efforts to addressing problems, and the necessity of forging partnerships was highlighted by the ICPD. Our experience corroborates the centrality and relevance of the approach.

What is lacking, however, are practical strategies to ensure women's empowerment. There is very little in the design of the reproductive and child health programme that envisages genuine participation of women. Although efforts are underway to assess community needs, women's roles in making such assessments are not clear. In this respect, the programme appears in practice to be almost as much top-down as the earlier programme, with more of a horizontal spread in coverage to include reproductive and child health issues, rather than a qualitative transformation in the design of the programme. Our experience clearly suggests that a top-down process cannot be empowering. Even if the health needs of women are adequately addressed, a top-down approach is not likely to promote empowerment.

Another related area in which the programme appears to fall short is in information dissemination, and the subsequent process of conscientisation that enables women to use such information so that they can make informed choices in reproductive matters.

Our project shows how basic information on the health status of the community, including the reproductive health status of women, can be obtained in a cost-effective manner by using local resources. Although such information is based on self perception, and may vary considerably from information based on clinical examination, it does give an indication of the problems confronting the community. Since it is reported by the women themselves, it also reflects their perceived health needs.

Our experience in all the three locations where the project has been implemented shows that such information provides an excellent basis for initiating discussions in community groups on the health needs of women. The survey results, which were taken back to the women, were used as talking points on reproductive health related discussions in focus groups, *mahila mandal* meetings and meetings involving *panchayat* members and health officials at various levels. The programme has to start this process of bottom-up deliberations to be truly participatory.

Further, our experience can complement the reproductive and child health approach by locating the programme within established institutional structures to ensure sustainability. This role is deemed to be played by the *panchayat* in the project design. In our experiences, the functional stability and effectiveness of these local structures ensures success. The programme is still designed as a vertical one and is unclear about its location within the local scenario. This may create problems in the long run in terms of sustainability as well as legitimacy within the existing federal structure in the country.

Thus, from all indications it appears that while the reproductive and child health programme has put in place some basic ingredients of a reproductive health approach, it has to supplement the effort with greater attention to articulation and management of needs emerging from the grassroots. It also has to locate itself within existing institutional structures at the local level so that it is more responsive to needs as perceived by the community. An institutional structure must be in place for disseminating information back and forth to ensure that women's empowerment is operationalised in a meaningful way. Future efforts should be directed to promote such initiatives so that the goal of enabling women to make informed reproductive choices can become a reality.

Note: The Reproductive Health Through Panchayat (RHTP) project funded by the John D. and Catherine T. MacArthur Foundation is being carried out in three states in collaboration with three grassroots non-governmental organisations. These are: Child in Need Institute (CINI) in West Bengal, Leading Organisation for Rural Development (LORD) in Karnataka, and Social Uplift Through Rural Action (SUTRA) in Himachal Pradesh.

References

Government of India. 1998. Manual on Community Needs Assessment Approach in Family Welfare Programme. Ministry of Health and Family Welfare, New Delhi, India.

Institute of Social Sciences Trust. 1994. Status of Panchayati Raj in the States of India 1994. New Delhi: Concept Publishing Company.

Institute of Social Sciences Trust. 1998. *Panchayati Raj Update.* September, 57: 6.

Pachauri, S., 1995. Defining a Reproductive Health Package for India : A Proposed Framework. The Population Council, South and East Asia, Regional Working Papers No. 4, New Delhi, India.

United Nations. 1995. Programme of Action of the International Conference on Population and Development. Cairo, September 5-14, 1994. Reprinted in *Population and Development Review,* 21(1&2).

PART THREE

Addressing Reproductive Health Problems

1

HIV/AIDS in India: Gulf Between Rhetoric and Reality

Radhika Ramasubban

This paper was published in the *Economic and Political Weekly* on November 7, 1998

Background

India is the second most populous country in the world after China (over 900 million). The majority of the population (around 75 percent) live in rural areas and practise agriculture and allied occupations. India also has a large and well developed industrial sector. Although the urban concentration is relatively small, the rate of growth of big cities and small towns and, therefore, of the urban population has been rapid over the last few decades, mainly due to rural stagnation and industrial growth. The problems of urban development, therefore, have already begun to assume considerable significance in economic, environmental, social, and political terms.

Income and social inequalities continue to remain high and the incidence of absolute poverty is widespread. Economic status determines life expectancy at birth, access to food, education, career opportunities, health care, housing and even basic amenities such as drinking water and sanitation. There is no state provision for social security. Economic disparities, evident everywhere, are the most glaring in the cities, where between 40 and 60 percent of the population is forced to live in overcrowded and unhygienic slum settlements, with poor access to infrastructural facilities such as water and sanitation. The quest for livelihood propels considerable migration from rural to urban areas. While earlier, migration was directly to the metropolitan centres, the rapid growth of smaller towns and cities in recent years reveals a step-by-step pattern of migration, as individuals and households seek to improve their earnings. While some cultural/regional or landless groups may migrate with their families or acquire families once they come to live in a city, several regions of the country have a tradition of male migration only, where urban networks are used to further income-earning opportunities, in order to repatriate money home to the village.

The Indian state is committed to providing free access to health and educational facilities for the vast majority of the population, which does not earn enough to purchase good quality education or health care. However, in quantity, quality, and gender sensitivity, these public facilities fall short of real needs. Huge social inequalities, based on caste and gender relations, exacerbate the role of economic disparities in making for unequal access to important development inputs. In terms of literacy alone, India has the largest number of illiterates in the world, with little signs of any improvement. The overall literacy rate is around 52 percent, with around 64 percent for males and 39 percent for females. These rates are higher for the urban areas, but gender disparities remain strong. Although the public sector for health care is large, it is the thriving private sector, which is the preferred option even for the very poor who see it as more efficacious than the overcrowded, politicised, bureaucratised, and inefficient government sector. In effect, therefore, private expenditure on health and education is estimated to be around three times the public expenditure (World Bank, 1995).

India is a country of continental proportions. It is divided into 26 self governing linguistically organised states, and 6 union territories that are directly administered by the central government. The states vary considerably on all major human development and economic indicators, depending on their social, political and developmental history. It is a complex society, which is multi-lingual (over 16 languages and several hundred dialects), multi-religious (Hindus constituting over 80 percent, Muslims 12 percent, Christians 2.5 percent and Sikhs, Jains, Buddhists, Jews, and Parsis being the other important religious groups), with a multitude of castes, ethnic groups and cultures. But irrespective of these differences, every Indian citizen enjoys equal status in the eyes of the law. The country is a sovereign, democratic and secular republic, governed by a Constitution, which guarantees significant fundamental rights to every citizen, regardless of caste, religion, race, language, sex, or place of birth. It is in the access to and exercise of the law that the social and economic disabilities outlined above act as constraints.

Introduction

The AIDS epidemic in India is referred to in official documents as being in its "early stages" (NACO, 1996). This, is a euphemistic description of an epidemic whose real epidemiological and social dimensions are even now inadequately understood, and this, 12 years after the first case of AIDS was isolated in a woman commercial sex worker in Chennai (originally Madras), the capital of Tamil Nadu. It would be more accurate to describe India as being at an early stage of social learning and policy formulation with respect to AIDS, even as the epidemic itself threatens to get out of hand.

According to WHO estimates, today India reportedly has the largest number of HIV positive individuals in the South and South-East Asian region (along with Thailand, India accounts for an estimated 95 percent of the reported cases of AIDS in the region; WHO, 1992). There are an estimated three million HIV positive cases in India. Given the size of its population, India is expccted to have the largest concentration of AIDS affected individuals in the world, if the present rate of transmission continues unchecked.

During the 1980s, when Africa was the negative centre of attention with respect to AIDS, India took refuge in postures of denial on the grounds that AIDS was a foreign disease. It was believed that the traditional socio-cultural norms of monogamy, universal marriage and, therefore, heterosexual relations and virtual non-existence of homosexual behaviour, mother goddess worship, and societal proscriptions against an explicit focus on sex and sexuality in public social interactions and discourse, provided the necessary shelter from a predominantly sexually transmitted disease (STD). The fact that STDs were the third most important group of diseases in the country, next only to malaria and T.B. was glossed over (Ramasubban, 1990). Also, international scientific evidence to support the link between pre-existing STD infection and vulnerability to AIDS had not yet been firmly established.

The first AIDS case, isolated in 1986, drew an official response of treating AIDS as a problem of vigilance by the law and order agencies – suspicion of foreign visitors, incarceration by some state governments of individuals (e.g. blood donors, sex workers) found to be HIV positive to prevent them from infecting the rest of society and, in some other states, deportation of commercial sex workers by the government of their state of domicile to their state of origin, in an attempt to transfer the problem.

By the early 1990s, denial had given way to an attempt to contain "AIDS control" within the medical establishment. The viewing of AIDS as an exclusively medical problem was prompted as much by ignorance of the changing socio-cultural context of sexual behaviour, as by the fact that it came naturally to a medical establishment that had a long experience of running national (i.e., top-down, centrally administered) curative-oriented disease control programmes. Of the several national disease control programmes initiated since the early 1950s (including a national STD control programme), none had a clear strategy for disease prevention or an understanding of health behaviour. Disease prevention calls for predominantly non-medical, i.e., social, political, public health, and administrative solutions, all requiring complex, sensitive and politically controversial interventions. These included localised and differentiated social education strategies, public participation, policy planning to effect structural changes in the socio-economic linkages of communicable diseases, and integration into primary health care. With the exception of small pox (for which a vaccine existed) and malaria (where the DDT technology was available), all other control programmes for diseases such as T.B., leprosy, etc., have been curative in approach. Poor coordination between the central and state governments and the low priority accorded to public health by the state governments along with poor attention to public participation in disease prevention, have negated the effectiveness of these programmes (Ramasubban, 1984). Today, among these diseases, malaria has resurged, leprosy eradication still remains a major challenge, and the high rates of T.B. and STDs have become the greatest ally of the AIDS epidemic.

The positive aspect of this medical definition of AIDS was the concern for the mode of transmission through blood and blood products and organ transplants, a real concern in a country where resort to blood transfusions is high and where quality control of blood banking is poor.

But the negative aspect was the neglect of the socio-cultural, behavioural and economic dimensions of HIV transmission in favour of moral condemnation and victimising of high risk groups. This resulted in the failure to develop the necessary technical and administrative skills to raise awareness about the disease, high risk behaviour and primary prevention among these groups and in the larger society, or to develop support structures for those suffering from the disease.

In the ensuing chaos, AIDS funding became a politically contested issue, as both the Government of India and all manner of NGOs attempted to jump onto the AIDS bandwagon, resulting in ineffective and counterproductive use of international donor funds. Studies in selected areas among certain groups now reveal that the epidemic has developed as rapidly in India as was observed in some African countries in the mid-1980s.

For India, AIDS has been and continues to be a social learning experience (as it has been for all the countries of the world in lesser or greater ways). The Indian AIDS policy has taken a long while to come to terms with the challenges required and even today is, still at an incipient stage. Much of its evolution has been a process (a slow and contradictory one) of responding to pressures both from outside the country and from within, to move in a more coherent and integrated direction. The former have been mainly international donors, who have been an important impetus for policy change, and who have also been bringing in new scientific knowledge and technical skills, and methodologies for research in both medical and social and behavioural sciences. The latter, i.e., forces within the country, have been health and legal NGOs, who have been pressing for more space and funding for NGO participation, more enlightened legislation with respect to AIDS, and more evidence of political will to tackle the disease.

Starting from an exclusionist stance, the AIDS policy is now very slowly incorporating a more inclusive and cooperative element into its structure, making space for involvement of other sections of civil society. These sections, as of now, are only a few isolated NGOs working with specific target groups (and even they have to struggle consistently for the security and expansion of their space). They do not include people affected by the disease or other marginalised groups at high risk such as sex workers or drug users. Such a wide ranging partnership with civil society does not come easily to a traditionally top-down system of governance, or to a society where topics such as sexuality and substance abuse have tended to be pushed underground, and where stigmatising of any degree of deviance from dominant social norms is widely practised, among rich and poor, high and low caste alike.

It is only since 1992 that there has been a serious effort to put into place an infrastructure at the central and state levels for tackling the problem of AIDS. That year, the National AIDS Control Organisation (NACO) was set up and the Control Programme expanded into a National AIDS Prevention and Control Programme, acknowledging that all sections of society had to be addressed rather than the "high risk" groups alone. The period 1994-96 witnessed a more systematic move in the direction of epidemiological surveillance, although the dearth of credible surveillance data continued to be a major constraint to policy planning and programme formulation. In Tamil Nadu alone, policies and programmes for sentinel surveillance, risk behaviour assessment, primary prevention, and organisational and managerial reforms involving partnership with NGOs and people affected with AIDS (PWA) began to be put into place in 1994. Today, Tamil Nadu has become a model for other states to emulate. In 1996, judicial activism led to a landmark Supreme Court directive making HIV screening mandatory in all blood banks. Several organisational reforms in the matter of collection, testing and handling of blood have since been set into motion. Since 1997, a further process of overhauling NACO has been initiated to enable it to consolidate some of the reforms mentioned above, and to spearhead changes at the state level. Today, in mid-1998, a draft National AIDS Prevention and Control Policy is under consideration. A beginning, therefore, has been made.

The AIDS Situation

As of May 31, 1997, the seropositivity rate per thousand screenings was 18.6 or around 1.9 percent (NACO, 1997 b). Seropositivity increased from 2.5 per 1,000 in 1986 to 11.2 per 1,000 by 1992, to 16.3 per 1,000 by end-1996. A cumulative total of 3,551 AIDS cases have been reported to NACO. This is estimated to be barely 1-2 percent of the actual cases and it is believed that at least 150,000 AIDS cases and around 2.5 to 3 million infections must have occurred.

The reason for this huge discrepancy is that disease surveillance is among the weakest links in the health infrastructure and planning chain. It is only in the context of AIDS that this weakness has come to be squarely confronted.

Until 1994, surveillance was based on data from 62 surveillance centres situated in different parts of the country. Data from different target groups were pooled and was cumulative in nature and, therefore, did not lend itself to monitoring trends of infection. Again, HIV infected individuals were detected only in states where testing facilities were available for surveillance, blood testing or research. The more urbanised states, with their greater concentration of facilities and technical skills, therefore, showed higher rates. These included Maharashtra, Tamil Nadu, Karnataka, and Gujarat. In 1993-94, the sentinel surveillance system was adopted. But epidemiological data remains a major weakness affecting policy planning and even today, tells us virtually nothing about what is happening in the rural areas.

The deficiencies in data notwithstanding, some major trends can be discerned. The major concentration of AIDS cases is in

Maharashtra and Tamil Nadu, with Maharashtra alone accounting for almost half the number. Along with Manipur (in north-eastern India), these three states account for 77 percent of the total cases in the country. Despite this concentration, HIV is present in all states with the exception of only one state.

The 55 sentinel sites established in 1994 to monitor trends in specific "high risk groups" (CSWs and STD clinic attenders) and in "low risk groups" (women attending antenatal clinics), and the rounds done so far reflect the rapid increases in seropositivity among all three groups (NACO, 1996). STD clinic attendees are almost all married, or are adolescents set to marry soon, given the cultural norm of universal marriage. Therefore, the spread to the general population is very likely. About 1 percent of the HIV cases, according to current estimates, are antenatal mothers, normally considered a low risk group. But these figures do not reveal anything about women, particularly in the urban areas, who are not married, pregnant or who are sterilised and who would not be attending antenatal clinics. This does not account for the fact that antenatal clinic attendance is not universal, given the low awareness of hazards to reproductive health and women's poor financial, logistic and social access to facilities. Recent studies of sex workers reveal an increasingly complex picture of this group (Voluntary Health Services, 1996). While these are overwhelmingly women driven into the profession due to destitution, and are without stable marital family ties as in the brothels of the big cities, in small towns and major truck halts along inter-state routes, there is a growing trend for married women living in marital unions to take to this activity as a means of coping with poverty.

There are clearly several ongoing HIV epidemics in India. The epidemic among sex workers has been the most alarming, with seropositivity rates there climbing steadily and exponentially. Patients attending STD clinics come next with rising rates among them too, followed by recipients of blood/blood products. These trends are all India in character, although the rates are the highest in Tamil Nadu and Maharashtra, followed by Gujarat and Karnataka. Other discernible epidemics are among injecting drug users (this is localised in one state at present – Manipur where 54 percent of intravenous drug users (IVDUs) are estimated to be HIV positive (NACO, 1996; 1997 b).

The data suggests that the majority of infections are contracted through the sexual route (around 75 percent), followed by unmonitored blood transfusions (8 percent) and unsterilised needle sharing by drug users (around 8 percent). Almost 90 percent of the cases were reported from those between 18 and 40 years of age. Higher HIV prevalence was being found along major truck routes. Migrant workers and rapid transport facilities have increased the chances of spread of HIV from urban to rural areas and from one state to another. (NACO, 1996; 1997 b).

The male to female ratio is 3:1 as discerned from reported AIDS cases. The credibility of this figure, too, suffers from the same disability as described above, since women are even less likely than men to access a medical facility. While within the sexual mode of transmission, heterosexual unions are the norm, and a culturally sanctioned definition of homosexual identity is conspicuous by its absence, bisexuality tends to be commonly practised by men who or may not be in marital union. Considerable numbers of HIV positive men, particularly, report to be practising bisexual preferences (*Maniar*, pers. comm.). *Hijras* (or third sex members) have generally been known to provide such avenues in the form of receptive anal sex, but there is growing evidence that homosexuality may be a more common practice than is acknowledged. This may be particularly true of situational homosexuality in unequal (i.e., exploitative or potentially exploitative) relationships, defined by age (older men with adolescent boys, particularly restaurant/hotel workers), occupation (truck drivers with boy cleaners), or power (jail inmates). Sexual abuse meted out to the millions of street children in cities has yet to be tackled in the context of AIDS. A 65-city sexual behaviour study initiated by NACO in the early 1990s, revealed that men who have sex with men were among the hardest to reach groups (along with IVDUs).

In sum, it may be said that since AIDS is not a notifiable disease (for obvious reasons of confidentiality), and since the official figures reflect only cases reported by public hospitals with testing facilities, and since these hospitals may be expected to be accessed by barely 10-20 percent of the population, the figures do not convey the full magnitude of HIV/AIDS infection.

We know even less about the actual morbidity due to HIV, since the majority of patients are believed to be succumbing to opportunistic infections such as TB long before they reach the stage of full blown AIDS, given general conditions of poverty, ignorance on the part of sufferers and providers alike, and rapid depletion of immunity. Studies have yet to tell us whether the incubation period of immune suppression attributable to HIV is the accepted average of 10 years. A number of cases go underground, both private and public hospitals generally refuse to accept HIV positive patients, with some notable exceptions. Also there is a tendency on the part of patients to go treatment shopping, and for practitioners to offer widely different drug regimens even in cases of those diseases for which standard multiple drug regimens exist (such as TB, leprosy), and there is no reason to believe that this might be different in the case of HIV.

Impeding and Fostering Factors

AIDS, as no other disease before it, holds up a mirror to Indian society, compelling both policy makers and members of the civil society to bring on centre-stage policies, social processes, social groups and behaviour that had hitherto been relegated to the margins.

These are, on the one hand:

a) sexuality (a taboo topic about which no clear, unambiguous information exists in the public domain and which, therefore, spawns a host of misconceptions);

b) promiscuity (differential sexual freedom norms for men and for women, permitting degrees of freedom for men without knowledge of how to prevent disease, but enforcing through severe moral and religious strictures pre- and post-marital chastity for women, leaving women powerless to negotiate safe sex with their husbands or partners);

c) prostitution (grinding poverty which forces huge numbers of women into commercial sex, where they are again powerless to negotiate safe sex or ensure early treatment);

d) intravenous drug use (which is a legal offence and, therefore, inhibits the possibilities of needle exchange programmes, counselling and care; a high proportion of such persons in Manipur are in jail);

e) homosexuality (again, a morally proscribed behaviour, forcing men underground); and,

f) the private domain of the patriarchal family, which is based on the subordination of women, leaving them in a poor state of reproductive health, silent victims of a range of reproductive tract infections, and with little autonomy to seek and purchase timely and effective health care for themselves (Ramasubban, 1995).

How these marginalised social spaces are confronted would determine the successful mounting of an enlightened and timely response for prevention and management of AIDS.

On the other hand, are the longstanding disabilities and anomalies arising from the current stage in the country's socio-economic developmental history; disabilities that have serious implications for the sustained success of management of the epidemic.

These are:

(a) the low priority accorded to health generally in national planning and resource allocation;

(b) the relative neglect of primary health care, and the resultant weak health infrastructure in the states and people's alienation from it, encircled by a huge and variegated private sector which is accessed by over 80 percent of the population and is not easily amenable to reform and control;

(c) failure in coordination between the central and state governments in the funding and management of disease control programmes; mainly the inability/unwillingness on the part of states to sustain commitment of financial and manpower resources for the programmes once the central and international donor sponsorship has run out;

(d) inefficiencies and bureaucratic inertia in the administration of the programmes at the state level, resulting in failure to maintain consistent drug supplies and inability to integrate the programmes with the primary health care system;

(e) lack of supporting preventive work at the level of local communities, and patient counselling work by health outreach workers;

(f) the history of neglect of elementary education, resulting in continuing high rates of illiteracy and low levels of school education, and the lack of sensitivity to the need for health education and sex education, both through the educational system and the mass media;

(g) the high incidence of STDs in the country (40 million new infections a year, and an estimated incidence rate of 5 percent), and historical neglect of both prevention and facilities for diagnosis and treatment, due both to ideological barriers, low status accorded to the scientific speciality and bureaucratic apathy;

(h) widespread poverty and the survival strategies of the poor, which forces whole sections of women into prostitution and ignorant migrant workers into unsafe sex,

(i) the exclusive focus in the national family planning programme on women's sterilisation and failure to focus on men and on counselling/educating them in the direction of behavioural change such as condom use and more equal sexual and contraception negotiation;

(j) patriarchal structures and taboos on the open discussion of sex and sexuality which make for gross ignorance and impede public acceptance of such a disease; and,

(k) the late arrival of the sexual revolution in India in the context of such widespread ignorance and the threat of AIDS.

In this sense, AIDS has been a major political challenge to ongoing health and educational policies, and to state-society dialogue. Inability to come up with a coherent response to this challenge has led to AIDS being related to the recesses of the NACO in the Ministry of Health and Family Welfare, rather than being brought into the public arena for debate and social policy.

The very low levels of literacy and education, and of health awareness generally mean that HIV awareness-raising interventions will take longer to have effect, will require more innovative instruments for conceptualisation and dissemination, and will have to ensure that women, who are the most disadvantaged with regard to education and who cannot be easily reached in any institutional context, get access to HIV-related information. There is strong evidence to suggest that direct health-related information can be more effectively absorbed and retained when there is a pre-existing basis of general education. This could well become the crucial marker of how consistently HIV prevention awareness will actually be practised.

The emphasis so far on surveillance of marginalised high risk groups such as sex workers, STD clinic attenders and drug users is, admittedly, one of the necessary attempts to understand the dimensions and behaviour of the disease, and to establish AIDS-related infrastructure – primarily for surveillance and testing – in the states. However, this preoccupation has tended to overshadow the development of policy thrusts in the direction of legislative and ethical issues such as testing, freedom of movement, right to livelihood, messages for condom use, and access to treatment and care. The AIDS epidemic has come in the wake of a dawning sexual revolution and rapid economic and social change. Neither the state nor the civil society have as yet been able to overcome ideological barriers, to be able to come up with wide-ranging interventionist tools to deal with this sensitive area of behavioural change. What is required is a whole new paradigm for public discourse.

From the foregoing discussion, it would seem to suggest that the only progressive way ahead for the AIDS policy is to forge close working partnerships between the state and civil society. Given the ideological barriers, this is bound to be a slow process. But it could be an effective one if planned sensitively and holistically.

Among the major societal factors present in the Indian context that could foster such partnerships are:

a) The open nature of the polity, theoretically leaving space for debate, and for pressure groups safeguarding human rights;

b) An active judiciary, which in recent years has taken the initiative to set off political and administrative reforms in public interest to circumvent a stonewalling executive;

c) Given the long history of governmental interventions in social sectors, the state can play an active role in AIDS prevention, if there is political and administrative will;

d) There is a growing sector of NGO-led developmental activism, particularly in states which, coincidentally, are also among the most affected by the epidemic, e.g., Tamil Nadu, Maharashtra, Gujarat and Karnataka. Although few NGOs are engaged in exclusively AIDS-related work, with more active state involvement, these numbers may be expected to grow;

e) In the last five years, there have been considerable social and behavioural science inputs into understanding the prevailing patterns of sexual behaviour. Given the neglect of this area of research in the traditional academic preoccupations in the country, much of the impetus for this has come from international donors. They have been instrumental in bringing together research and advocacy NGO groups into the AIDS and reproductive health domain;

f) Today, a growing body of evidence exists to show that notwithstanding traditional prescriptions and proscriptions, there is considerable sexual mobility within the subcontinent. Apart from visiting commercial sex workers, who are by far the most ubiquitous avenue for pre-and extra-marital sexual gratification, particularly among the poor of all ages and among adolescent youth, there is much partner change that is not paid for among relatives, neighbours, friends and acquaintances. The fact that this takes place within the context of universal marriage, and within a framework of gross ignorance about sexually transmitted diseases and how these may be prevented, suggests the plethora of channels of HIV transmission into the general population. Genital ulcer disease is very high in the country, women have lower knowledge about methods for STD prevention than men and this cuts across educational differences, and male students, who will go on to marry, account for the highest proportion of non-treatment seekers for STDs (as compared with even commercial sex workers and truck drivers) (Ramasubban, 1990; Voluntary Health Services, 1996);

g) The Indian government's positive response to the deliberations at the Cairo International Conference on Population and Development, has culminated in the recasting of the National Family Planning Programme into a reproductive and child health programme, incorporating STD and reproductive tract infections (RTI) diagnosis, prevention and treatment, safe hospital practices and safety of blood and blood products (World Bank, 1997).

Case Studies

State led interventions – the case of Tamil Nadu

The first initiative that the Government of India has taken in light of the new draft AIDS policy is to assume leadership for the fight against AIDS and in this, its first step has been to overhaul the NACO structure. Simultaneously, efforts are on to communicate this philosophy to the states; and to encourage them to set up and strengthen state-level AIDS cells. Technical and financial assistance for AIDS-related work is coming entirely from the central government at this point, which in turn is aided by several bilateral and multilateral donors (mainly World Bank, USAID, DFID).

But the moot question is how the states will generate the necessary political and administrative will to overcome their historical inertia in the area of public health, and indifference to participation from the civil society in government sponsored programmes. This would also determine the prospects for the integration of AIDS prevention into primary health care.

Tamil Nadu, in southern India, has been the first state to show the way since 1994. It is the state with the second highest incidence of HIV after Maharashtra, where the first HIV positive case was isolated in the country. It is one of the most urbanised states, with an acknowledgedly large population of commercial sex workers in big cities and small towns, as also a large concentration of medical research groups and a tradition of NGO activism.

The main thrust of the Tamil Nadu Government's initiative is in three directions: organisational reform, media involvement, and state-NGO partnership

The Tamil Nadu State Aids Control Society (TNSACS) uses an organisational paradigm (which has also proved to be effective in other government-led social sector interventions in the country), whereby a state government sponsored body sets itself up as an NGO structure for the purposes of effective non-bureaucratic functioning in order to achieve time-bound results. The main features of this model are: self-governance, ease of receipt of foreign assistance, experimentation with organisational innovations, coordination with other crucial government departments (such as finance), and establishing partnerships with other NGOs.

TNSACS, with the financial and technical backing of NACO and international donors, has shown in its three years of functioning that governments can take the initiative in controversial and morally charged areas like AIDS prevention. TNSACS agenda has been: blood safety, STD control through better equipped (including counselling services) government clinics, high visibility campaigns through the mass media and film celebrities for AIDS prevention awareness, skill formation among government health sector personnel in the care of AIDS patients, plans to start such training for private medical and paramedical personnel, financial support to NGOs, and care for people with AIDS.

Of these, the government-funded media campaign – which involved training of English and regional language print journalists in AIDS coverage, and deployment of private advertising agencies – is what brought AIDS into the public arena. Aimed at reaching beyond "high risk" groups of sex workers and STD patients, the open advertising of and regular newspaper coverage to a sexually related theme was an unprecedented government-led initiative, and created shock waves, generating protests and controversies. But, the result was that people's knowledge of the disease underwent a major change.

For example, in 1994, a survey among married women had found that only 23 percent had heard of AIDS, around 27 percent thought it was transmitted through heterosexual relations, and only 9 percent felt that it was transmitted through blood. A Family Health Survey conducted in the state in 1996, three years after the launch of the campaign, found that awareness had gone up. By now, 46.5 percent of married women had heard of AIDS, 60 percent knew of the heterosexual mode of transmission and 29 percent had become aware of the blood transfusion route. Tamil Nadu claims that it is the only state which, while continuing to witness steadily rising rates of HIV among commercial sex workers and STD clinic attenders as in other states, has been able to bring down HIV incidence among the general population (using women attending antenatal clinics as a proxy), from 1 percent to 0.5 percent (Ramasundaram, 1997).

Notwithstanding the political legitimacy given to AIDS prevention, which is the most important contribution of this initiative, the experiment admittedly raises several questions. Even now, what we know from the above data regarding awareness levels pertains only to urban areas and even there, only to the educated middle class and the better off – going by the number of private clinics that have come up in the capital alone, at least 22 percent of the patients are married women, believed to be in monogamous relationships (Business India, 1997/98). Thus, little is known about the impact on the urban poor and rural populations, who have no recourse to high-quality counselling and care.

Another question pertains to the impact of media campaigns upon illiterate or poorly educated populations, who are bereft of a tradition of reasoned enquiry or the back-up of counselling/face-to-face information communication channels. There is reason to believe that the poor may be becoming the victims of irrational fears, leaving "AIDS patients" with heightened prospects of being discriminated against through witch-hunts and violence against them as messengers of death and destruction of local communities. There have been recent media reports from Tamil Nadu of known HIV positive patients being driven out of their villages/localities and beaten or burnt to death by fear-driven mobs afraid of contagion (Natarajan, 1998). The government's media campaign may thus be stressing morality over, more importantly, the consistent practice of protected sex whatever the circumstances (the more critical message for AIDS prevention), since it might be reluctant to be seen as condoning promiscuity. In a culture where stigmatisation – on the basis of colour, gender, disability, caste, widowhood, divorce/desertion, pale skin patch – is deeply ingrained (applicable to large parts of the country and not to Tamil Nadu alone), an HIV positive identity may be full of dangers. Indigenous health beliefs, which stress acceptance of particular states of the body as being "in one's nature" and which associate presence of disease only with a calamitous or life-threatening consequences, may also serve to bolster resistance to behavioural change in the ordinary course, while setting off panic reactions in the face of suspected or confirmed HIV presence.

That the rich are not free from the fear of stigma is also evident from the fact that large private hospitals in Chennai still do not accept HIV positive patients. Public admission of a personal problem, particularly one with possible moral overtones, may open a person, family or institution to all manner of speculation, and may evolve into degrees of neglect, rejection or even ostracism. Tamil Nadu has made a bold attempt to involve celebrities in AIDS awareness media campaigns, as part of its effort to legitimise the problem of AIDS. However, at this point in time, celebrities endorsing AIDS campaigns may still be a culturally dissonant import of the western model, at least in relation to poor audiences. The openness that one witnesses in the West in the matter of personal lives even among celebrities is missing among elites in predominantly tradition-bound societies, where the latter's legitimacy and mystique depends upon their distance from the ordinary people. This leaves the poor unable to identify with celebrities in non-fantasy roles, and may thus, reduce AIDS endorsements into condescending gestures.

India has yet to witness a member of the elite social groups publicly admitting to have contracted AIDS and willing to talk about it. Until this begins to happen, celebrity endorsements notwithstanding, counselling and face-to-face support as a back-up to media messages is inescapable. This is particularly true of resource poor environments, where low levels of education make absorption and retention of complex information through impersonal communication channels difficult. The strengthening of the health and education infrastructure, with the important component of counselling – a hitherto neglected area of social skills and provisioning – is an essential adjunct of efforts to induce and sustain behavioural change. In the long run, Tamil Nadu's ability to sustain the gains made in direct AIDS control will depend on reforms in these allied areas of social policy.

NGO-led interventions – the case of the STD/HIV Intervention Project, Sonagachi, Calcutta

This sexual health project was initiated in 1992 by NACO through the All India Institute of Hygiene and Public Health, with assistance from international donors. Begun in order to tackle the AIDS issue among commercial sex workers, the project has grown from its initial view of AIDS as a public health and medical problem into one that recognises the complex sociological and environmental ramifications of sex work and the inevitability of confronting these for a sustainable sexual health programme.

Sex work in Calcutta is predominantly brothel-based. There are an estimated 6,000 sex workers, who live in the Sonagachi area, and an estimated 20,000 men who visit them; the women thus averaging around four customers a day. The women are drawn from India, Nepal and Bangladesh, and over 90 percent of them come to this trade as victims of destitution, desertion/ divorce or other lack of family support. The women are powerless, controlled by the madams who run the brothels, with the active assistance of pimps, and who are broadly supported by a network of policemen, politicians, landlords, and other underworld elements.

At the start of the project in 1992, less than 3 percent of the women used condoms. STDs were found to be high amongst them – over 80 percent were found to be infected with one or more STD causative agents, and HIV positivity rate was 1.1 percent. The main thrust of the project, therefore, was condom use promotion and AIDS awareness-raising through peer educators. For the purpose of STD control, a clinic was set up in the heart of the area.

By 1995, condom use had gone up to 82 percent, of which 50 percent was habitual condom use and 32 percent was frequent condom use. Whereas knowledge of STDs and AIDS, respectively, had been 70 percent and 31 percent in 1992, by 1995 it had gone up to around 97 percent in both cases. Prevalence of genital ulcer disease, which had been around 6 percent in 1992 had come down to 3 percent in 1995; syphilis alone had witnessed a decline from around 25 percent in 1992 to 14 percent in 1995.

While the positive response to the intervention project is testimony to the will of the women to safeguard their own health, the project has begun to encounter limits to further improvements, both in condom use and STD prevalence. These limits were found to arise mainly out of the power structures within which the women have to practise their occupation, complemented by the infrastructural constraints within which they operate, and the continuous influx of new sex workers. The women are bonded to the madams, who are unwilling to permit insistence on condoms, and brothel rules and client insistence on sex without condoms are upheld through the violence meted out by the pimps, police and the local mafia. The competitive nature of the trade and resulting insecurity among the women was also found to be a constraint on adopting behavioural changes. Infrastructural constraints such as lack of space and the shared nature of the space available further impeded condom use negotiation. The easy availability of all manner of private practitioners for treatment of STDs, the widely differing drug treatments practised by them, and the resistance of clients, particularly from habitual partners of the women, to use condoms even while they indulged in multiple partners, have kept the STD rate reasonably high (AIIHPH, 1997).

The community mobilisation process, however, has had unexpected effects of a wider nature. The sex workers have begun to undergo an increase in self esteem and have begun a search for a professional identity and better work environment, and towards this end, they have begun a process of self organisation. Among the ingredients of this new self awareness is the knowledge about and ability to protest against uninformed blood testing and unethical vaccine trials, and demand for repeal of the Prevention of Immoral Traffic Act which, they argue, actually strengthens the police and further victimises the sex workers.

In keeping with these demands from the sex workers themselves, what began as an AIDS intervention project has begun undergoing the following changes:

a) the collaborative base is now a broad one, comprising both governmental and non-governmental organisations;

b) the Sonagachi Sex Workers Forum has begun networking with other sex workers forums within the state and outside to feel part of the larger democratic process;

c) there is a demand for the legalisation of the sex trade in order to ensure health, hygiene and safety of the women and to prevent children and adolescents from being brought into it;

d) advocacy at the policy-level is underway for change and modifications in oppressive legislations;

e) STD management has changed from laboratory-based diagnosis to syndrome-based management; and,

f) Follow-up of cases is through peers.

Lessons Learnt

1. The early stages of the evolution of the Indian AIDS policy – denial, precedence accorded to medical solutions over behavioural ones – have parallels with responses in other parts of the world. While faith in the traditional socio-cultural norms proscribing private behaviour provided the basis for denial in the early stages of the epidemic, the open nature of the polity facilitated the flow of foreign

assistance and the stimulus for critical investigation of actual patterns of sexual behaviour. The result has been the growing evidence that sexual behaviour is not in keeping with the traditional stereotypes.

2. One of the major factors impeding the assertion of an "effective, efficient and equitable" AIDS policy has been the lack of political commitment on two fronts. First, to collect and disseminate information and foster a public debate on HIV prevalence, risk behaviour, effectiveness of alternative programmes, their costs, etc. Second, to work constructively with those at greatest risk of contracting and spreading HIV. There would seem to be a fear of formulating policies that might be seen as facilitating socially deviant or immoral behaviour, such as teaching people how to use condoms irrespective of the nature of the sexual union. Both the case studies presented earlier have attempted to do this in limited ways, i.e., created space for discussion about HIV and sexual behaviour, and shown that it is possible to do so in the Indian socio-cultural context.

3. The above-mentioned case studies notwithstanding, a major obstacle to a coherent AIDS policy has been the lack of frank and public discussion of sources of risk. Public discourse about sexuality is lacking in Indian society, although emerging studies show considerable partner change beneath the veneer of monogamy. The absence of frank public discussion means that open and validated sources of knowledge about sex and about sources of infection are unavailable. Personal behaviour, doubts and agonies have no "safe" spaces to be aired in. A recently set up hotline in Delhi by an NGO reveals the exponential growth of demands for accurate knowledge. Even now, these demands are made by only men, as women are not supposed to evince public interest (a hotline is a public space) in sexual matters.

4. One of the greatest challenges is how to formulate an AIDS policy that integrates into more general public health and primary health care programmes. One of the obstacles to mounting an adequate policy response to AIDS in India has been the lack of knowledge and skills in public health management, borne largely out of the historical lack of political will to generate such skills in

what has been a low status, residual area of social policy. In a country where the majority are poorly educated and live in poor physical and socio-economic conditions, there is need for interventions to take the form of multi-faceted programmes in which mutually amplifying public health and social policies play an integral role. Success in the AIDS sphere will depend upon complementary reforms in the larger spheres of health and education policies, since a sustainable AIDS policy must aim at integration, especially in the area of treatment and care of those affected, and must base its prevention strategies on education and awareness raising for consistent behaviour change.

5. One of the major cultural and political challenges posed by AIDS is that men's behaviour is being called into question for the first time. Indian population control/ family planning programmes have consistently targeted women and have left men well alone. AIDS is showing up men's attendance at STD clinics; men engaging in pre- and extra-marital sex with multiple partners without thought for the health consequences of their actions; and, youth engaging in casual sex in gross ignorance. Women are emerging as powerless – whether as sex workers or as unmarried adolescents or as wives – with little or no knowledge of sex or of STDs or RTIs and in no position to negotiate condom use. It is becoming clear that women's powerlessness and vulnerability arising out of the prevailing gender inequalities are among the most deep-rooted and resilient of the factors impeding effective implementation of AIDS policies. Reaching into the private domain of men in order to effect far-reaching behavioural change is the major challenge of any AIDS policy. Media campaigns (as in Tamil Nadu) will have to be bolstered by direct mobilisational strategies to reach men in an effective way.

In conclusion, it may be said that what is happening in India is that there are a growing number of projects, mainly with high risk groups, which are doing some very useful work. However, HIV/ AIDS prevention and care is not yet part of the mainstream social process. The main factors inhibiting this have been the resilient socio-cultural norms and stereotypes. These have combined with organisational inefficiencies and weaknesses, and the lack of political will, particularly at the state level, to undertake major public health and educational reforms or tackle the intractable problem of poverty. This is the stage at which we are today, despite the presence of an open political system, an active judiciary, the role of international funding and scientific collaboration bridging the gap between scientific developments worldwide and in the country, and the drafting of a National AIDS Control and Prevention Policy.

The Tamil Nadu case is one illustration where HIV/AIDS has been mainstreamed and where things are beginning to work, largely due to certain inherent advantages that the state enjoys. However, even that experience suggests that with all the good intentions and resources, it is still uncharted territory. The constraints upon open discussion of sex and sexuality inhibit the emergence of safe spaces wherein enough information may be obtained. We still do not have the methodology to formulate messages that can be correctly interpreted by ordinary people, so that they may protect themselves. Underlying these are the patriarchal structures and gender relations that constitute the most enduring obstacles.

Bridging the gap between women's powerlessness and the uncharted terrain of men's private behaviour is one of the major cultural and political challenges posed by the AIDS epidemic. Bridging the gap between AIDS control measures and primary health care strategies is an area requiring immediate attention. The challenge of AIDS prevention and control should act as a stimulus to other bridging processes as well – such as between the central and state governments with regard to health policy formulation and programme implementation; between socio-cultural stereotypes, on the one hand, and the real world within which sexual behaviour actually takes place, on the other, through a more concerted process of knowledge generation; between telling people what they should do and listening to what they say are their needs; through skill formation in the area of counselling; and, between what is happening in people's bodies and people's own understanding of and ability to cope with it, through the tool of both education and counselling.

References

All India Institute of Hygiene and Public Health. 1997. Five Years Stint of STD/HIV Intervention Programme at Sonagachi 1992-1997, Calcutta, India.

Business India, December 29, 1997 - January 11, 1998.

Nataraj, S. 1998. Testing Positive for Ignorance on HIV, *Times of India,* June 9.

National AIDS Control Organisation, Ministry of Health and Family Welfare, Government of India. 1997 (a). HIV/AIDS in India, A Status Report, June. Mimeo. (b). Draft National AIDS Control and Prevention Policy. Mimeo.

National AIDS Control Organisation, Ministry of Health and Family Welfare, Government of India. 1996. National AIDS Control Programme, India: Country Scenario and Update, New Delhi. June.

Ramasubban, R. 1984. The Development of Health Policy in India. In: T. Dyson and N. Crook (eds.). India's Demography: Essays on the Contemporary Population. New Delhi: South Asian Publishers.

Ramasubban, R. 1990. Sexual Behaviour and Conditions of Health Care: Potential Risks for HIV Transmission in India. In: T. Dyson (ed.), Sexual Behaviour and Networking: Anthropological and Socio-cultural Studies on the Transmission of HIV. Liege: International Union for the Scientific Study of Population.

Ramasubban, R. 1995. Patriarchy and the Risks of HIV Transmission to Women. In: M. Das Gupta, T.N. Krishnan and L.C. Chen (eds.). Women's Health in India: Risk and Vulnerability. Mumbai: Oxford University Press.

Ramasundaram, S. 1997. Tamil Nadu: Blazing a Trail, *Nexus*, March-May.

Voluntary Health Services. 1996. AIDS Prevention and Control Project: HIV Risk Behaviour in Tamil Nadu: Sentinel Surveillance Survey, Report on Baseline Wave -1996, Chennai, India.

World Bank. 1995. India: Policy and Finance Strategies for Strengthening Primary Health Care Services, Washington DC, USA.

World Bank. 1997. Appraisal Document, India: Reproductive and Child Health Project, April.

World Health Organisation. 1992. AIDS in South East Asia: No Time for Complacency. WHO Regional Office for South East Asia, New Delhi, India.

Select Country Profile – India

Total population (in million) *		850
Proportion of population in sexually active age group (15-49 years) **		50.0%
Proportion of adolescent population ~		20.0%
Urban population *		26.0%
Rural population *		74.0%
Population below poverty line: #	Combined	29.2%
	Rural	32.7%
Crude death rate <>	All India	9.8%
	Urban	10.6%
	Rural	7.1%
Literacy rate *	All India	52.2%
	Female	39.3%
	Male	64.1%
Literacy rate (urban) *	Female	64.0%
	Male	81.0%
Literacy rate (rural) *	Female	30.6%
	Male	57.0

Sources:

* Census of India, Series 1, Paper No. 2 of 1992, Final Population Total, Brief Analysis of Primary Census Abstract.

** Office of the Registrar General, India (Vital Statistics Division), Ministry of Home Affairs, New Delhi, "Sample Registration System 1988".

<> Office of the Registrar General, India (Vital Statistics Division), Ministry of Home Affairs, New Delhi, "Sample Registration System: selected demographic indicators 1991".

~ Office of the Registrar General, India 1993 (Fertility and Mortality Survey Division), Ministry of Home Affairs, New Delhi. "Sample Registration System: Fertility and Mortality Indicators, 1992, IIPS, National FHS, 1992-93".

Government of India, "Family Welfare Programme in India, Year Book, 1989-90", Ministry of Health and Family Welfare, New Delhi.

AIDS Profile – India

Seropositivity rate per thousand screened (May 1997) *			18.6
Cumulative total of AIDS patients (May 1997 as reported to NACO) *			8551
HIV present in all states except one, principal concentration in Maharashtra, Tamil Nadu, Manipur **			77%
Trend in seropositivity rate: # (per thousand screened)	September	1993	6.89
	March	1994	7.32
	March	1995	7.25
	July	1996	15.97
	May	1997	18.60
Main routes of transmission:	Sexual		75%
	Blood transfusion		8%
	IVDU		8%
Main affected groups:	Commercial sex workers		
	STD clinic attendees		
	Clients of CSWs		
	IVD users		

Sources:

* National AIDS Control Organisation, Government of India. 1997. HIV/AIDS in India: A Status Report (June).

** National AIDS Control Organisation, Government of India. 1997. Draft National AIDS Prevention and Control Policy.

National AIDS Control Organisation, Government of India. Reports for relevant years.

2

Government Response to HIV/AIDS

Geeta Sethi

The views expressed in this paper are entirely those of the author and do not necessarily reflect official policy or positions of the United Nations Development Programme

Introduction

A National AIDS Control Programme was initiated in India in 1987, soon after a few individuals tested positive for HIV in 1986. This was seven years before the International Conference on Population and Development (ICPD) was held in Cairo, in 1994. By that time, the National AIDS Control Organisation (NACO), an apex body under the Ministry of Health and Family Welfare, was into its second year, with a well thought out strategic plan underway. What were the implications of the ICPD for AIDS related policy and programmes in India? Did the debate and the globally endorsed reproductive health approach influence the national response to the HIV/AIDS epidemic? This chapter seeks to explore these questions by providing an overview of the first phase of the National AIDS Control Programme and its operation; drawing out the parallels and linkages between the reproductive health approach and HIV/AIDS prevention strategies; and examining the proposed second phase of the National AIDS Control programme.

In 1985, the Indian Council of Medical Research (ICMR) established a task force on AIDS, to screen sera from high risk groups at two sites in the country. The first detection of HIV in 1986 in Chennai, led to strategic thinking and programme planning. A Central AIDS Cell was established in New Delhi and cells were set up within each state. All states were encouraged to design their own plans for AIDS surveillance. A network of laboratories and surveillance units was established, with at least one in every state; these were linked to referral centres for confirmatory testing. The Ministry of Health and Family Welfare along with the Indian Council of Medical Research, developed a programme to train laboratory scientists, managers, and others. In addition, special emphasis was placed on the creation of awareness.

In 1986, a National AIDS Committee was formed under the chairmanship of the Secretary of the Union Ministry of Health and Family Welfare, to formulate, plan and implement a preventive programme. Members from health and other ministries and NGO representatives were included. Limited surveillance in areas and groups perceived to be 'risk-prone', screening of blood and blood-products, and health education and information activities were planned.

The National AIDS Control Programme was established in 1987 to implement this plan which was reviewed in 1990 in consultation with the World Health Organization (WHO). As a result of this consultative process, a medium term plan for three years with an estimated cost of US $ 20 million was prepared. Its focus was on the four identified high-risk metropolitan cities (Mumbai, Delhi, Chennai and Calcutta) and the states of Maharashtra, Manipur, Tamil Nadu and West Bengal. The basic strategy remained the same with an added emphasis on interventions through health education and condom promotion among identified risk-behaviour groups.

In 1991, a comprehensive nation-wide plan, the Strategic Plan for the Prevention and Control of AIDS in India, was drawn up with seven distinct programme components: (1) strengthening programme management; (2) surveillance and research; (3) information, education and communication (IEC); (4) control of sexually transmitted diseases; (5) condom promotion; (6) blood safety; and, (7) reduction of impact. The projected budget was US $ 265.5 million for a five year period (1992 to 1997). Phase I of the project, with a US $ 84 million soft loan from the World Bank evolved from this proposal (NACO, 1993).

National AIDS Control Programme (1992-1998)

Operationally, the programme aimed at developing HIV/AIDS preventive activities nationally, but with a special focus on the epicentres of the epidemic. Its major components were: 1) strengthening the management capacity for AIDS control; 2) promoting public awareness and community support; 3) improving blood safety and promoting rational use of blood; 4) building surveillance and clinical management capacity; and, 5) controlling sexually transmitted diseases.

Project activities were to be implemented through the existing government health infrastructure, private sector, non-governmental organisations, and the mass media institutions. The role of the Government of India was co-ordination of the project, a procurement, and development of policies and technical guidelines. Implementation was the responsibility of state governments and non-governmental organisations (NGOs) funded by the Government of India. Recognising the epidemic raises several social, ethical and legal issues, a sub-committee was established to examine these and make recommendations to the government.

Programme strategies

The government reacted fairly quickly to the HIV/AIDS epidemic, even though there was scepticism about the need for a programme in several quarters and the disease was perceived as one pertaining 'foreigners' and marginalised risk groups. Information from early testing and surveillance was taken seriously enough to review the programme and to formulate a strategic plan. The government was prompt in negotiating a soft loan from the World Bank and setting up the National AIDS Control Organisation. There was also commitment to a multi-sectoral approach demonstrated through the establishment of a high-powered muti-sectoral National AIDS Committee.

The strategic plan was well prepared and made provisions for focusing activity at the state level (since health is a state subject). It recognised the immense variations in culture and behaviour and stressed the importance of working in close co-operation with local bodies, NGOs and community based organisations. It also recognised the need to work with other sectors such as education, transport and tourism, industry, and information, broadcasting and the media. The plan drew positive interest and commitment from international donors, sections of the scientific community and selected NGOs across the country. After considerable efforts, all states signed an undertaking agreeing to implement the programme. Some activity is now underway in all the states in the country.

Programme implementation

Anonymous and unlinked surveillance of persons at higher risk at selected STD clinics, as well as those representing the general population at antenatal clinics, was initiated. Blood samples (and not individual persons) were screened at places where blood was routinely drawn for other tests. This enabled the collection of valuable data essential for advocacy, programme planning and implementation.

To generate widespread awareness at all levels, an advertising agency was commissioned to handle mass media. The National Aids Control Organisation produced an information, education and communication training manual, and initiated capacity building for NGOs and staff at the state level. Free time was negotiated on television networks for broadcasting HIV/AIDS messages. To reach the maximum number of people and to provide a regular channel of communication for states and interested persons, a newsletter titled 'AIDS in India' was published.

Sensitisation workshops were conducted for the mass media, small media and folk media. Some efforts were made to encourage newspapers and other print media to develop peer-guidelines for reportage of stories related to HIV/AIDS, and to be sensitive and considerate of the privacy and dignity of infected and affected persons. Generic packages of information, education and communication materials were developed through collaborations with NGOs, media experts and others.

Interventions for HIV/AIDS prevention and control required dealing with extremely sensitive and personal aspects of human behaviour and relationships as well as with marginalised groups, like drug users, sex workers and men who have sex with men. As these groups were unlikely to be reached by the government, the implementation of the programme was seen as largely being in the NGO domain. NGOs were encouraged to integrate HIV/AIDS activities within their ongoing programmes instead of setting up exclusive AIDS prevention projects. They were provided basic information on HIV/AIDS and offered training to strengthen capacity for designing interventions. The government prepared a set of guidelines to facilitate the application for, and release of funds to NGOs. Simultaneously, efforts were made to equip government staff within states to work more effectively with NGOs.

Efforts were also made to promote collaboration with the Department of Youth Affairs and Sports, through the Universities Talk AIDS project, a peer-education programme for colleges and through the Department of Women and Child to integrate an HIV/AIDS component into their work. The Confederation of Indian Industry and the Federation of Indian Chambers of Commerce and Industry were approached to involve industry and discussions were held with the railways, the border security force to involve them in the programme.

There is a gross lack of information on sexual behaviour. The traditional ideal of a woman who is a virgin at marriage and is always faithful to her husband along with double standards that tacitly permit men to have pre-marital as well as extra-marital sex, had led to a situation where the existence of sex outside marriage is so well camouflaged as to be virtually invisible and definitely not discussed or acknowledged. Other risky behaviours, like male to male sex, were also not acknowledged. These were seen as alien to the culture of the country and therefore not meriting attention. The ideal of sexual purity for women included 'innocence' regarding sex which translated itself into lack of information, inability to negotiate sex, and lack of initiative in communicating even with the spouse or sexual partner. In spite of these assumptions about sexuality, the high STD rates and anecdotal evidence pointed to the large gap between public pronouncements and individual behaviour. To prevent HIV, it was essential to change sexual behaviour, therefore more data on sexual and other risk behaviours were urgently needed.

The National AIDS Control Organisation supported several studies to explore the patterns of risky behaviours in the major cities in the country to identify areas needing intervention. This was a pioneering initiative, as methodologies for research were not well developed, and there was reluctance to undertake serious research on sexuality and sexual behaviour. Conducting research therefore forged a new understanding, and built trust and relationships with partners so that a foundation for effective interventions could be formed.

Recognising the importance of adequate information and understanding, and acceptance of sex and sexuality for healthy sexual behaviour, the National Council of Educational Research and Training developed an AIDS education training package for teachers (NACO, 1995). Through co-curricular activities, this package provided an acceptable way of reaching schools, and formed the basis for plans to include sex education in schools that were submitted by 15 states.

Facilities and trained manpower for sex counselling were found to be inadequate, particularly for handling counselling for HIV/AIDS. Counselling was essential while revealing test results; in helping infected and affected persons to cope; in changing to safer behaviour by those who were at risk; and for those who had doubts, queries, or fears regarding HIV/AIDS. The plan envisaged training a cadre of counsellors, by drawing upon persons already in service, and in a position to offer counselling services such as health professionals in blood banks, nurses, and teachers, social workers and psychologists. Training manuals were prepared for training of counselling trainers, and for self-learning of grassroots level counsellors. A country-wide plan for training counsellors through regional counselling training centres, academic institutions and NGOs was operationalised.

Initially, the strategic plan did not have a gender perspective. However, it subsequently attempted to address the specific needs of women as well as men. NGOs, women's health activists and women's-studies-centres were consulted to identify priority issues, to prepare a plan of action, and to define research questions.

Recognising that early detection and treatment of STDs was essential for preventing the transmission of HIV, the syndromic approach was promoted. Guidelines and flow-charts were prepared, and training programmes to use these guidelines were organised for both private and public sector physicians. STD clinics around the country were up-graded through the provision of equipment and training of laboratory technicians.

Transmission through infected blood and blood products accounted for about 12 percent of reported cases in the country (NACO, 1996). To provide safer blood, more rigorous screening of blood and blood products was promoted by amending the existing legal framework. Blood banks were up-graded by providing equipment and training personnel. More rational use of blood was advocated with special emphasis on doing away with single-unit transfusions which accounted for a high proportion of the transfusions in the country. Making the most of every unit of blood through the use of components rather than whole blood whenever possible, was also emphasised.

Improving quality, access and availability of condoms, as well as educating people on the importance of using condoms to protect themselves from sexually transmitted diseases including AIDS, is critical for HIV/AIDS prevention. The unlubricated condoms supplied through the Family Welfare Programme were not suitable for HIV prevention as they had a high breakage rate and were not comfortable, especially for use during anal sex and for multiple sexual encounters in a relatively short time-span. The Schedule "R" of the Drugs and Cosmetics Act was therefore changed to ensure that quality condoms could be distributed through the health infrastructure in the country. The system of distribution was also changed to make it more flexible. In addition, the social marketing of condoms was stepped up.

Some successful targeted interventions were initiated for the prevention of HIV/AIDS: the intervention in the sex industry in Calcutta (which included sex workers, brokers, regular partners, madams, and clients); with clients engaging in male to male sex in Chennai; and with injecting drug users in Manipur. First steps were taken to set up systems for a continuum of care from home to hospital in Manipur and in Maharashtra.

Simple and practical guidelines for hospital infection control were prepared. These guidelines were aimed at reinforcing universal precautions that all health providers should follow irrespective of the threat of HIV/AIDS. The message was that HIV infection does not require any unusual precautions, and that this infection can be handled much like any other.

These 'achievements' did not come easily. Continuing and intensive effort had to be made to garner support from those who should have been partners – such as the state governments, allied sectors and sceptics within the government – who did not see HIV/AIDS as a problem meriting serious concern. The shortfalls of the programme were so serious that the achievements, although hard won, could not keep pace with the epidemic.

Programme shortfalls

Although the strategic plan was comprehensive, operationalising it was not easy. The programme failed to generate commitment and a sense of urgency. A decade after the first cases were detected and five years after the National AIDS Control Organisation was established, denial of the problem continued. Denial persisted even as the reported number of persons tested positive for HIV crossed 66,000 (NACO, 1997) and the Joint United Nations Programme on HIV/AIDS estimated the number of positive persons in India at 3-5 million. A gap in communicating with the general public and with key stakeholders remained.

Denial impeded the implementation of the programme. Staffing at national and state levels reflected the low priority it had received. Several key positions were not filled over long periods of time. There was a swift turn-over of officials at the state level resulting in lack of continuity and inadequate time and opportunity to grasp the subtle nuances required for an effective response. Many officials were given the responsibility for this programme in addition to their other responsibilities. Mechanisms to systematically strengthen capacity and provide technical support were inadequate.

A strange paradox in the programme concerned money. While in theory adequate funds were available, utilising these funds was extremely difficult. Procedural paper work made the disbursement of money slow and hard. This constrained responses and frustrated those who were eager and ready to initiate activities. The inability to release funds on time placed officials at the state level in a defensive position with NGOs and others, which strained relations that should have been mutually supportive and based on trust. In an innovative attempt to overcome the difficulties in accessing and disbursing money, the Government of Tamil Nadu set up a society through which funds could flow more easily. This worked well and has now been adopted by other states.

Although there was an understanding of the importance of a multi-sectoral approach, and some attempts were made to develop linkages, the programme actually remained largely a vertically oriented health programme. The response to HIV/AIDS, therefore, could not be contextualised. This was a major drawback in India where vulnerability is determined by social, economic and cultural factors rather than by individually selected behavioural options. There is ample evidence to show that gender, poverty and lack of education and employment opportunities severely curtail sexual decision making, and the option of practising safer sex is not available to women, to the poor, and to those with little access to information and services. The socially compromised position of women, along with traditional notions of modesty, present serious barriers. The fact that women have to prove their fertility and the high premium placed by society on producing a male child, further pressures young women to have unprotected sex.

Finally, the possibility and experience of sexual abuse and violence makes refusing unsafe sex near impossible. The rising rates of HIV in antenatal mothers in some states – five states have reported HIV positivity of over 1 percent among antenatal mothers (NACO, 1998b) – clearly shows that women are unable to protect themselves and their unborn children. Similarly, migration in search of jobs, or due to natural or man-made disasters, and the lack of access to information and services, result in vulnerability and risk behaviours that require larger macro-economic and social policy interventions.

The procurement and distribution of essential equipment for blood banks, testing kits and even condoms were uneven and often delayed. These delays damaged the credibility of the programme and undermined its urgency.

Another major shortfall was that research findings were not used for advocacy, nor were they used to design interventions. Early efforts focused only on so called high-risk groups. For example only sex workers and drug users were tested for HIV. The conclusions were that infection in these surveyed groups was increasing rapidly, which strengthened the prevailing stigma and negative feelings about the risk groups and reinforced the notion that HIV/AIDS is restricted to these 'risk groups'. This fortified denial, and countered efforts to make HIV/AIDS everybody's concern. Confronted with this intensified denial, the approach that 'everyone is at risk' did not ring true in the minds of the general public.

Research findings were often quoted without adequate reference to the context, and sometimes distorted to make assertions that were not adequately supported by the data. This led to an overall discrediting and scepticism regarding research. Although some very interesting studies were undertaken, the National AIDS Control Organisation was shy of owning the results of these studies and sharing them. Important research results of high risk behaviours undertaken in over 30 cities in the country, and of the preventive indicators survey in five sites, were for instance, not disseminated.

Even though there was agreement on the need to share and use research findings prudently, data was not fed back into the programme.

Another major difficulty was that ten years into the epidemic, and twelve years after surveillance started, there was still no consensus on the epidemic. There were widely differing estimates about the magnitude of the problem. Information on sero-surveillance, STD studies and behavioural studies was not collated to construct a picture of the likely situation. This hesitancy in making a projection was an immense hurdle in efforts at advocacy and in programming. The epidemic remained hidden and invisible. Instead of deepening understanding, creating a readiness for action, and countering the widespread denial, the manner in which research findings were handled led to further denial.

Although the creation of awareness about HIV/AIDS was a primary goal of the programme, the overall awareness in various sections of the population still remained very low. This could be attributed to a combination of factors, including cultural sensitivities and inhibitions that hindered open discussion about sexuality; inability to see the epidemic as directly relevant to oneself; and limitations of the approach and the methods and materials used for information, education and communication.

Not enough attention was given to monitoring the quality of the material produced and even less to assessing the impact of different materials, media and approaches. Experience shows that most visual material failed to make the link between what was seen as a blood-borne infection (due to the emphasis on safe blood and information about testing) and the use of condoms. Similarly, there is a gap in assessing the short and long term impact of fear based messages.

The socio-cultural context; values, customs and social status; and the socialisation process and concepts of sexuality were not adequately explored. Programme staff did not understand how all of these affect relationships, interpersonal communication, sexual decision making, and hence sexual behaviours and practices. The approach seemed to be based on the tacit assumption that the programme knows what is best; it tells the people how to behave; and the desirable course of action is to follow its recommendations. Insufficient attention was paid to the underlying developmental factors that shape and constrain behaviours, such as poverty, gender and inequalities based on class and caste, or to accepting that often, individuals have little control over their sexual lives. Similarly, there was insufficient exploration of what idiom works in different cultural settings and with different groups. The approach relied on the government being seen as a credible source of information, and on the assumption that appropriate information would lead to a change in behaviour – an assumption widely held globally in the earlier phases of the epidemic.

This approach is particularly surprising, because at one level, there was recognition of the significance of the local context, of the importance of preceding information, education and communication campaigns with formative research, and of the necessity of involving communities (the prime guardians of behavioural norms and peer influence) in all stages of the intervention process. At the same time, there was little effort at the local level to create an 'enabling environment' that would facilitate and support behaviour change as well as the practice of safer sexual behaviours. The programme seemed more concerned with doing what was politically correct than in taking risks and experimenting with a variety of strategies to reach people in a manner that would make a difference to the way they perceived HIV/AIDS in relation to themselves.

The programme did not really accommodate the range of existing perspectives or attempt to address each one on its own turf, starting with where people were in terms of understanding, beliefs and behaviour. It tried to overcome the barriers imposed by cultural double standards and subterfuges by drawing attention to their existence, rather than understanding them and working within the situation they represented.

The media can play a significant role in creating public opinion and shaping public reactions. The sporadic, tentative initiatives with the media did little to genuinely inform reportage or editorial policies.

The media continued to sensationalise and stigmatise HIV/AIDS and infected persons (Pioneer, 1996).

The NGO guidelines formulated in 1993-94 did not effectively mobilise NGOs to participate in the national programme. There were difficulties in identifying suitable organisations to review and accept proposals for funding, in the timely release of funds, and in building capacity for work in the area of HIV/AIDS. Further, the 'nodal agency' model adopted for the selection of NGOs at the state level did not work, probably due to the lack of trust and networking between the NGOs themselves. There was a lack of clarity on the roles and linkages between the central and state governments and NGOs. There was a lack of a transparent, participatory process of role definition so that each was aware of its contribution and that of others, which was essential for the smooth functioning of what was designed as a collaborative effort. Mutual support and building of capacity was inadequate. Instead, blame and mistrust between different sectors continued to hamper coordination.

This is a long list of shortfalls. However, the genuine efforts and commitment of several government functionaries who worked with passion and tenacity in an extremely harsh environment to keep AIDS on the agenda, and who tried to make a difference to the lives of the millions affected and infected, should not be discounted. In substantial part, the shortfalls were due to the lethargy of a system which took much too long to respond. The initial responses, strategies and activities were framed and designed when far less was known about the epidemic and how to handle the many complex questions it raised. In the time taken for those initial plans to be implemented, the epidemic raced ahead. The situation is now dramatically different. So also is the state of the art in understanding what is necessary to impact the epidemic, and what is required to enable people to protect themselves. The government's response in India has now moved into a higher gear in an attempt to catch up with, and bring into control the fast growing epidemic. The past eighteen months have seen a dramatic change to a more mature, and well rounded developmental initiative.

AIDS Response and Reproductive Health Approach

Although the government's response to HIV/AIDS preceded the clear articulation and endorsement of the reproductive health approach by several years, there are similarities between the two. There are several shared concerns and similar ideological underpinnings. While it is not possible to clearly state how, and to what extent one influenced the other, it may be more accurate to say that both are products of the same process of evolution of social change and the intersection of health, women's rights and democratic self-determination at the individual as well as at community level. More important, both are firmly based on a strong acknowledgement and assertion of human rights.

The reproductive health approach envisages a situation where people have the right to reproduce and regulate their fertility; women are able to go through pregnancy and child birth safely; the outcome of pregnancy is successful in terms of maternal and infant survival and well being; and couples are able to have sexual relations free of the fear of pregnancy and of contracting diseases (Fathallah, 1988). This approach encompasses "all aspects of human sexuality and reproductive health needs during the various stages of the life cycle. ...(and) enable(s) clients to make informed choices; receive screening, counselling services and education for responsible and healthy sexuality; access services for...the prevention and management of reproductive morbidity" (Pachauri, 1995). In emphasising individual needs against larger societal goals, as a basis for action, the approach calls for a decentralised, responsive programme. The inclusion of sexual health within reproductive health brings in sexually transmitted diseases. HIV/AIDS is a part of reproductive health concerns.

Sexuality and sexual behaviour

Reproductive health legitimises sexuality as an important concern, and recognises that men and women have sexual needs which must be addressed. It provides a sense of credibility to research on sexuality related issues. Prevention and management of STDs is a major concern for both programmes. The reproductive health approach recommends the integration of STD services with other reproductive health services.

Thus, reproductive health extends the boundaries of the traditional family welfare programme which addressed the needs of married couples only, to all persons who are, or may become sexually active. The approach of the HIV/AIDS control programme is similar. The latter addresses the needs of sex workers, men who have sex with men, and persons with multiple partners. It also recognises that behaviour is often outside the immediate control and decision making of individuals, and that changes in the larger context can bring about and sustain changes in individual behaviour (Correa and Petchesky, 1994). Finally, both reproductive health and AIDS control programmes emphasise the importance of providing information to all, as the basis for promoting responsible behaviours.

Need for partnerships

The preparatory process as well as the follow up of the ICPD brought together several groups with significantly varied perspectives and demonstrated that diverse constituencies can find common ground to work together. In addition to health professionals, the role of human rights activists, women's health advocates, behavioural and social scientists, and community representatives was particularly important. The process also emphasised the need for listening to the people and decentralising decision-making. The definition of participation was enlarged and NGOs, and other community groups were seen as equal partners in defining priorities and not merely as implementers of programmes designed by those in positions of authority and power. The importance of putting people affected by

HIV/AIDS at the centre of the response, of genuinely empowering sex workers, injecting drug users, and others who are usually viewed as recipients of services, was strongly supported.

This experience of being more inclusive, of bringing in and bringing together various stakeholders, was especially significant for both the reproductive health and HIV programmes in India. In the past, both were top-down vertical programmes. The population programme was seen as imposed from above by the government and not as one formulated in response to the people's need (Jain, 1998). Similarly, the response to HIV was also seen as a top-down reaction to a problem that did not really affect the larger population of the country (Priya, undated). The ICPD proposed a comprehensive reproductive health framework. It provided a strong foundation of partnerships and solidarity on which the HIV response can be built. There is now growing political commitment to prevent and control HIV/AIDS. In December 1998, the Prime Minister addressed a meeting of members of parliament, NGOs and donors where he eloquently described AIDS as 'the most serious public health challenge that the country is facing today' (Vajpayee, 1998). Thus, both the reproductive and HIV/AIDS control programmes have begun to secure a high level of political commitment.

Human rights framework

The importance of human rights as a bed-rock, is emphasised by both programmes. There were several attempts to make HIV testing compulsory and segregate risk groups in the so called larger interest. However, the programme has been able to withstand these pressures and has been successful in promoting voluntary counselling and testing. In its approach to different marginalised and vulnerable populations, the programme has also shown considerable sensitivity and maturity. Thus, respect for human rights is at the core. Both programmes aim at ensuring that equity, dignity and rights are upheld.

Addressing the needs of youth

The reproductive health approach has drawn attention to the urgency of addressing the special needs of adolescents and youth. While the HIV/AIDS programme took the first steps in initiating sex education in schools and peer education in colleges, these attempts were tentative, and could not progress due to lack of popular support. The reproductive health initiative has contributed substantially to the impetus for informed, responsible sexual behaviours among youth. From a situation where schools were unwilling to implement sex education programmes for fear of parental opposition, and authorities were unwilling to take a stand, we are now at a point where the prime minister states:

> *"Information about sexual and reproductive health and right sexual behaviour can help the children in developing a necessary value system and face any eventuality, with courage and understanding. I do not think we should hesitate to tell the children about the process of growing up and its implications. The growing threat of HIV/AIDS in the country points to the urgency of doing this sooner rather than later"* (Vajpayec, 1998).

The experience gained from reproductive health programmes can show effective ways of how young people can be reached with information and necessary services (Hawkins and Meshesha, 1994). This is a gap in the HIV/AIDS control programme that the reproductive health programme can help to bridge.

Phase II of the National AIDS Control Programme (1999-2004)

The Government of India estimated the total number of HIV infected persons at about 4 million in early 1998 (NACO,1998).

Acknowledging the changing epidemiology of HIV/AIDS in India, the trend is summarised as follows:

> *"HIV is prevalent in almost all parts of the country. HIV/AIDS is spreading from urban to rural areas. HIV/AIDS is also spreading from high risk behaviour groups to the general population, since early 1990. One in every four cases reported is a woman. About 89 per cent of the reported cases are from the sexually active and economically productive age group of 15-49 years."* (NACO, 1998).

The increasing numbers of antenatal women testing positive for HIV raises questions regarding the use of prophylactic drugs to reduce mother to child transmission, and a review of recommendations for breast-feeding. Factors contributing to this rapid spread are identified as labour migration and mobility from economically less developed areas to more developed ones; low literacy leading to low awareness; gender disparity and the prevalence of STDs.

Other problems that require serious attention are stigma and rejection, which manifest into refusal of health care, denial of employment and education, and even violence leading to death. There are limited treatment options due to the prohibitive cost. There is also the danger of exploitation of naive and inadequately informed people by those promising a quick cure. Summing up the present situation, the National AIDS Control Organisation asserts that:

> *"because of the behavioural nature and strong socio-economic implications, the disease requires to be treated as a developmental issue which impinges on various economic and social sectors of government and non-government activity"* (NACO, 1998).

Lessons learned

These proposed implementation strategies for the second phase are derived from lessons learned from the first phase of the programme. These include recognising the importance of HIV/AIDS as a development issue; the creation of ownership at the state level and building capacity at local level; decentralisation of the programme with adequate back-up for states with limited capacity; ensuring that reliable surveillance data are available for policy and programme formulation, advocacy, and monitoring and evaluation; designing targetted interventions to address the special needs of people who are most vulnerable to infection; addressing issues related to people living with HIV/AIDS, especially human rights and care; securing the participation of communities in the national response; providing appropriate technical support; promoting bio-medical research for vaccines and treatment, and behavioural and operations research for programming; and strengthening intersectoral links.

Strategies and objectives

Clearly, the understanding and definition of HIV/AIDS as an issue has changed considerably during the past five years. The programme has also expanded substantially in partnership with the central and state governments, the World Bank, bilateral donors, the United Nations system and others. The proposed budget is US$ 244 million. A National AIDS Policy document was recently submitted for approval by the Cabinet. The policy framework emphasises behaviour change rather than more awareness creation; decentralisation with substantial ownership by states and the municipal corporations of large cities; an evolution of the role of National AIDS Control Organisation to provide policy and technical leadership; strengthening partnerships between the government, private sector, NGOs, and donors; and incorporating monitoring and evaluation systems.

Two key objectives of the programme are to: i) reduce the spread of HIV infection in India; and ii) strengthen India's capacity to respond to HIV/AIDS on a long-term basis (NACO, 1998b). To achieve these objectives of reducing spread and strengthening capacity, the following activities are proposed:

- reduce HIV transmission among poor and marginalised sections of the community at the highest risk of infection by targetted interventions, STD control and condom promotion;

- reduce the spread of HIV among the general population by reducing blood-based transmission, information, education and communication and voluntary testing and counselling;

- strengthen implementation capacity at the national, state and municipal levels through the establishment of appropriate organisational arrangements, training and increasing timely access to reliable information;

- develop capacity for community-based, low cost care for people living with AIDS; and

- forge intersectoral linkages between the public, private and voluntary sectors (NACO, 1998b).

The following initiatives have been taken to promote NGO involvement and strengthening capacity.

NGO mobilisation

To facilitate greater involvement of communities, a social and NGO assessment made recently, provides a more complete understanding of vulnerability in different contexts and suggests strategies to reduce vulnerability. The strategy proposed is co-ordinated and collaborative action by the government, NGO and private sectors. Several measures to accelerate the pace of NGO involvement, include appointing NGO advisers in each state; implementing an open and transparent process for the selection of NGO proposals for funding; establishing NGO representation on government committees; convening state NGO forums to provide mechanisms for dialogue and collaboration between national and international NGOs, donors, and the government; and creating links between NGOs and proposed technical resource groups.

Strengthening capacity

Given the focus on developing capacity and recognising the need for technical inputs at the local level, technical resource groups have been formed to focus on different thematic areas e.g., blood safety; law and ethics; STDs and condom programming; counselling; workforce and industry; and research and development. Each group is located in an institution which is recognised for its excellence in that field. The group is chaired by an eminent person and members include experts with proven track records in the field of specialisation. Technical resource groups will document best practices, make recommendations for action plans, inform the programme of new knowledge, and provide technical services to the states. A secretariat for coordinating the training resource groups will be established and funded through a trust-fund mechanism. The secretariat will facilitate technical and financial linkages with training institutions and donors.

Concluding Comments

The AIDS control programme and the reproductive health approach have developed side by side, with strong mutual support and interaction as well as definite areas of intersection. The ideological underpinnings of both – a commitment to upholding human rights, informed choice, gender equity, and people-centred, need-based services in an enabling, positive environment – are virtually the same. The non-judgemental inclusive attitudes and openness to sexuality are also similar. The National AIDS Control Programme created the environment for initiating a much needed dialogue on sexuality and on providing the services relating to sexual health. And concurrently, the reproductive health approach has played a vital role in mainstreaming sexual health into the family wefare programme. Programmatically also, there are several areas of convergence related to STDs, safe motherhood, child survival, and safe sex. The strategies and approaches of both are based on the same philosophy – multisectoral focus, involvement of NGOs, in both programme implementation and policy development, decentralisation, and capacity building. There is a strong, mutually supportive relationship between the processes and philosophy globally endorsed at the ICPD, and the direction in which the national response to HIV/AIDS is developing.

References

Byron, J. 1996. A Dialogue Between the Sexes: Men, Women and AIDS Prevention. The AIDSCAP Women's Initiative, Family Health International. Arlington, USA.

Correa, S., and Petchesky, R. 1994. Reproductive and Sexual Rights: A Feminist Perspective. In: G. Sen, A. Germaine, and L.C. Chen, (eds.). Population Policies Reconsidered: Health, Empowerment and Rights. Harvard Series on Population and International Health. Boston: Harvard University Press.

Fathalla, M. 1988. Research Needs in Human Reproduction. In: E. Diczfalusy, P.D. Griffin, and J. Kharlna, (eds.). Research in Human Reproduction. Biennial Report (1986-87). Geneva: World Health Organization.

Family Health International Symposium Panel on Women and AIDS. Undated. Statement of the Caucus. In: M. Dadian, and M. O'Grady, (eds.). Cairo and Beijing: Defining the Women and AIDS Agenda. AIDSCAP Project. Family Health International. Arlington, USA.

Germaine, A., Nowrojee, S., and Pyne, H. H. 1994. Setting a New Agenda: Sexual and Reproductive Health and Rights. In: G. Sen, A. Germaine, and L.C. Chen, (eds.). Population Policies Reconsidered: Health, Empowerment and Rights. Harvard Series on Population and International Health. Boston: Harvard University Press.

Government of India and World Health Organization. 1990. Medium Term Plan for the Prevention and Control of AIDS in India. Directorate General of Health Services, Ministry of Health and Family Welfare, New Delhi, India.

Government of India and World Health Organization. 1992. Strategic Plan for the Prevention and Control of AIDS in India: 1992-1996. Ministry of Health and Family Welfare, New Delhi, India.

Hawkins, K., and Meshesha, B. 1994. Reaching Young People: Ingredients of Effective Programs. In: G. Sen, A. Germaine, and L.C. Chen, (eds.). Population Policies Reconsidered: Health, Empowerment and Rights. Harvard Series on Population and International Health. Boston: Harvard University Press.

Jain, A. 1998. Population Policies That Matter. In: Jain, A. (ed.). Do Population Policies Matter? Fertility and Politics in Egypt, India, Kenya, and Mexico. New York, Population Council. USA.

Lamptey, P. Undated. Preface. In: M. Dadian, and M. O'Grady, (eds.). Cairo and Beijing: Defining the Women and AIDS Agenda. AIDSCAP Project. Family Health International. Arlington, USA.

Measham, A. R., and Heaver, R. A., (eds.). 1996. Supplement to India's Family Welfare Program. Moving to a Reproductive and Child Health Approach. World Bank. Washington D.C., USA.

National AIDS Control Organisation. 1993. Country Scenario. Ministry of Health and Family Welfare, Government of India, New Delhi, India.

National AIDS Control Organisation. 1996. Country Scenario Update. Ministry of Health and Family Welfare, Government of India, New Delhi, India.

National AIDS Control Organisation. 1997. Country Scenario. Ministry of Health and Family Welfare, Government of India, New Delhi, India.

National AIDS Control Organisation. Undated. A Guide for the State AIDS Control Programme Managers for Collaboration on HIV/AIDS Programme. Ministry of Health and Family Welfare, Government of India, New Delhi, India.

National AIDS Control Organisation. Undated. Guidelines for Planning HIV/AIDS in the Community. Ministry of Health and Family Welfare, Government of India, New Delhi, India.

National AIDS Control Organisation. Undated. Revised Guidelines for the NGOs for Collaboration on HIV/AIDS Programme. Ministry of Health and Family Welfare, Government of India, New Delhi, India.

National AIDS Control Organisation. Undated. Guidelines for the Involvement of NGOs in National AIDS Control Programme. Ministry of Health and Family Welfare, Government of India, New Delhi, India.

National AIDS Control Organisation. 1995. AIDS Education in School: A Training Package. Ministry of Health and Family Welfare, Government of India, New Delhi, India.

National AIDS Control Organisation. 1998. Project Implementation Plan. National AIDS Control Project Phase II (1999-2004). Ministry of Health and Family Welfare, Government of India, New Delhi, India.

Pachauri, S. 1995. Defining a Reproductive Health Package for India: A Proposed Framework. Working Paper No. 4, South and East Asia Regional Office, New Delhi, Population Council, New Delhi.

Priya, R. Undated. Contextualizing AIDS: An Indian Perspective. In: M. Dadian, and M. O'Grady, (eds.). Cairo and Beijing: Defining the Women and AIDS Agenda. AIDSCAP Project. Family Health International. Arlington, USA.

Sen, G., Germaine, A., and Chen, L. C. (eds.). 1994. Reconsidering Population Policies: Ethics, Development and Strategies for Change. In : G. Sen, A. Germaine, and L.C. Chen, (eds.). Population Policies Reconsidered: Health, Empowerment and Rights. Harvard Series on Population and International Health. Boston: Harvard University Press.

Vajpayee, A. B. 1998. Address at the Meeting on National Programme for Prevention and Control of HIV/AIDS. New Delhi, India. December 12.

3

NGO Response to HIV/AIDS: A Focus on Women

Ravi K. Verma, Asha A. Bhende
and Purnima Mane

Introduction

The Joint United Nations Programme on HIV/AIDS (UNAIDS) and the World Health Organization (WHO) estimate that of the 32.2 million adults with HIV/AIDS worldwide as of December 1998, 13.8 million (43 percent) are women; and, of the 5.2 million adults newly infected with HIV in 1998, 2.1 million (40 percent) are women (UNAIDS and WHO, 1998). As of January 1998, 28 percent of the AIDS cases in India are reported to be women (NACO, 1998). This proportion is on the increase, mirroring the global situation. In this paper, we focus on the problem of HIV/AIDS in women in developing countries. We do not focus only on women in the sex trade, which is critical in itself and merits special attention and discussion, but on women in the general population who are also vulnerable but whose needs have not been adequately addressed by past programmes.

According to the National Family Health Survey conducted in 13 Indian states, where HIV is thought to be especially prevalent, only one in six women had ever heard of AIDS (Lahiri et al, 1995). The survey included the largest nationally representative sample of ever-married women and can, therefore, be taken as a benchmark for information during 1992-93. In India, currently-married women in the reproductive age group have been the targets of family planning interventions for several decades. They have been reached with contraceptive information and services. However, other important subgroups of the population, i.e., men and adolescents have not been adequately addressed by this programme.

The importance of designing interventions for HIV/AIDS prevention among women in the general population has begun to be recognised only recently. It is, therefore, heartening to note that some efforts are now underway in India. In the past, targetted interventions focussed on providing information, promoting condom use and providing services to populations at risk. More recently, efforts are being made to raise awareness, provide information, and strengthen women's capacity through empowerment processes. In this paper, programmes undertaken by non-government organisations (NGOs) to address women's needs are discussed.

Methodology

Several methods have been utilised for collecting information on HIV/AIDS interventions. We reviewed published material and sought information from organisations active in the field of HIV/AIDS. Our coverage is by no means exhaustive. The innovative and unique features of select NGO programmes are highlighted. No attempt is made to evaluate the intervention programmes or to assess their effectiveness. The objective is to paint a broad picture of the range of HIV/AIDS interventions focussing on women, that are being carried out by NGOs in India. Some government initiatives are also discussed.

Interventions for Adult Women

We discuss these interventions in four categories: (1) interventions designed to empower women; (2) interventions that address the problems of HIV/AIDS; (3) interventions that employ a need based approach; and, (4) HIV/AIDS prevention in the context of reproductive health.

Interventions designed to empower women

Within the context of women's empowerment, two approaches can be discerned. In the first approach, women's empowerment is the ultimate goal and HIV/AIDS prevention is an important intervention. The second approach is based on the assumption that no HIV/AIDS intervention can be successful unless it also deals with the issue of women's empowerment. The latter approach views empowerment as key to successful HIV prevention in women while the former focusses on empowerment and includes HIV prevention as one strategy.

The Women's Health Development Training and Service Programme of the King Edward Memorial Hospital Research Centre in Maharashtra exemplifies the first approach. This programme covers 30 villages in Pune district. Its objective is to improve the status of women by making them self reliant and confident. HIV/AIDS prevention is one of the many activities that are organised (Rao and Ranade, 1994). A similar approach is adopted by the government and NGOs who integrate HIV/AIDS prevention within education and family planning programmes for women.

The second approach deals with the problem of HIV/AIDS in the broader context of women's empowerment but with a difference. It focusses on the problem of HIV/AIDS as it affects women and sees it as stemming from their powerlessness. For example, the Mahila Sarvangeen Utkarsh Mandal (MASUM) initiated a programme in 30 villages of Pune district, Maharashtra, in 1994. This programme is broad based and uses a feminist approach to health care. It aims to strengthen women's sexual negotiating skills. MASUM treats HIV/AIDS as a broader socio-cultural problem that has its roots in sexuality. This NGO aims to promote women's sexual health and sexual rights in its widest sense; it helps women understand sexuality and sexual behaviour so that they can define their own sexuality from their perspective and modify their behaviour to ensure safe sex and to enjoy sex (Shreedhar and Colaco, 1996).

The AIDS/STD Health Action (ASHA) programme of the Mumbai Municipal Corporation is another effort to reach women in the general population. Initially ASHA focussed on women in prostitution but it now provides a platform for all women. It deals with sexual health problems as one way to empower women (Pawar et al, 1996). Women's empowerment also finds a place in the programme implemented by the Centre for AIDS Research and Education of the Y. R. Gaitonde Medical, Educational and Research Foundation in Chennai. The goal of this NGO is to provide quality medical care and relief to the poor. The objectives of the Centre are to: (1) decrease the stigma and fear associated with AIDS in the community by providing information, education and communication and increase the capacity of individuals and the community to cope with HIV/AIDS; (2) slow the spread of HIV through education and counselling; and, (3) empower HIV positive women to minimise the violence they face at home and in the community. The last objective clearly focusses on the needs of HIV positive women.

Interventions that address the problem of HIV/AIDS

The primary concern of several NGOs is to create widespread awareness about HIV/AIDS and sexually transmitted infections (STIs). Several government programmes are trying to reach the general public with information. Hoardings, posters, newspapers, advertisements, and radio and television spots bear testimony to this approach. The sole purpose of this approach is to inform one and all about the problem of HIV/AIDS without paying attention to the needs of any particular segment of the population.

Combating AIDS is a major concern of most NGOs and government organisations in the North East, particularly in the state of Manipur where HIV prevalence is the highest in the country. Although injecting drug use is the major mode of HIV transmission, the virus is now spreading rapidly to the general population because of risky sexual behaviour. A large number of NGOs have started community based intervention programmes to address women's needs. The Continuum of Care Project in Manipur has prepared a directory of resource organisations that work with married and unmarried men and women to prevent HIV/AIDS transmission, including those that provide services such as de-addiction rehabilitation, counselling, education and training. In addition, several NGOs are attempting to change the negative attitudes of the people and their misconceptions about HIV/AIDS in general, and among injecting drug users and their sexual partners in particular. These programmes aim to promote safer sex through community based interventions.

Interventions that employ a needs based approach

NGOs have always taken a lead in setting up HIV/AIDS intervention programmes in response to the special needs of the areas where they work. For example, the Mother Sardadevi Social Service Society in Tamil Nadu works in a temple town that attracts thousands of women, as it is a centre of a large vegetable producing area. This NGO implements a programme that aims to: (1) provide information on HIV/AIDS and STIs to women in prostitution and to women living in urban slums; (2) increase women's knowledge about safer sex; (3) increase condom use; (4) heighten women's health consciousness; and, (5) provide prevention and support services for women. The Society covers a range of health, environment and economic development programmes for women of different religious faiths and HIV/AIDS prevention is one of them. (Shreedhar and Colaco, 1996).

Several NGOs also report that there is no real 'felt need' for HIV/AIDS interventions in the areas where they work. For example, Myrada, an NGO that works in rural Karnataka found that the response from most people was, *"Why are you telling us about AIDS when we have so many other problems?"* The Myrada/ Plan AIDSCAP project established in 1994 is perhaps the first large scale rural initiative; it covers 492 villages. Its objectives are to: (1) create awareness; (2) provide education and services for STIs; and,

(3) promote condom use. This NGO believes that caste is an important factor in rural India:

> *"Women of lower caste, who work as labourers in the field, are often subject to sexual abuse. There have also been reports of upper caste landowners soliciting unprotected oral sex from their lower caste female labourers. The prestige attached to male promiscuity also adds to the vulnerability of rural women to HIV infection."*

HIV/AIDS prevention in the context of reproductive health

HIV/AIDS prevention is one of the services provided under the broad umbrella of reproductive health which include services for contraception, maternal and child health, safe abortion, infertility, reproductive tract infection and sexual health. The Government of India is now committed to adopting this approach (Government of India, 1997). The following are some examples of NGO programmes that have experimented with this approach.

The Family Planning Association of India (FPAI) has attempted to demonstrate the feasibility of such an integrated approach in three districts of Madhya Pradesh. This programme covers 4.35 million people in 3,901 villages and 20 towns. The Small Family by Choice (*Parivar Pragati Pariyojana*) project established in 1994, focusses on promoting the use of spacing methods within the broader context of reproductive health. AIDS prevention is one of its activities (Zamir, 1996).

Some limited experience of working with this approach in a tribal area is reported by the Society for Education, Welfare and Action Rural (SEWA-Rural) in Gujarat. SEWA-Rural's Community Health Project works with the government's primary health services and the Integrated Child Development Services programme. The project covers about 30 villages with a population of around 38,000. It is attempting to integrate prevention of HIV/AIDS and STIs within its community health programme.

Strategies for Operationalising Programmes

In analysing the strategic framework used to operationalise programmes for HIV/AIDS prevention, we find that most NGOs aim to involve the community in different ways so that it can become a partner in programme planning and implementation. Another strategy NGOs employ is to organise health services and programmes to spread awareness about HIV/AIDS and STIs in the general population.

Involvement of the community

Targetted interventions focus on changing individual risk behaviour. However, when working with the general population, it is necessary to mobilise the community to take action. The aim of involving the community is to have a longer lasting impact. For example, MASUM organises rural women in Maharashtra so that they can deal with various forms of exploitation and sexual abuse. Its health programme is based on the principle of self-help. Women learn to diagnose their infections with guidance from a nurse. They examine their own genitals with the help of a speculum and a mirror. This programme encourages women to talk about their sexuality and to place the problem in the context of their domestic and working lives. The goal is empower women so that they can eventually take charge (Shreedher and Colaco, 1996).

Myrada, in rural Karnataka, uses a similar approach by working with people's organisations such as youth clubs and *mahila mandals* (women's clubs). In this programme, peer educators play an important role in creating awareness about HIV/AIDS and STIs. They produce special information, education and communication material suited to local needs and also organise street theatre and other social and cultural activities. Similarly, the Mother Sardadevi Social Services Society works in a temple town in Tamil Nadu and uses animators who are locally recruited married women to create awareness of HIV/AIDS. Animators establish a rapport with the community.. They study sexual behaviour and help to change high risk behaviour, in a non-judgmental manner. In the opinion of the project co-ordinator, the animators are successful because they have credibility with the people.

In this temple town, many women have more than one sexual partner. They live with their families and sell sex without the knowledge of their family members to supplement their meagre family income. Though these women do not strictly fall in the category of 'sex workers', they are exposed to high risk. It would have been difficult to identify these women without the help of the animators. The NGO organises a one-week training programme for the animators to help them understand their own sexual behaviour and their attitudes to sex and sexuality as well as the special problems women face.

The operational strategy is to form women's groups. Women work together and develop confidence so that they can have a greater say in decisions affecting their lives. These groups meet regularly to discuss problems related to health, income, children, sexuality and sexual behaviour, and the attitudes of their husbands and sexual partners. A participatory rural appraisal approach is used to enable the community to participate in designing, implementing and evaluating the HIV/AIDS prevention programme.

While implementing its Small Family by Choice project, the FPAI, also depended heavily on reaching the community through local women's groups. These groups are empowered through skills development and income generation activities. It is expected that these groups will become the focal points of change at the village level. It is also expected that such an approach will enable the programme to extend its coverage to a larger population. ASHA, in Mumbai, is another NGO that reaches out to women through the formation of women's organisations. ASHA observes *"this was the first platform made available on issues related to sexual health"* (Pawar et al, 1996). Thus, we find that several NGOs are now adopting this approach. However, its long term impact has yet to be assessed.

Strengthening service provision

SEWA-Rural, an NGO that works with tribal people, is aware that high risk behaviour is widely prevalent in that community. It is, therefore, organising a programme that aims to modifying sexual behaviour of tribal people. SEWA-Rural began this work by creating general awareness but since it implements health services, it has now begun to focus on training health personnel and strengthening its referral system. A special programme for increasing the awareness of newly married couples about health, including reproductive and sexual health, is also being implemented.

Some NGOs focus on providing counselling services for HIV/AIDS and sexuality either through telephone services, which target only a limited section of people and are not always accessible to women, or through face-to-face services. The Naz Foundation and Talking About Reproductive and Sexual Health Issues in New Delhi, the Y.R. Gaitonde Medical Education and Research Foundation in Chennai, and Counselling and Allied Services for AIDS in Mumbai, are some examples. It is not known, however, whether women who are difficult to reach actually avail of these services.

At present, there are very few NGOs that provide comprehensive programmes; most provide limited services. It is, therefore, important for NGOs to review their own programmes and strengthen referral links so that women's multiple needs can be met more effectively.

Interventions for Adolescent Girls

Interventions for adolescents are classified according to the setting in which these programmes are implemented. These interventions are either community based or are based within educational institutions.

Community based interventions

Community based interventions are characterised by two approaches. Some NGOs undertake educational activities that are targetted at adolescent girls in the community. Others organise networking services for the entire community. For example, while the World Vision project in Mumbai focusses exclusively on adolescent girls, several NGOs in Manipur implement education and service programmes, where girls' needs are addressed along with other target groups in the community (Help Line, 1995).

In 1992-93, the World Vision of India initiated a project in the suburbs of Mumbai that aimed to evolve a model for AIDS prevention among low-income, urban adolescent girls. The objective was to design and test a sex and family life education programme for AIDS prevention. Quantitative and qualitative methods were used to collect data (Bhende, 1994). Several lessons learned from this experience were used to design and implement interventions. First, it became clear that for girls to participate in the programme, the support and co-operation of their parents and the larger community is essential. Second, because they carry a heavy workload, support services such as child care for their younger siblings must be provided to enable them to attend the educational sessions. Third, in addition to providing information, it is necessary to incorporate mechanisms to encourage adolescent girls to talk to each other, express their opinions freely, and build their self-confidence. And finally, for the educational interventions to be effective and relevant to the needs of this population, they should be designed to address issues related to women's status and rights rather than be restricted only to HIV/AIDS prevention.

Drawing from these lessons, World Vision of India developed an educational intervention programme to cover the following themes: being a women, puberty, human sexuality, sexual exploitation and harassment, human immune system and health problems, (specially STDs and HIV), women and AIDS and how to develop a plan of action to protect oneself against HIV infection. An AIDS awareness programme was implemented simultaneously in the community. It included meetings with community leaders, mothers of the adolescent girls, young men and adolescent boys. Street plays were organised to dramatise the status of women at different stages of the life cycle. Using the same model, a similar programme for adolescent girls and boys in the urban slums of Mumbai was later implemented by a government institution (Family Welfare Training and Research Centre, 1997).

Institution based interventions

While community based interventions require community support and involvement, intervention carried out in institutions, specially educational institutions, need the support of policy makers, decision makers and administrators. Institution based programmes have the advantage of getting a captive audience of students. These programmes try to reach adolescent boys and girls, high school students, and undergraduate college students. The programme of the BrihanMumbai Municipal Corporation and the Universities Talks AIDS programme that have been ongoing for some years reach large populations. Other small scale programmes have had a limited reach.

The experience of these programmes shows that there is growing need among adolescent girls and boys for sex education and that opposition from the parents and the community can be overcome if educational authorities take a lead in organising these interventions. Reaching out-of-school adolescents is more difficult. NGOs have made some efforts to reach them through organisations such as local sports clubs, recreational youth clubs, community centres, and shelters for street youth. Since adolescent girls have limited access to institutional services, their needs may have to be met by innovatively combining institutional and community based strategies.

Addressing the Needs of School Children

Since 1994, the BrihanMumbai Municipal Corporation has implemented an AIDS prevention programme in secondary schools. The strategy is to train the medical officers who work in these schools and involve the principals, teachers, parents and students. This programme aims to sensitise 50 percent of the municipal secondary school population – about 24,000 children in the ninth and tenth standards and all teachers and the principals (2,300) of these schools, as well as the parents. Although the programme is primarily targetted at school children, it also reaches out to women by involving parents and teachers (Nadakarni et al, 1994).

In 1995, a similar AIDS prevention programme was started by the government's health department for secondary schools in rural Maharashtra. It aims to reach rural adolescents in the ninth and tenth standards. It also involves teachers, principals and parents. The strategy is to develop a cadre of peer communicators among the students. Peer communicators – a boy and a girl – are selected from each school and are given an orientation on AIDS prevention through a one-day training programme (Verma et al, 1995). They then, along with selected teachers, organise lectures and question-answer sessions in their respective schools. This experience highlights that there is a widespread need for such programmes in rural areas. Contrary to expectations, parents do not oppose educational efforts if the teachers and principals are involved.

Addressing the Needs of University Students

Students in universities are reached through extra-curricular and co-curricular activities. For example, the National Service Scheme, an all-India programme of voluntary community service and education for students in colleges and universities, started the Universities Talks AIDS programme in 1991. This programme aims to provide AIDS education and to promote healthy lifestyles and positive attitudes (University Talks AIDS, 1993). The strategy is to spread AIDS education to the entire student community using student peer leaders as communicators. The programme relies heavily on training for leadership development. The Department of Youth Affair and Sports, Ministry of Human Resources Development, Government of India, has prepared an elaborate training manual for youth. The manual has six modules that cover: HIV/AIDS; the issues and medical facts; human sexuality; psycho-social impact of HIV/AIDS; prevention of HIV/AIDS; communication skills; and, action plan development.

The University Grants Commission, an apex administrative body for universities in India, also includes AIDS education as an integral part of its population education programme. Population Education Resource Centres produce educational material on HIV/AIDS. Several universities have organised counselling services for young people as well as a hotline (University Grants Commission, 1996).

NGOs are also reaching out to young people in colleges and universities through educational sessions on AIDS prevention and sexuality. For example, the Continuum of Care Project in Manipur has prepared a directory of resource organisations and has listed several NGOs that are working among youth in colleges (Continuum of Care Project, 1995). The Bangalore Medical Trust, an NGO in Karnataka, covers approximately 23,000 students. Since 1993, this NGO has organised educational sessions, games, quizzes, play-acting, and other activities to enhance HIV/AIDS awareness, sex and sexuality, the reproductive system, sexual abuse, risky and responsible behaviour, and condom demonstration (Bangalore Medical Trust, 1996).

Concluding Comments

Although, there is a growing momentum in efforts to address women's needs, many questions requiring urgent attention remain unanswered:

What steps should be taken to ensure the sustainability of interventions?

What indicators and criteria can be used to evaluate interventions?

How can successful interventions be replicated and upscaled?

How can lessons learned from these experiences be shared and disseminated?

How can more NGOs be encouraged to implement HIV/AIDS interventions? What financial, technical and professional support is required?

How can NGOs be encouraged to address the needs of women with AIDS? How can issues related to home-based care be addressed?

How should services be organised to address the emerging problem of mother to child HIV transmission?

The following are some patterns that emerge from the experience of NGO programmes. Some of the lessons learnt through these initiatives may have relevance for developing HIV/AIDS interventions for women:

- The fear of HIV/AIDS has led to the development of programmes that focus not only on sex workers but also on women in the general population.

- Women have started receiving attention not just in the context of childbearing and childrearing but also as sexual partners with their own needs and rights.

- The problems of STIs have not received attention in the past but is now included in many HIV/AIDS prevention programmes, even for women.

- The need to address the problem of HIV/AIDS within the larger context of sexuality is beginning to be recognised, especially by NGOs that work with women.

- Although not always explicit, there is a growing recognition that empowering women is an essential pre-requisite for preventing HIV in women.

- The importance of reaching adolescent girls and boys with sex education and information on HIV/AIDS is being increasingly realised. Such information is being included in the formal educational system.

- Although the need for comprehensive approaches is recognised, there are not many such programmes. However, when linkages are established with health care systems there are better chances of success.

- The support and involvement of the community is essential for the success of these interventions.

Gender disparities are a major barrier in efforts to enhance women's capacity to protect themselves. While gender issues are difficult to deal with in HIV/AIDS programmes, it is important to design strategies to address these problems for a meaningful long term impact.

References

Bhende, A. 1994. Evolving a Model for AIDS Prevention Education among Low Income Adolescent Girls in Urban India. International Center for Research on Women, Washington, USA.

Bangalore Medical Trust. 1996. Personal Communication from Lalitha Jaggannathan, Managing Trustee, Bangalore Medical Trust, Bangalore, India.

Centre for AIDS Research and Education. 1996. Personal communication from Suniti Solomen, Director, Y.R. Gaitonde Centre for AIDS Research and Education, Chennai, India.

Continuum of Care Project. 1995. A Resource Directory for Continuum of Care Project, Manipur, India.

Government of India. 1999. A Research Study to Develop a Programme for AIDS Prevention Education Aiming at Under Privileged Adolescent Boys and Girls in Urban Slums of India, Mumbai. Family Welfare Training and Research Centre.

Institute of Social Diseases. 1995. HIV/AIDS Intervention Amongst Injecting Drug Users and their Sexual Partners. The Helpline Centre, Singjamei Parking, Manipur, India.

Joint United Nations Programme on HIV/AIDS and World Health Organization. 1998. AIDS Epidemic Update, December 1998. Joint United Nations Programme on HIV/AIDS, New York, and World Health Organization, Geneva.

Joint United Nations Programme on HIV/AIDS. 1998. Young People and HIV/AIDS. Background Discussion Paper on the Elements of a Global Strategy. UNAIDS/PCB (7)/98-3.

Lahiri, S., Balk, D., and Pathak, K.B. 1995. Women in 13 States have Little Knowledge of AIDS. National Family Health Survey Bulletin No.2. (October). International Institute of Population Studies, Mumbai, India, and East West Center, Honolulu, USA.

Nadakarni, V., et al. 1994. Monitoring and Evaluation Study of the AIDS Prevention Programme. Tata Institute of Social Sciences, Mumbai, India.

National AIDS Control Organisation. 1998. Epidemiological Information 1998. New Delhi, India.

Rao, S.S., and Ranade, M. 1995. King Edward Memorial Hospital Research Centre, Annual Report 1995-96. Pune, India.

Shreedher, J., and Colaco, A. 1996. The Mahila Sarvangeen Utkarsh Mandal, Maharashtra. In: Broadening the Front: NGO Responses to HIV and AIDS in India. New Delhi: Actionaid, The British Council and United Nations Development Program.

Shreedhar, J., and Colaco, A. 1996. The Mother Saradadevi Social Service Society, Oddanchatram, Tamil Nadu. In: Broadening the Front: NGO Responses to HIV and AIDS in India. New Delhi: Actionaid, The British Council and United Nations Development Program.

University Grants Commission. 1996. Report of the Population Education Sub-committee on Population Education for University Students. September. New Delhi, India.

University Talks AIDS. 1993. AIDS Education for Students Youth: A Training Manual. Department of Youth Affairs and Sports, Ministry of Human Resource Development, Government of India, New Delhi, India.

Verma, R.K., et al. 1995. Evaluation of AIDS Prevention Education Programme in Rural Maharashtra. International Institute for Population Sciences, Mumbai, India.

Zamir, J. 1996. Operationalisation of Sexual and Reproductive Health Services in Small Family by Choice Project. Family Planning Association of India, Bhopal, India.

4

Management of Reproductive Tract Infections in Women: Lessons from the Field

Masuma Mamdani

With Assistance from:
Souhaila Abdulali, Sashwati Bannerji, Bishakha Datta, Renu Khanna, Sandhyarani Mohanty, Rukmini Rao, Sangeeta Subramanian Sokhi and Aleyamma Vijayanan.

This monograph is the outcome of a project funded by the Ford Foundation (New Delhi) to document the experiences of community-based programmes in addressing reproductive health needs of women in India.

Introduction

Recent policy and programme changes evidenced in many low income countries toward a more comprehensive reproductive health care approach at the primary health care level have been primarily due to the recommendations of the 1994 United Nations International Conference on Population and Development (UN/ICPD, Cairo:1994). The management and control of reproductive tract infections (RTIs), including sexually transmitted infections (STIs), at the grass roots level, is one such example.

The results of a number of community-based prevalence studies of gynaecological morbidity undertaken in the last decade, both in India (Brabin et al,1998; Koenig et al, 1998), and in other developing countries such as Nigeria, Turkey, Bangladesh and Egypt (Brabin et al, 1995; Bulut et al, 1997; Wasserheit et al,1989; Younis et al, 1993), have led to an increased awareness among researchers and policy makers, of the magnitude of reproductive tract infections and their grave consequences among poor women. In India, these have been instrumental in placing the neglected issue of RTIs on the national policy agenda (Measham and Heaver, 1996; Government of India, not dated).

The impetus for improved management and control of STIs in particular, and the resultant shift in focus, from special treatment and referral centres, to primary health care clinics, follows the advent and rise of the Human Immunodeficiency Virus (HIV) infection and the Acquired Immunity Deficiency Syndrome (AIDS) during the last decade (Chen, Sepulveda, Amor and Segal, 1991; Mann, Tarantole and Netter, 1992). Current evidence strongly supports the facilitating role of genital ulcerative diseases – chancroid, syphilis, or herpes – in HIV-1 transmission (de Schryver and Meheus, 1990; Finger, 1992). The recent results of a study carried out in Zaire, also suggest trichomoniasis to be a risk factor for HIV-1 transmission (Laga et al, 1993).

On the whole, the relationship between nonulcerative STIs, such as gonorrhea, chlamydia, and trichomoniasis, and HIV-1, has yet to be assessed. Nonetheless, as about 80 percent of HIV-1 infection is spread by the sexual route, experts agree that in order to prevent the spread of HIV-1, a global initiative would be required in the prevention and control of STIs, at the primary health care level (Adler, 1996).

While there is greater knowledge and awareness of RTIs in India, significant gaps nevertheless persist in our understanding of how to address these most effectively at the community level. India has had a national programme for the prevention and control of STIs since the 1960s, but services are either of poor quality, inaccessible, or socially unacceptable (Luthra et al, 1992; Nag, 1993; Ramasubban, 1996). On the whole, the public sector health programme, which is the largest source of health care in India, is not need-based or gender-sensitive. Most existing services are not designed to reach women (Starrs and Measham, 1990; Jejeeboy, 1996). Those that are, such as maternal and child health and family planning services, have poor coverage, and have until recently, been preoccupied with meeting only contraceptive targets.

Women in India face constraints, not only in obtaining services, but also in expressing their reproductive health needs (Gittelsohn et al, 1994). Lack of awareness, cultural barriers and economic factors prevent them from seeking timely care. Women are relatively unlikely to seek advice when there is a tendency to view morbidities such as 'white discharge' as normal, and when the condition is often associated with shame or guilt, owing to its perceived link with promiscuity. Further, most women with a lower RTI, are asymptomatic. Pelvic examinations are strongly resisted by all women, but more so, if they are asymptomatic, and especially, if they are to be performed by health service providers who are not sensitive to their needs. Finally, given most women's limited mobility and their lack of autonomy in decision making, it is unlikely that they will take the initiative in obtaining health care for themselves.

All RTIs are preventable. Moreover, all, except some of those caused by viruses, are curable. But, the prevention, treatment and control of RTIs is unfortunately a complex issue. A multitude of factors – psychological, economic, political, and social – foster their spread and must be addressed, if RTIs are to be brought under control (Dixon-Mueller and Wasserheit, 1991). Health professionals in India meet considerable challenges in scaling up RTI services within the public sector. Several issues need to be addressed. For example, given limited resources and expertise, what can be done at the primary health centre level? What services can paramedical and non-medical workers realistically be expected to provide at the grassroots level? What is the rationale for women-focused programmes versus those that also address men? What are the trade-offs, between comprehensive provision of RTI services, versus selective or phased introduction for specific morbidities? What should be the balance, between interventions focusing on education, or awareness and curative care?

A useful first step in seeking possible solutions is to closely examine existing health programme models. Although at a relatively embryonic stage, there are a small but growing number of community-based programmes addressing the issue of RTIs. With few exceptions, these examples are found mainly within the voluntary sector (non-governmental organisations, or NGOs), as more comprehensive reproductive health services have yet to diffuse to the public sector programme. Owing to limited funds, and noting that women have few resources to access health services, most of these programmes started by targetting only women in their various activities. Realising that women's reproductive health needs cannot be addressed without the support of their male partners, some programmes are beginning to reach out to men, albeit with limited success. It is now important to understand how these programmes, designed to address women's reproductive health needs, have been conceptualised and implemented.

The purpose of this review is not to provide a blueprint for the development of future RTI programmes but to synthesise the lessons from existing programmes, primarily from the voluntary sector, in providing RTI services to the communities they serve, and thereby provide guidance for future activities in the public and private sectors. The objectives are to gain an insight into their approach, the difficulties encountered, the major operational factors involved, and the sustainability of such programmes in the long term. Much of the information was obtained from field visits, undertaken by a number of consultants over the last couple of years (see Appendix I for a brief summary of the scope and methods of the project).

This paper: (1) provides an overview of RTIs and their magnitude in India, highlighting some of the methodological problems encountered in assessing the prevalence of RTIs; (2) draws upon the experiences of a cross-section of programmes, and discusses some of the critical problems encountered in the effective management of RTIs in resource poor settings, especially at the community level and, (3) discusses some of the key issues that need to be considered when thinking about scaling up RTI services within the public sector. As policies increasingly embrace reproductive health as a central programme tenet, the question of how to cost-effectively and feasibly provide such services will increasingly emerge as a central issue for the next decade.

An Overview of Reproductive Tract Infections

Reproductive tract infections in women usually originate in the lower tract – external genitalia, vagina, and cervix (Dixon-Mueller and Wasserheit, 1991). These may be sexually transmitted; or they may be endogenous infections, resulting from an overgrowth of organisms normally present in the reproductive tract. There is usually some overlap between each of these two modes of transmission. Without early treatment, certain RTIs – gonococcal and chlamydial infections and bacterial vaginosis organisms – can spread to the upper genital tract (uterus, fallopian tubes, and ovaries) and cause pelvic inflammatory diseases (PID). This spread may be spontaneous. It may also be facilitated by the introduction of instruments through the cervix during poor quality medical procedures, such as when inserting an intra-uterine device (IUD), during procedures such as sterilisation, or unsafe abortion and delivery practices.

A majority, but not all STIs are also RTIs. Some STIs, such as syphilis and HIV/AIDS are also systemic infections (Adler, 1995). Further, only a minority of the 40 or so different microbial agents, which can be sexually transmitted, have sexual transmission as their sole or dominant route of spread. For example, HIV is mainly transmitted sexually, though it may also be transmitted perinatally, and via infected blood or blood products (as in intravenous drug users). Likewise, the transmission of the syphilis pathogen is usually by the sexual or transplacental route, but it may also be through contaminated blood.

Women are recognised to be vulnerable, both biologically and socially. In most societies, because of their sexual behaviour – unprotected sex with multiple partners and/or with female sex workers – men are usually at a higher risk of initially contracting STIs, and subsequently transmitting them to their wives or sexual partners (Brabin, 1993). Nonetheless, once infected, the clinical management of STIs in men is usually simpler than treating comparable infections in women (Hawkes, 1998). In contrast to men, a greater percentage of women with STIs – gonorrhoea and chlamydia, in particular – are asymptomatic; consequently, they do not seek treatment and are at an increased risk of developing PID (Schulte,1994). In addition, for reasons previously noted – lack of awareness, fear of social stigmatisation and poor access to appropriate services – even symptomatic women often fail to seek timely care. Women also tend to suffer more because of the synergistic effects of infection, malnutrition and reproduction.

The consequences of untreated RTIs in women range from acute distress to death (Elias, 1991). Women with PID are at an increased risk of tubal infertility, ectopic pregnancy, recurrent urinary tract infection, considerable pain during coitus, menstrual irregularities and chronic pelvic pain. The incidence of PID-caused infertility in developed countries is estimated at 15-25 percent of all gonorrhoea and chlamydia cases, increasing to 70 percent after three episodes (Schulte, 1994). The percentages are thought to be higher in developing countries, because PID treatment is usually very delayed, of insufficient duration, or completely unavailable (Germain et al, 1992). For example, around 50-80 percent of female infertility in Africa, is thought to be due to RTIs (Wasserheit and Holmes, 1992). Little is known about the levels, patterns and determinants of infertility in India. Figures of 6 to 7 percent have been quoted, though these are thought to be under-estimates (Jejeebhoy, 1995). Infertility can be a devastating social handicap for women in India, and often leads to marital discord and social ostracism.

In addition, accumulated data strongly suggest that STIs such as genital warts, that are caused by certain types of human papilloma virus (HPV), are the primary causal agent of cervical cancer (Luthra et al, 1992; Richter, 1990). Though most HPV infections are symptomatic, they are difficult to treat. Finally, the fact that certain STIs facilitate the transmission of HIV-1 adds substantially to the total health impact of RTIs.

Failure to diagnose and treat RTIs in pregnant women can also adversely affect child health and child survival. For example, if a pregnant woman infected with early syphilis, remains untreated, her foetus has about 40-50 percent chance of perinatal death or prematurity (Adler, 1995). Infants born to mothers infected with chlamydia and gonorrhoea, are at risk of congenital infections which manifest as sepsis, pneumonia or ophthalmia neonatorum. Recent data also show an association between bacterial vaginosis and preterm labour and delivery, though the evidence is not conclusive (McCoy et al, 1995; McDonald et al, 1997; Joesoef et al, 1995; Morales, Schorrs and Albritton, 1994).

Magnitude of RTIs in India

Till recently, little was known about the extent of RTIs among women in India. Much of the available data was limited to high-risk, or, clinic-based populations, and, as expected, indicated a relatively high prevalence of many RTIs. For example, a survey of 370 female sex workers in West Bengal (referred to as the Sonagachi study from here on), revealed that 13.2 percent of these women were suffering from gonorrhoea, 58.8 percent from syphilis, 11.1 percent from trichomoniasis and 23.2 percent from candidiasis (Singh, 1995). In all, 80.6 percent of these women were infected with single or multiple RTI pathogens. Though the prevalence of HIV infection in the 442 FSWs tested was found to be quite low (1.1 percent), conditions are highly favourable for the rapid spread of infection (Pal et al, 1994).

Likewise, reports of men and women attending government sexually transmitted disease (STD) clinics, point to an increasing trend in the number of cases seen at the clinics, from 1981 to 1991 (Luthra et al, 1992). The actual numbers are likely to be an underestimate, largely because a substantial number of cases resort to private practitioners or pharmacies for treatment and therefore go unreported. Interpretation is also made difficult by the fact that this increasing trend may be the result of an actual increase in STI rates, but could also be due several other possible factors: for example, a growing susceptible population; more people resorting to STD clinics for treatment; improved diagnostic skills; and/or, better reporting procedures.

In general, information pertaining to high-risk, or clinic-based populations, is useful, but of limited value, since it is atypical, and not totally representative of the population. However, in the last few years, a number of community-based prevalence studies of gynaecological morbidity among women have been undertaken in India. The study findings have provided invaluable insights into the problem of gynaecological morbidity in general, and RTIs in particular, in what may be termed as 'low-risk' women. The results of six of these studies are shown in Table 1. A marked variation is

TABLE 1: Prevalence of Self-Reported and Clinically Diagnosed Gynaecological Morbidity Among Women: Community-Based Studies in India

Location	1	2	3	4	5	6
			Percentage of women			
SELF-REPORTED SYMPTOMS:						
Sample size	654	500	756	840	440	1103
Menstrual problems	60	33	41	58	65	59
Excessive discharge	13	50	31	22	22	57
Lower abdominal pain	13	17	21	9	16	NA
Lower backache	30	5	39	24	NA	30
Dyspareunia	7	2	NR	NR	1	NR
One or more conditions	55*	65	74	65	NA	84
CLINICALLY DIAGNOSED MORBIDITY:						
Sample Size	650	500	756	548	385	324
Vaginitis	62	4	15	11	13	10
Cervicitis	48	14	40	13	24	8
Cervical erosion	46	2	21	5	10	20
PID	24	1	16	8	11	8
Prolapse	0.5	17	18	5	3	NA
One or more conditions	NA	43	74	26	70	43

NR = not recorded; NA = Could not be ascertained from available data

Source: *Koenig et al. (1996)*

* Does not include lower back and lower abdominal pain.

1 = SEARCH's (Society for Education, Action and Research in Community Health) Study in Rural Maharashtra, 1989 (Bang and Bang, 1996; Bang et al, 1989)

2 = CINI's (Child in Need Institute) Study in Rural West Bengal, 1990-91 (BCC et al, 1995; Bhattacharya, 1994)

3 = Streetakarini's Study in Mumbai, 1988-89 (BCC et al, 1995; Parikh et al, 1996)

4 = BCC's (Baroda Citizen Council) Study in Baroda, 1990-91 (BCC et al, 1995; Latha et al, 1994)

5 = Study in Karnataka undertaken by a team of researchers, 1992 (Bhatia and Cleland, 1995; Bhatia et al, 1995)

6 = SEWA-Rural's (Society for Education, Welfare and Action-Rural) Study in Rural Gujarat, 1988-89 (BCC et al, 1995; SEWA-Rural Research Team, undated)

evident across these studies regarding the patterns and levels of both self-reported symptoms, and clinically diagnosed RTIs. The percentage of women reporting excessive discharge, for example, ranged from 13 to 57 percent. Overall, the percentage of women reporting one or more symptoms, indicative of RTIs, or related morbidity (PID) ranged from between 55 to 84 percent.

The prevalence of clinically diagnosed conditions, ranged from 4 to 62 percent for vaginitis, 8 to 48 percent for cervicitis, 2 to 46 percent for cervical erosion and 1 to 24 percent for PID. By and large, conditions such as vaginitis, cervicitis and PID affected more than 10 percent of women in most sites.

In contrast, the recent findings of another community-based study, carried out among women living in Mumbai slums (reffered to as the Brihan Mumbai Municipal Corporation Study, or the BMC Study, hereafter), shows a relatively low prevalence of all RTIs (Brabin et al, 1998). As seen in Table 2, even common endogenous infections, such as candidiasis, which may have been expected of women from such poor socio-economic background living in unsatisfactory housing conditions, were not that common, as was also observed among women from a similar background in the Streehitakarini study. The BMC study was one of the largest detailed microbiological studies ever undertaken in a low-risk population in India, involving 2,879 non-pregnant women. Using sensitive culture and polymerase chain reaction (PCR) techniques and a very stringent criteria for defining RTIs, the findings from this study suggest that STIs are not a major factor contributing to reproductive morbidity, or PID, in this population of Indian women.

With reference to the three studies considered in Table 2, the relatively high prevalence of RTIs among women examined in the rural Maharashtra study for example, may, to some extent, be due to their poor access to appropriate health facilities. In general, much of the observed variability (Tables 1 and 2), may be attributed to the use of widely varying sampling designs and diagnostic procedures for RTIs. These include possible selection bias, variations in questionnaire wording and the extent of probing, variable reference periods, as well as the lack of standardisation in clinical definitions

TABLE 2: Prevalence of RTIs Based on Laboratory Investigations

Location and Year of Study	Sample Size	Chlamydia	Gonorrhoea	Syphilis	Trichomoniasis	Candidiasis	Bacterial Vaginosis	Pelvic Inflammatory Disease
Gadchiroli, rural Maharashtra, 1989[3]	558 ever-married women	n/a[4]	0.3	10.5	13.98	34.05	62.19	n/a
Mumbai, urban Maharashtra, 1988-89[5]	569 (exc. chlamydia)	n/a	1.1	0.2	7.7	16.5	8.3	n/a
	399 (inc. chlamydia) ever-married women	14.5	1.5	0.3	9.8	17.3	8.3	0.1 (0.5)[8]
Mumbai, urban Maharashtra, 1993-95[6]	2,433 controls	0.2	0.1	2.8	0.9	0	0.5	
	446 cases[7]	0.5	0	0.5	0.5	0.9	2.2	7.1 (11.9)
	295 infertility cases	0.3	0	4.1	0.3	0.3	0.3	3.8 (10.7)
	151 suspected PID cases, ever-married women aged < 36 yr.	0.7	0	0.7	0.7	2.0	6.0	24.0(18.0)

[3] Community-based prevalence study undertaken by SEARCH (Bang et al, 1989) [4] n/a: not assessed [5] Community-based prevalence study undertaken by Streehitakarini (Parikh et al, 1996) [6] Community-based prevalence study undertaken by Briham Mumbai Municipal Corporation (BMC) and the Liverpool School of Tropical Medicine, UK (Brabin et al, 1998)

[7] Cases are women who presented for gynaecological investigations either with symptoms of acute PID (suspected PID), or a history of infertility (excluding those women with an infertile male partner); controls were fertile women seeking tubal ligation and who had no symptoms of gynaecological disease.

[8] percent women with acute salpingitis, percent women with chronic PID in parenthesis; diagnosis based on laparoscopy findings; no. of women examined - 2425 controls and 311 cases (50 suspected PID cases and 261 infertile women).

and criteria for RTIs (Brabin et al, 1998; Koenig et al, 1998). For example, on clinical grounds, Brabin et al. classified 74.8 percent of the suspected PID cases as having PID; whereas, only 42 percent of the suspected PID cases were in fact confirmed by laparoscopy. In the Sonagachi study mentioned earlier, endocervical pus was found in approximately 12 percent of the women (Singh, 1995). Of these, only 16 percent were found to be positive by the Gram smear, and 10 percent by culture. On the whole, less than 20 percent were positive by either of these laboratory techniques. With regard to the six prevalence studies considered in Table 1, Koenig et al. also indicate the possibility of under-reporting of certain STIs, and over-reporting of others, such as white discharge, due to lack of specificity in asking questions. Reporting also appears to have been strongly influenced by the background of the interviewer : morbidity levels reported to medical practitioners, or to interviewers, shortly preceding clinical examinations, tended to be significantly higher than those reported to interviewers in home visits.[2]

On the whole, the above results emphasise two important facts: first, the low levels of correspondence among the three commonly used modes of assessing RTIs – self reported symptoms, clinical diagnosis and laboratory examinations; and second, the difficulties entailed in comparing prevalence rates from studies, in the absence of standardised criteria for the diagnosis of RTIs, even when these may be using the same source of information.

In brief, based on available data, it is difficult to draw any firm conclusions on the extent of RTIs amongst women in India. The lack of standardisation in defining RTIs has resulted in extremely variable estimates of prevalence, and there is no readily discernible pattern to indicate which women are most in need of services.

---

[2] Similar observations were made by a study carried out in Istanbul, Turkey, where 81 percent of the women reported experiencing one or more symptoms associated with reproductive morbidity when interviewed by a physician; and 65 percent when interviewed at home by an interviewer (Bulut et al, 1995). Both, the Turkish study and another study undertaken in Egypt (Zurayk et al, 1995), indicate little agreement between self-reported symptoms and clinical or laboratory diagnostic status.

Management of RTIs at the Community Level

Non-governmental organisations (NGOs)

A number of NGOs deal with the problem of RTIs in women at the community level. This report is based on a detailed assessment of seven of them. Their approach may be broadly categorised into the following three groups, though there are some significant variations within each of them:

Clinic-based programmes

These are undertaken by the Ashish Gram Rachna Trust and Sonagachi. All RTI cases (mainly women, in the case of Ashish Gram; and female sex workers and their clients at Sonagachi), are diagnosed and managed by a doctor (who may also be a qualified gynaecologist) at the clinic. Both programmes have community-based health workers who are trained to disseminate information, raise awareness and refer symptomatic cases to the clinic.

Clinic cum community-based programmes

These are undertaken by the Action Research in Community Health and Development (ARCH), the Bhansali Trust, the Rural Women's Social Education Centre (RUWSEC), the Society for Education and Action Research in Community Health (SEARCH), and the Society for Rural Education and Development (SRED). All their programmes train and support community-based health workers in symptomatic or syndromic management of RTIs (mainly vaginitis) in women, using allopathic or herbal remedies. Recurrent cases (usually STIs) are supposedly referred to a doctor or a qualified gynaecologist at the programmes' clinic. Except for SRED, which refers cases in need of laboratory tests to the nearest government facility, the remaining four programmes have laboratory facilities, though there is a wide variation in the range of services they are able to offer. There is a significant difference in their approach at the community level. At the Bhansali Trust, for example, the focus is on pregnant women where the community health workers (CHWs) conduct home visits for antenatal care. Health workers at SEARCH, ARCH and SRED attempt to raise awareness in their project area, and provide services to all women seeking assistance, either from their homes or at the patient's home. RUWSEC's health workers conduct routine home visits and according to a standard check list, probe for symptoms indicative of RTIs.

Community-based programmes

These are mainly done at Aikya. Here, community-based health workers are trained as 'barefoot gynaecologists cum counsellors' to identify and treat the most common RTIs (mainly vaginitis) in women, using herbal remedies. Cases which require specialist care are referred to the nearest government or private health facility.

The principal aim of all these programmes is to prevent the development of RTIs, their complications, and sequelae, and to interrupt and reduce the transmission of RTIs. This can be attained through the two approaches of primary and secondary prevention (see Box).

Strategy for the Management of RTIs: Some Examples

Primary Prevention

Health Education/ Information, Education and Communication: Promote safe and responsible sexual behaviour – partner reduction or selection; use of condoms and female barrier methods; reduction of non-consensual sex (rape, violence against women); promote hygienic practices; minimise use of intravaginal products which may be harmful; minimise infection prevailing practices and improve overall quality of health care/ family planning; and, increase access to safe abortion practices.

Secondary Prevention

Improve reproductive and health-seeking behaviour; identify established infections; manage symptomatic infections; and, detect and treat asymptomatic infections through case finding and screening.

Source: Elias 1996

This section mainly draws upon the experiences of the seven programmes in discussing some of the major obstacles encountered in effectively managing RTIs at the community level.

Case management

Asymptomatic Women

Many women with RTIs are asymptomatic. For example, 82 percent of the 151 asymptomatic females examined in the Sonagachi study, were infected with at least one RTI pathogen (Singh,1995). Screening programmes are important if these women are to be found and treated. Active case detection is generally difficult, especially in settings where facilities and materials for laboratory testing are limited or non-existent. It is financially not viable. Experience has also shown that asymptomatic women are most unlikely to undergo invasive screening procedures, such as a pelvic examination. However, where facilities are available, the screening of asymptomatic women, presenting for antenatal care or family planning services, for example, is more feasible. With the exception of SEARCH, which screens all antenatal cases presenting to their hospital for bacterial vaginosis, the focus of all programmes is on diagnosing and treating symptomatic women. Thus, a significant number of women, especially those with STIs, remain untreated and will therefore continue to transmit infection.

Symptomatic Women: Health Care Seeking Behaviour

Except for RUWSEC, where community health workers undertake regular home visits, and routinely probe for symptoms indicative of RTIs, the diagnosis and treatment of RTIs in all programmes is usually limited to women who are aware of, and present with, symptoms perceived to be related to RTIs. There is some evidence which reveals that even when services are available, women fail to use them (Bang et al, 1989; SEWA-Rural ,1994). Often, women only seek assistance when they are suffering from the secondary complications of the infection – such as PID, ectopic pregnancy or infertility. Why do women not utilise the available services? The reasons are not clear but, as earlier mentioned, may be manifold: lack of awareness, cultural and economic barriers, etc.

It is all the more important therefore, to implement appropriate educational strategies towards raising awareness and changing health seeking behaviour. This necessitates outreach efforts to women with limited access to health services, and to those who might not consider themselves at risk for RTIs. Various strategies have been adopted by these programmes, in their attempt to ensure that women recognise symptoms associated with RTIs, and realise the importance of presenting themselves for treatment. A number of programmes have also undertaken exploratory in-depth studies to understand women's and men's perceptions of morbidity, and in establishing local terms and expressions for describing gynaecological complaints. A couple of them have also documented their findings: SEARCH (Bang and Bang, 1991; 1994), and, SARTHI – Social Action for Rural and Tribal Inhabitants of India (Amin, Fatula and Grenon, 1996; Amin, Fatula and Khanna, 1997; Grenon, 1996; Grenon and Mawji, 1996). These studies show that several synonyms are frequently used to describe white discharge. People have their own intricate classification, each with distinct characteristics, and different significance; there is a hierarchy of perceived severity among them. These findings have been crucial for the delivery of appropriate and acceptable health education and counselling.

The process of modifying beliefs and practices is always a slow one. But, women at Aikya, SARTHI, RUWSEC, SEARCH, SRED and Sonagachi for example, are gradually beginning to view RTIs as genuine health problems. Given a supportive environment, they are opening up and coming forward with their concerns. For example, at Aikya, at a recent session held by a trained health worker, for local women on vaginal infections, the women sat around openly discussing problems they had endured in silence all their lives.

Diagnosis of Symptomatic Women

The most important aspects of management are accurate diagnosis and effective treatment. Diagnosis needs time and skill, in taking a detailed sexual history from the patient (number and type of sexual contacts in the last few weeks, symptoms in partner), and in carrying out a comprehensive physical examination. But above all, microbiological and serological facilities are essential, initially, and at follow up, for all patients, to differentiate between the various infections, and exclude more than one occurring at a time; this holds especially true for STIs.

On the whole, few community-based programmes have laboratory facilities and the required specialist staff. The logistics and infrastructure required are often beyond the means of most programmes. Further, due to financial constraints, even programmes with basic laboratory support provide minimum services for RTIs, or at times, none at all, as for example, at the Ashish Gram Rachna Trust. In general, there appears to be no standard protocol. Laboratory tests are often undertaken on an ad-hoc basis, usually for detection of suspected gonorrhoea and syphilis, and only when the doctor or the community health worker in charge is in doubt. Further, there is increasing variability between the different laboratory tests. Typically, both culture and rapid nonculture tests differ in their sensitivity and specificity, depending on the population being studied – high or low risk, male or female, genital or extragenital sites. The more sensitive techniques are usually not available in the field. For example, the standard test used for the diagnosis of gonorrhoea is the microscopic examination of a Gram stained specimen, a technique which has very poor sensitivity, especially in women, and particularly in low prevalence areas. Sole reliance on this test results in about 50 percent of cases being missed. None of the programmes is able to provide routine culture services for the detection of chlamydia, which cannot be identified by direct microscopy, although it may occur concurrently with other STIs, in particular, gonorrhoea. The diagnosis of syphilis can be confirmed by one or all of the following four tests – dark ground microscopy, serology, examination of cerebrospinal fluid, and radiology (TPHA test). Which of these tests appear as positive will depend on the clinical stage of the disease. Dark ground microscopy is a vital test, since, in primary syphilis, it may be the only positive means of establishing the diagnosis. But considerable experience is required to recognise the pathogen. Currently, the recommended best combination of tests for the screening of syphilis is the VDRL test and the TPHA test (Adler, 1995). However, none of the programmes with laboratory facilities is able to provide the TPHA test; all rely solely on the VDRL test implying that as many as 20 percent of women may end up receiving treatment for a condition they do not have, and just as many cases of primary syphilis will go untreated. The diagnosis of vaginal infections on the other hand, can be made relatively easily with a microscope, although none of these programmes do this routinely.

Syndromic management

In the absence of diagnostic laboratory support, and the lack of clinical expertise in many resource poor settings, and acknowledging the difficulties inherent in accurate clinical diagnosis, the World Health Organization (WHO) has placed increasing emphasis on the use of a syndrome-based approach for the diagnosis and treatment of RTIs in symptomatic patients, especially at the grassroots level (WHO, 1991). These algorithms are advocated for use by trained community-based health workers, particularly in high prevalence areas, and rely on the manifestation of the most common symptoms which include: urethral discharge in men; genital ulcers in both men and women; abnormal vaginal discharge in women, and lower abdominal pain in women. The algorithm for genital ulcers assumes that the two commonest causes of such a sign are syphilis and chancroid, and that it is appropriate to give therapy for both conditions. Likewise, the algorithm for urethral discharge assumes that the etiology could be gonococcal and/or chlamydial, and that the therapy appropriate for both should be utilised. The algorithm for vaginal discharge recommends therapy for four conditions: gonorrhoea, candidiasis, trichomoniasis and bacterial vaginosis. The one for lower abdominal pain recommends therapy for PID.

In order to contain costs, improve women's access and treatment at an earlier stage, most community-based programmes have adapted the WHO algorithms and trained their health workers in syndromic management of RTIs in women, in particular vaginitis. Health workers at SEARCH are also trained to diagnose and treat PID in women. Unfortunately, none have really tried to evaluate its effectiveness in their particular setting. Nevertheless, it is clear from the findings of the studies cited earlier that symptoms and signs in women are poor predictors of most RTIs.

Results of studies carried out elsewhere – Turkey (Bulut et al, 1995; Filippi et al, 1997), Egypt (Zurayk et al, 1995), Tanzania (Mayaud et al, 1995) and Zaire (Vuylsteke et al, 1993), for example, have also shown that the algorithm for vaginal discharge, usually the most common presenting symptom in women, is not that discriminating and its usefulness appears to be limited, especially in the diagnosis of STIs. In the case of Tanzania also, the results demonstrate that it performed poorly in screening pregnant women with symptoms of vaginal discharge and/or genital itching for gonococcal and/or chlamydia infections; the sensitivity was 43 percent and the specificity was 58 percent. The results from Kinshasa and Zaire indicate a weak relationship between the classical symptoms and signs, with the eventual diagnosis of gonococcal and/or chlamydial infection in both high prevalence (prostitutes) and low prevalence (pregnant women) populations.

From a public health point of view, the priority is to identify and treat the largest proportion of women who have a RTI. The syndromic approach may ensure that all women presenting with an abnormal vaginal discharge, and clinically diagnosed to have a possible RTI, are receiving the required treatment. However, in addition to the fact that the approach misses out on a significant proportion of asymptomatic women in whom RTIs occur without abnormal vaginal discharge, the studies cited above have demonstrated that even in symptomatic women, the approach performs poorly; both in high and low prevalence areas. Many women suffering from a RTI are being missed out; also, many are being treated for conditions they may not be suffering from. Apart from the obvious fact that the approach is not cost-effective, it also results in overtreatment, with potentially negative side effects, and possibly poor compliance by patients.

To address this problem, the WHO has developed a simple risk score system[9] for the identification of chlamydia and gonococcal infections in women complaining of vaginal discharge (WHO/GPA, 1993). Accordingly, all women with an abnormal vaginal discharge, should receive treatment for vaginitis (candidiasis, trichomoniasis and bacterial vaginosis); in addition, women with a positive risk assessment should also receive treatment for gonococcal and chlamydial infections. The objective is to increase the specificity of the algorithm by restricting treatment of cervical infections to those who are at highest risk. The usefulness of the new WHO risk assessment algorithm has not as yet been evaluated in India, though health workers at some of the programmes – the Ashish Gram Rachna Trust, RUWSEC, SEARCH and SRED – do intuitively apply a form of risk assessment, albeit an unstandardised approach, when assessing the need to refer a patient for further diagnosis. Although these health workers are to a certain extent able to discuss, and procure information, that may be sensitive in nature, in the absence of any data that would allow for an assessment of the validity of the information obtained, it is not possible to know if the women are telling the truth.

The findings of a number of studies carried out elsewhere are mixed. For example, the results of a recent study performed among pregnant women, with or without vaginal discharge, in Kenya, suggest that none of the demographic or behavioural factors of the WHO score were associated with cervical infection; the sensitivities were found to be very low for both the WHO score (13 percent) and the syndromic management (20 percent) (Thomas et al, 1996).

The results of another recent study, undertaken in Tanzania, demonstrate that this new approach in dealing with women complaining of vaginal discharge and/or genital itching, can considerably reduce overtreatment of gonococcal and chlamydia

[9] The following five questions comprise the WHO risk score: Are you aged less than 21 years? Are you single? Have you had a new sexual partner in the last three months? Have you had more than one sexual partner in the last three months? Has your partner experienced urethral discharge and/or dysuria within the last month?

infections, in both pregnant and nonpregnant women (Mayaud et al, 1998; Mayaud et al, in press): 63.5 percent of non-pregnant women and 80 percent of pregnant women would be correctly treated (i.e., receive treatment, if infected, or not receive treatment, if not infected). However, it failed to identify 38 percent of nonpregnant and 54 percent of pregnant women with these infections, leaving many women with potentially serious infections untreated. The results from Tanzania also suggest that, as a screening tool among pregnant women, who often do not recognise, or report symptoms related to STIs, the WHO score system performs poorly, and is not a cost-effective option: only 10.2 percent of cervical infections were identified; the specificity was 92 percent and the predictive positive value was 9.8 percent.

The results of an international study on family health in Jamaica showed that in symptomatic women, the new WHO algorithm had a sensitivity of 84 percent, a specificity of 39 percent, and a positive predictive value of 42 percent (Family Health International, 1994).

Several other scoring systems have also been developed and evaluated in different setting, as for example, in Kinshasa (Vuylsteke et al, 1993), rural Tanzania (Mayaud et al, 1995), Gabon (Bourgeois, 1996) and Kenya (Daly et al, 1994). Once again, the findings are mixed, and imply that a considerable refinement of vaginal discharge algorithms is still required. They also indicate that the risk determinants may vary in different settings; cultural inhibitions, particularly, in countries such as India, to some of the questions which require disclosure of the respondent's sexual practices could be a challenge, and may need to be evaluated. The challenge exists to find rapid, reliable and inexpensive diagnostic tests, that can be used for widescale screening purposes for most STIs, especially chlamydia.

Treatment

Through Herbal Remedies

Most NGOs located in remote rural areas, face tremendous problems in recruiting and retaining well-trained professionals who share their 'women-centred' perspective. To make health care more accessible, affordable and sustainable in the long-run, a growing number of programmes without the necessary infrastructure – SARTHI, Aikya, SRED and Deccan Development Society (DDS), for example – are encouraging traditional health practices, especially for women's health.[10] They are working with herbalists or traditional healers, and are documenting their current practices, attempting to evaluate the use, their acceptability amongst potential users, and encouraging these practices when they work (Shodhini, 1997). To ensure ready availability of basic herbs that are routinely used, these groups have planted herbal medicine gardens which hopefully will become a resource to the health workers in each village. The health workers are trained to provide a range of services (see Box). But, as pointed out by Rukmini Rao of DDS (1997), though these health workers are able to identify reproductive tract infections, they are unable to provide further refined categorisation of the problems. Treatment is symptomatic, and it is not clear if these cures are permanent, or of a reasonable duration, or the extent to which women use the herbal remedies. Without a systematic reporting system, it is impossible to ascertain their effectiveness. This notwithstanding, experience does suggest that herbal remedies are popular and often the first choice of treatment as they are culturally more acceptable and prescribed by accessible healers.

---

[10] SARTHI, DDS and Aikya, have been key participants in the Shodhini project which was carried out from 1987 to 1990 (Khanna, 1996). Shodhini was working for alternatives in women's health, based on the self-help methodology and plant-based medicines. Central to the project was the object of empowering women to take greater control over their bodies and health, and train local women to recognise and treat common gynaecological problems.

Poshamma, a Village Health Worker (VHW) at DDS

Poshamma is approximately 30 years old, and has been working as a health worker for the last eight years. She mainly provides herbal medicines and referral services. Poshamma's story is best told in her own words.

"I am a member of the DDS *sangam*, and have been working as a health worker for the last eight years. In the beginning I did not know anything. We started meeting regularly and learning about herbal medicines from each other, particularly from older women from nearby villages, who were experts. We were a group of 40 women. Now, I provide medicines for a number of problems women suffer from. For example: for white discharge, I suggest 10 varieties of herbal medicines; for red discharge, I suggest two plants that work very well. If there is a vaginal infection, I suggest the use of boiled neem leaves to wash the vagina. Usually, I have a detailed discussion with the women to identify the exact problem. For example, if there is any smell in the white discharge, we identify this as an infection and give appropriate treatment. If the problem appears serious, I insist on an internal examination. If cervical cancer is suspected, I refer the patient to a regular gynaecologist in Hyderabad , who helps us by providing cross verification. I have been able to cure women with vaginal blisters, etc., by giving them the appropriate treatment. In some cases, surgery is carried out. Many women in the villages suffer from prolapse of the uterus. If the problem is at the initial stage, I recommend exercises and teach the women how to do them. I also suggest the use of two or three herbal medicines... Though I am a *Dalit* woman (untouchable), I go into all the households in the village...In the last few years, I have treated over 60 cases of white discharge, about 15 women with red discharge, about 23 cases of prolapse of the uterus and 10 with other gynaecological problems. Most have been cured, but few remain uncured. Shiva Kala for example, has had white discharge for the last three years – her husband is not cooperative, and does not allow her to go to the city for referral. Though she has had a tubectomy, her problem continues, and has not been resolved. Then, there are five cases of prolapse of the uterus, but the patients are either very afraid to be operated on, or, are suffering from extreme poverty, and are not able to pay for the surgery. And, Santa, whom I identified some months ago, does not want to talk about her problem. Chandramma, from Pastapur village, died because she had cancer. She had been referred to government hospitals in Hyderabad... I also give treatment to men, if they come forward. Usually, we need to refer them to other doctors. I provide couples information about family planning. Men also come to me for condoms; very often however, it is the women who do. I visit the Permaculture school twice a week, and teach the children about herbal medicines. I also advise adolescent girls on how to deal with menstrual cramps... The nearest PHC is at Jharasangam, and to go there, I have to pay Rs 2.50 as bus fare. I now know the Medical Officer very well. The auxiliary nurse midwife, and three other health staff are all my friends now. Emergency cases or difficult deliveries, are referred to Zaheerabad or Bidar. I usually accompany the patients... Abortion cases are also referred to the local doctors. Usually, I don't like to be involved with abortions, but I help occasionally, particularly if the girls are unmarried... Over the years, people's belief in herbal medicines has grown... Although we dispense medicines at home, we find that people are not willing to pay, because they are not used to it. Initially, we used to give free herbal medicines, but now, we ask people to pay. I find it difficult not to give medicines when people need them, and I occasionally get Rs 2 or 3 for the medicines dispensed... This programme has helped me a lot. I used to be impatient and reluctant to conduct deliveries, but now I am more patient... I have learnt to do deliveries, and support women who have a number of problems. My husband is very supportive of my work, which is what enables me to carry on... I feel we are now stagnating and need to develop our skills further. Not having literacy skills is a major problem for us."

Sexually Transmitted Infections

The most difficult issue is the effective management of STIs. To prevent the spread of STIs, the treatment must be effective, and be seen to be effective. This means selecting the correct dose of medication for the disease, carefully monitoring its administration, and carrying out regular follow-up microbiological tests. The patient's sexual contacts must be traced, so that they also can be treated, and thus prevent re-infection.

Recurrent infections are reported to be quite common. To what extent are these recurrences due to women genuinely becoming re-infected because of inadequate tracing and treatment of sexual contacts? To what extent are they re-infected due to an incorrect diagnosis made in the first instance? Or are the strains resistant to the prescribed antibiotic? Or due to poor compliance with the full course of treatment? Following are some of the constraints programmes face, in not only trying to trace and treat sexual contacts of all women with STIs, but also in ensuring cure in the women themselves.

Constraints

Inadequate Information System

It is important to acknowledge the immense difficulties involved in implementing an effective supervision and follow-up system at the community-level. To begin with, it would be quite impossible to follow-up on all RTI cases to ensure they have been cured, especially in instances where programmes are reaching out to a large and scattered population – as for instance, in the case of the Orissa Institute of Medical Research and Health (OMRAH), or the Bhansali Trust. A simple but efficient reporting system however, which includes a symptoms check-list and the results of previously carried out tests, might enable a more efficient and methodical assessment of the diagnosis made, and of the treatment given by the health workers, whether it is allopathic, or herbal in nature.

A common feature of most of the community-based programmes is a weak or non-existent information system.

Traditional birth attendants at SEARCH routinely refer patients to the out-patient department, but information from these patients is usually obtained orally and informally, and much of it goes unrecorded. Women health workers at SARTHI record a patient's history, and their diagnosis of the illness, the treatment prescribed and the outcome, but systematic information on the accuracy of their diagnostic skills, or the outcome of the treatment is not available. Community health workers at RUWSEC usually advise herbal remedies as the first course of treatment. Despite RUWSEC's attempts to implement a standardised monitoring and reporting system, the scrutiny of one of the family folders revealed the following: '...the course of treatment and advice offered by the health worker was comprehensive. In addition to the herbal treatment that she advised for white discharge, she also suggested that the woman wash the area with a salt solution. Further, she advised her to clean her underskirt, boil it and not bathe in the pond to prevent spreading the infection. However, the suggested herbal remedy appeared to be standard for all types of white discharge. Besides, each visit was treated as a separate episode and even after two months of a woman having the same complaint, no referral advice was given; the same herbal treatment was repeated.' This observation has been made possible because RUWSEC had a detailed record-keeping system. Similar problems probably exist in all programmes but, in the absence of accurate patient records, it is not possible to make any comments. ARCH is one of the few programmes which has maintained a patient's case history over the last three years, though it is not clear if this data base was used as a monitoring tool. A prerequisite would obviously be to make use of these records, and systematically review them on a periodic basis.

Further, if the available resources are to be optimally used, it is important to ensure that programmes have adequate monitoring and evaluation systems. This can be achieved through routinely collected statistics, supplemented by ad hoc surveys. It is important to appreciate that the collection of reliable and relevant statistics will require resources. People responsible for collecting routine statistics will need to receive adequate training and supervision, if the quality of the data that they collect are to be maintained.

Referral Care

The second constraint revolves around the accessibility of appropriate referral services, and the ability and willingness of women to take time off and seek care. Only the clinic or clinic cum community-based programmes are able to provide referral services, and that also only to a limited extent. As previously noted, most such programmes provide basic laboratory facilities and have yet to develop effective linkages with the government health services. Moreover, with programmes which look after a large and scattered target population, as in the case of the Bhansali Trust, women come from quite a distance, and rarely return for a follow-up visit to ensure cure, let alone bring their husbands.

Most community-based programmes do not provide referral care – as is the case at Aikya, SARTHI, DDS, and SRED. Their health workers however, do encourage the use of referral services available at the local primary health care clinic and hospital, especially for STIs. Unfortunately, the public sector health programme is not need-based, and 'women-friendly' services are not available to most women, especially rural women. Often, facilities are located at a distance and women do not have the means to pay transportation costs to the referral facility, or fees for private care. A number of patients at DDS, for example, need to be referred to hospitals or private practitioners. The consultant gynaecologist charges Rs 25 per patient; abortion services cost Rs 400; emergency transport (by private taxi) to the referral hospital in Hyderabad would cost them another Rs 4,000, etc. This raises the issue of having appropriate and affordable referral services at a reasonable distance. Accordingly, some of these programmes are considering the possibility of liaising with private pharmacies and private doctors.

Social Repercussions

The third constraint common to all programmes, is the fear of social repercussions (in particular of being labelled as promiscuous) as a result of prevailing social norms which prohibit extra or premarital affairs. Thus, married women are usually not willing to report the existence of any partner(s) other than their husbands. Likewise, single, widowed or divorced women will rarely provide information on their sexual contacts. Besides the fact that it is difficult to reach out to the clients of female sex workers, the sex workers will usually not inform their 'regular partners' that they are suffering from a STI, given the possibility that the source of infection could be one of their casual contacts.

Limited Male Involvement

The fourth constraint is the reluctance of husbands or partners to seek assistance, especially if they are asymptomatic. To a large extent, this may be because most programmes are targetted mainly at women, and are unavailable to men at risk. There are a couple of programmes which have tried, but failed to involve men, because they did not have male health workers, and cultural considerations preclude female staff from treating any man presenting with sexual problems. Several programmes are gradually beginning to address and involve men in their activities. Their approaches may be broadly categorised as follows:

Education and Motivation

A number of community-based programmes are attempting to involve men where sexual and gender education are provided. The focus is on sensitising men (and at times adolescent boys) to gender issues, and on promoting safe and responsible sexual behaviour. They reach out to men through male health workers. Reports from Aikya and SARTHI for example, note an increased awareness amongst men regarding STIs and a visible change in their attitude. But in the absence of clinical services for men, it is not clear if these men receive appropriate care for STIs.

Educational Sessions and Clinical Services

Of the clinic-based programmes, a few are attempting to actively involve men by raising awareness and by providing clinical services as in the case of RUWSEC, SEARCH, Sonagachi and SRED. Two distinct approaches have been tried. One is raising awareness informally, at the individual level, by the male health workers, peer educators, village-based male activists and at times, through mass awareness raising campaigns, such as cultural fairs or health festivals. This has met with some success. For example, as a result of SEARCH's intensive health education campaign, the men sent a memo demanding that their needs be studied. However, even at SEARCH, where clinical services are available, men prefer not to seek advice or treatment from male health workers, and usually opt for private or traditional care for their sexual problems. In addition to the fact that traditional remedies continue to be popular, men are reluctant to approach someone who may be from their village and possibly a social acquaintance; confidentiality is obviously a key issue. Sonagachi has opened an evening clinic for clients of female sex workers, but it is not clear to what extent these facilities are being used.

A much more structured and comprehensive approach has been adopted by RUWSEC. Activities focusing on men are carried out in about 30 villages, and include informal counselling and referrals for STIs, from male health workers at the village level; separate gender sensitisation workshops for adult, married men, and unmarried adolescents, and for young married couples; condom promotion and diagnostic and treatment services for STIs. The reports are encouraging and positive. RUWSEC's experience also shows that it takes a long time for men to begin seeking services. One interesting aspect worth noting, is that RUWSEC does not have its own male health workers; it financially supports two local men's groups – the Social Development Trust (SDT) and the Social Education for Development Trust (SED) – to carry out its agenda in the villages. RUWSEC also provides relevant training to staff from these two organisations. Where SDT works intensively with men in RUWSEC's villages, SED conducts workshops in villages covered by other NGOs. Husbands of RUWSEC's health workers are actively involved in both SDT and SED, and provide the first point of contact between RUWSEC and the two organisations. On the whole, such an approach not only solves some of the constraints involved in managing a larger workforce and an increasing number of activities; it perhaps also offers men in the community a degree of anonymity or confidentiality, in the sense that the staff involved are not viewed as part of RUWSEC, and also may not necessarily be from the villages they are working in.

The provision of STI services to both men and women in controlling morbidity in the men themselves and in their female partners are essential. Moreover, an increased awareness in men will perhaps make it easier for women to seek treatment, when necessary. SARTHI, for example, admitted to making a tactical error when they did not involve men in the decision to broaden their women's health programme to include gynaecological care (Khanna, 1996). Many women were prevented by their husbands from attending the gynaecological camps. SARTHI has gradually been able to work through the fear and resistance among men, through its male community health workers, who have also participated in educational workshops on gender issues, including common reproductive health problems of men and women.

Prevention

Health Education/ Condom Promotion

Various efforts were made in health education programmes through *mahila mandals* (women's groups), modern mass media, workshops, through traditional modes of communication, peer groups and through individual contact and counselling. These attempt to promote hygienic practices and propagate safe and responsible sexual behaviour. Some target only women, while others have sought to reach out to men also; a few are beginning to involve adolescents. Depending on the target population, the messages tend to vary in content, emphasis and delivery. For example, at Sonagachi, peer groups provide special information, education and communication programmes focusing on HIV/AIDS, and promote and distribute condoms to female sex workers and their clients. At ARCH, information is disseminated at the antenatal clinics, at special health education sessions, and informally, by the community health workers, at the village level, albeit only to women.

Unfortunately, possible risk factors such as poor menstrual hygiene, are not a problem of awareness alone. They are related to affordability of better means of hygiene and water supply. The biggest problems facing many of these programmes – the Bhansali Trust, RUWSEC, Streehitakarini, and Krishan Nath Baba Memorial Trust and Health Centre, for example – are poor environment and sanitary conditions. Often, women have no place to take baths or have no latrines, and such conditions make it difficult to improve the women's well-being beyond a certain point.

A number of programmes are beginning to promote and encourage the use of condoms. Promising results are reported by a few programmes. For example, RUWSEC reports a steady increase in the demand for condoms, that are usually distributed at its sexual education workshops for married and unmarried men (RUWSEC, 1996). Evidence from Sonagachi shows that increased condom use has been accepted by the clients of female sex workers and this has an impact on the levels of infection also. Results of a repeat cross-sectional survey conducted among a sample of female sex workers, after 14 months of intensive health education campaign, including promotion of condoms by peer workers, showed that awareness of STIs and AIDS had increased greatly, and the regular use of condom was reported by 47.2 percent, as against 1.1 percent during the baseline survey (Singh, 1995). The prevalence of gonorrhoea was 3.9 percent as against 13.2 percent during the baseline survey; trichomoniasis was 9.8 percent as compared to 11.1 percent earlier; syphilis was 49.6 percent as against 58.8 earlier; and, candidiasis was reduced from 23.2 percent to 6.4 percent. In all, only 59.2 percent of the sex workers were infected with single or multiple pathogens as compared to 80.6 percent during the baseline survey. Some of this reduction may also be attributed to female sex workers (and perhaps their clients), seeking timely care as a result of their increased awareness, and also due to the availability of acceptable clinical services. Nevertheless, unsafe sexual practices remain a

The **MYRADA/PLAN AIDSCAP Project** working for Devadasis[11] in 525 villages of Belgaum district, in southern Karnataka has shown the importance of a community-based education process, and of community participation in promoting behavioural changes. The project did much work toward achieving its goal of increased awareness of HIV, and other STIs in their community. Although the project has ended, it is worth a mention, because of the ingenious ways the staff found in bringing a sensitive subject to the attention of the people, and helping them make informed choices about their lives. The project created awareness about transmission and prevention of STIs and AIDS, through training sessions held separately for men and for women; through *Gee Gee Melas* (old men who go from village to village, singing folk songs, on several themes including HIV and STIs); through separate all-male and all-female street theatre performers who disseminate information, and, through the local media, with occasional radio spots and newspaper advertisements. The project produced, and disseminated thousands of posters, stickers and pamphlets produced locally, mostly in Kannada and Marathi; and very colourful and attractive, with a focus on pictures rather than words. The project promoted condom use through education and marketing. And, though they had no doctors of their own, they upgraded the skills of registered medical practitioners, in diagnosing and treating STIs and AIDS, so that people in the more rural *taluks* had someone reliable to go to with their problems and questions. Most important, the project did not target 'high risk' groups alone, but the whole community.

---

[11] Devadaasi women in India live disseminated throughout rural villages where they typically maintain steady relationships with men often in exchange for monetary support (Sivaram, Gowda and Sogunro, 1995). Identified with their historical role as 'servants of Gods', these women are invited by the community to religious functions in their areas of residence. There are 2145 Devadaasi women in Belgaum district.

predominant cause of the continuing high levels of STIs among female sex workers, and recurrent infections are common.

Younger and inexperienced female sex workers are usually intimidated, and are unable to effectively negotiate the use of condoms by clients. Also, most female sex workers are not very successful in persuading their regular partners to use condoms. With the objective of reducing their dependency on the clients, and in an attempt to create a sense of security among female sex workers, a sexworkers' forum, which provides loans on easy terms, has been recently set up; arrangements have also been made with a centre for counselling and social support, that provides legal and paralegal advice. It is hoped that the psycho-social support provided by the programme will boost the morale of the sex workers, and empower them to resist abuse.

Overall, the success of such programmes is often difficult to assess, but it is clear that repeated reinforcement and monitoring are necessary, if initial modifications in behaviour are to be maintained over longer periods of time.

Alcohol Rehabilitation Programme

An interesting aspect of SEARCH's work with men has been the rehabilitation of alcoholics. SEARCH sees it as an integral component of reproductive health for two reasons: alcoholism inevitably affects the web of sexual, emotional, psychological and power relations between men and women; and they found that 75 percent of the alcoholics treated, suffer from STIs. The rehabilitation programme consists of a 15-day residential camp, held at the SEARCH campus; about 20 people attend each camp. After the camp ends, alcoholics commit to meeting once a month. Those who slip back into alcoholism, are allowed to attend a second time, but no more. SEARCH claims a sobriety rate of 50 percent.

Quality of care

To minimise possible morbidities, due to unsafe delivery practices, all programmes have trained their health workers – some of whom are traditional birth attendants, and others without this background

– in safe delivery practices and promote the use of safe delivery kits. In most, but not all instances, such health workers have also been trained in the symptomatic diagnosis of RTIs. The women in this way, are also being screened, and either treated by the health workers themselves, or referred to an appropriate facility, for pre-existing conditions. A few of the clinic-based programmes have also begun to provide safe and confidential abortion services for married and unmarried women, as for example, at the Ashish Gram Rachna Trust, RUWSEC, SEARCH and SRED. Some of these – ARCH, Ashish Gram, Bhansali Trust, RUWSEC, SEARCH and SRED – have started to screen women for RTIs before inserting an intra uterine device (IUD). Screening usually entails a physical examination. Along with the fact that asymptomatic women will not be detected, the limitations of diagnosing STIs, in particular on the basis of signs and symptoms, have already been discussed earlier.

Sustainability

The costs of RTI interventions, per se, are difficult to estimate. Nonetheless, it is evident that many programmes are constrained by their limited resources. Considering the difficulties involved in providing sustainable RTI services, several programmes have often opted for the sporadic camp approach. An inherent limitation of this approach is that not all women in need of care will seek advice. Another, is the quality of care provided. Women usually fail to receive appropriate follow-up care, in terms of suitable referral services, adequate health educational inputs, and the likelihood of treating sexual partners of women suffering from STIs. Adequate reproductive health services, including appropriate referral care, to meet the demand generated, and to provide comprehensive services to women, beyond the one RTI/STD episode that first brings them into the system, is not only important from an ethical perspective, but is also a prerequisite for the credibility of all these methods and programmes. Few women would agree to undergo a gynaecological examination, if effective follow-up treatment is not provided.

To improve access and make services economically viable, many programmes have opted for community-based management. Many have adopted the strategy of training locally recruited women. In some instances, the health workers are on the payroll of the programme (ARCH and Bhansali Trust); in other instances, they are gifted cash and kind[12]. At times, health workers rely solely on income they get from patients for their services. In most instances, salaries are not very attractive. Their motivation comes from the new skills they acquire over time, and the resultant increase in their credibility among the women they serve. There are, however, instances where health workers feel that they are paid a very small honorarium, and do not get due recognition for their work as at DDS, for example.

In order for any programme to succeed, there must be a level of interest in its development and sustainability on the part of the community members. A major problem is the very poor paying capacity of some of the patients. NGOs have an explicit mission to serve the disadvantaged. Although all programmes levy various user charges for services, considerable effort is devoted to providing partial, or full subsidies, to those who cannot afford the fees. However, even with fees fixed at nominal levels, a number of women at RUWSEC, for example, are not easily able to access services as a result of their inability to pay (RUWSEC, 1996). This was clearly evident when RUWSEC briefly experimented with providing free services once a month: hundreds of patients would turn up on the "free day".

Another problem encountered in some of the programmes is the patient's unwillingness to pay for services, especially if the same services have been available at no cost for some time. SARTHI, for example, has been experimenting with a participatory programme in some of its villages – the Sahbhagi concept (SARTHI, 1996).

---

[12] At Ashish Gram Rachna Trust for example, traditional birth attendants (TBAs) are permitted to charge for medicines and immunisations. These collections are retained and account for about 60 percent of the TBA's renumeration. TBAs, therefore have a strong incentive to seek out clients for immunisations, since they also benefit financially from increased coverage. In addition, TBAs receive an honorarium from the Trust, for delivering a complete package of antenatal and postnatal care, and child health services for three months.

Villagers are asked to contribute with funds and services. Initially, villagers were resistant, and did not wish to pay for medicines or medical services they could avail at no cost from the nearby primary health centres. Also, they simply could not come to terms with the fact that they could entrust matters related to their health to a volunteer who was far from their idea of a conventional doctor. Or take the example of DDS, where it is becoming increasingly difficult, and in the long run economically non-viable, to run the programme and develop it without people paying for herbal medicines. Raw materials have become quite expensive, and DDS has requested its health workers to charge a nominal fee for some of the services they provide. In some of the new villages where DDS has recently started working, people are willing to pay for herbal remedies, albeit on an ad hoc basis, but, there is increasing reluctance generally, from residents of the older villages to pay for herbal preparations, or for services, all of which they were till recently receiving at no cost.

Most groups aim for self-sufficiency, and have a very pragmatic approach to development, through integrating health with economic and social issues. However, health care requires huge inputs that no small organisation can afford. All programmes in the voluntary sector are, to a large extent, reliant on external funding. As a result of the increasing international commitment to RTIs, it is very likely that external resources will be available to support and expand RTI programmes for some time to come. Such funding could be put to good use – such as providing logistic and training support. But such support can also have repercussions. For example, external resources can also have considerable recurrent cost implications. Who is to be responsible for such long-term resource requirements? Are programmes generating a demand in the community which they may not be able to meet in the long term? In particular, one needs to consider the financial viability of clinic-based management. There is, on the one hand, the issue of possible over-medicalisation of services (tests and treatment) to justify the investment, and, on the other, the issue of its future ability to handle an increased case load. At present, it appears that only a fraction of the cases comes to the attention of the clinics concerned. In the long run, if numbers reporting for treatment increase, will the clinics be able to handle this increased case load? Additional financial inputs to cover treatment costs, and additional staff will most certainly be required. Furthermore, as programmes expand their range of activities and geographic coverage, can they still retain their level of efficiency, or will dilution inevitably take place?

While clearly woman-centred, woman-friendly clinical services are lacking in most parts of the country, and taking on the onus of starting such facilities within an NGO (which has other major agenda of community education and empowerment) may be putting too much burden on the organisation. The challenge of making the services truly woman-friendly, medically rational and radical in serving women's real needs, will bring up a host of conflicting issues that will need to be dealt with.

In summary, therefore, a number of programmes in the voluntary sector have attempted to address the issue of RTIs within their integrated approach to women's health. The approach has largely depended on the programmes' philosophy, available resources and their priorities in the light of other equally-pressing issues that may need to be addressed. Some are essentially clinic-based programmes, providing allopathic treatment. Others are exclusively community-based and have opted for various approaches: focusing on awareness raising, holding sporadic gynaecological camps, training their community-based health workers in the syndromic management of the common RTIs, such as using herbal remedies. The rest offer a mixture of both types of services.

The few programmes discussed in this paper, reflecting a variety of approaches, have shown that community-based workers can be trained to diagnose, and treat, some of the more common infections – candidiasis, bacterial vaginosis and trichomoniasis – among symptomatic women. Their experience confirms that the training of community-based workers in treating RTIs is a huge undertaking, and requires a substantial degree of on-going commitment over a period of time. Also, in the absence of a systematic reporting system, with a standardised check-list of symptoms, using a risk score driven approach, it is not clear if these women are receiving appropriate treatment, or if most women with STIs, are being identified, and referred, and also to what extent these cures, be they herbal or allopathic in nature, are permanent, or of a reasonable duration. In addition, the ability of health workers in making a correct diagnosis is very much hampered by the shortcomings of the syndromic approach in predicting RTIs in women. This notwithstanding, the experience of at least one these programmes, does confirm that health workers can also be trained to perform simple microscopic tests, that would enable them to make a more definitive diagnosis for these common conditions, but not many programmes have access to basic laboratory facilities. While several programmes have attempted to network with the nearby government facilities for appropriate referral care, often, such facilities are ill-equipped to address the issue.

In all instances, **effectively curing** STIs, leave alone preventing their recurrence, has proved to be a formidable task. To begin with, many women with gonorrhoea and chlamydia are asymptomatic, and although a few programmes attempt to screen all women seeking invasive family planning services (IUD, sterilisations, abortions), active case detection is generally viewed to be difficult, mainly because of poor diagnostic facilities available in detecting these STIs in women. Moreover, the impact of the treatment on the women is likely to be limited, unless, their sexual partner(s) receive concurrent treatment. Although a few programmes are attempting to reach out to men, they have met with varying degrees of success. Most are attempting to involve men, at the level of providing sexual and gender education, and promoting the use of condoms. Some are also attempting to provide clinical services. Their experience implies that for reasons of confidentiality, even where services are available, men often choose to seek assistance from pharmacies and private practitioners. Community-based workers can play a vital role in liaising with traditional healers, pharmacies and private practitioners, who are often a major source of care to many men and women.

All of the programmes discussed in this paper have chosen the more hopeful avenue of making people more health conscious through health education and awareness-raising, and through programmes aimed at enhancing women's self-confidence and self-image. Such interventions will perhaps encourage women to actively seek medical care when necessary. Most of these programmes have had some success with such efforts. There has been a perceptible increase in the level of awareness among both women and men about RTIs. Given a suitable setting, women are beginning to come forward and discuss issues of concern to them, issues that were once considered taboo subjects. There has also been a willingness to seek timely medical assistance, if available.

Scaling up RTI Services Within the Public Sector

The control of reproductive tract infection, including sexually transmitted infections, has been given high priority in India. The impetus comes from two sources. First, results of a number of community-based studies undertaken in the last decade, imply that RTIs are not limited to 'high-risk' populations, but are also prevalent within the general population, especially amongst those with poor access to appropriate health facilities. Second, it appears that STIs facilitate the transmission of HIV, which is one of the most important reasons for controlling STIs. Estimates of more than 1.75 million HIV-infected adults throughout India have been reported (Lalvani and Shastri, 1996). Recent results from studies carried out in Pune (Mehendale et al, 1995; Rodrigues et al, 1995) and Chennai (Solomon et al, 1994), demonstrate an increase in the incidence of HIV infection among STD clinic attenders. Both studies note the risk of HIV-1 infection in STD clinic attendees to be around 10 percent, per year. The results also suggest that this increase is not confined to people with high-risk behaviour, but is also gradually spreading into the population at large – antenatal mothers, voluntary blood donors and women who claim to be monogomously married.

Historically, STD control services have generally been implemented through vertical programmes (Pachauri, 1994). The emphasis has been on preventive efforts among targetted high-risk groups, and the treatment of individuals with disease symptoms and their sexual partners. Such services have been of poor quality, and not very accessible. More recently, as part of its recent shift in focus towards a reproductive health approach at the community level, the Government of India is planning interventions for the management of RTIs, including STIs, at all levels of the health system (Government of India, undated). It is hoped that fully decentralised STD services will not only be more accessible to the general population, but will also be less stigmatising than centralised services. Such efforts however, will also require greater inputs in terms of resources, both financial and personnel, and commitment – at the national and community level. Fundamental decisions will need to be made about the level at which laboratory support and diagnosis should, and can be provided.

At issue is how to identify and treat the maximum number of infected persons at the community level. Auxiliary nurse midwives, female health workers, and traditional birth attendants in rural India often serve as the initial source of contact to a majority of the women. What can they do? What can be done at the primary health centre level? To date, NGOs have been at the forefront of most integration efforts. The challenge is now to take the relevant experiences to scale and translate them to the government services.

The choice of strategies really depends on the prevalence of the different RTIs among women (especially STIs vs. endogenous RTIs); the level of infrastructure (laboratory, health facilities, trained staff); the access of women to these structures; and, the missed opportunities for the screening of such infections. Tables 3 and 4 give some possible options that may be considered. A mix of strategies is recommended: training community-based workers in diagnosing and treating certain endogenous infections in low-risk women, certain STIs in men, and developing a strong referral link

TABLE 3: Management of RTIs at Different Levels of the Health Care System: Some Options

Common RTIs	Community-based health workers – male & female	PHC/MCH-FP clinics	Referral clinics (STD clinics/ hospital out-patients department)
Candidiasis	+[1]	+	+
Bacterial vaginosis	presumptive diagnosis	+	+
Trichomoniasis	–	+	+
Syphilis	–	maybe[2]	+
Gonorrhoea	not in women, syndromic algorithm in men	in men	+
Chlamydia	–	–	maybe[3]
PID	–	–	+
Facilities	standard check list, speculum, litmus paper, potassium hydroxide	standard diagnostic criteria, microscope, technician trained in wet-mount & Gramstain techniques, possibly VDRL/ RPR tests	standard diagnostic criteria, microscope, technician trained in wet mount, Gramstain & culture techniques, VDRL/ RPR & TPHA tests & maybe laparoscopy for PID diagnosis

Issues: 1. Follow-up visit and contact tracing in case of STIs to ensure cure; 2. possibility of sending appropriate cervical specimens for culture test and of women returning for a follow-up visit; if not possible, may consider treating all female partners of STI infected men for similar infections; 3. at the community level, likelihood of low-risk women in whom symptoms persist returning for a referral.

---

[1] + denotes can be done at the stated level of health care; means it is not possible.

[2] where syphilis is known to be prevalent, every attempt should be made to equip the PHC clinic with VDRL test and staff should be trained accordingly.

[3] only possible at central referral laboratories

TABLE 4: Addressing RTIs at the Community Level – Possible Options

Female sex workers & clients	Pregnant women	General population
i). Encourage all symptomatic FSWs and clients to seek early assistance from adequately equipped clinics; for example, STD clinics, hospital outpatients; liaising with informal sources of care to ensure appropriate diagnosis and treatment. ii). Periodic screening of all FSWs for STIs.	i). Routine screening of all pregnant women in their first trimester for bacterial vaginosis; can be done at community level & with women presenting for antenatal care at MCH clinics. ii). Where syphilis is prevalent, consider routine screening of all pregnant women at clinic level for primary syphilis. iii). For parents of infants born with ophthalmia neonatarium, test for gonorrhoea where possible, otherwise treat for gonorrhoea and chlamydia iv). Other RTIs in symptomatic pregnant women: as for general population	i). Screen symptomatic women and treat accordingly for candidiasis; presumptive diagnosis for bacterial vaginosis (BV) at community level; refer women with a possible BV, 'high-risk' women and those with recurrent infections to clinic ii). Screen all women undergoing invasive procedures - IUD, sterilisation, abortion, etc. for possible RTIs iii). Screen symptomatic men and treat for STIs at community level; where necessary refer to clinic for confirmation.

Issues: i). Likelihood of tracing, diagnosing and treating all sexual contacts; ii). possibility of confirming VDRL positive cases using TPHA test and tracing and treating pregnant women with early syphilis; iii). problems inherent in identifying and screening all pregnant women for BV in their first trimester since women are often not aware of their pregnancy status in the first months; and also due to poor access to antenatal care; iv). likelihood of 'low-risk' women with recurrent infections returning for a follow-up visit; v). necessity of liaising with alternative sources of health care (traditional healers, pharmacists, private doctors) to ensure correct treatment regimen and with possibility of tracing sexual contacts.

with adequately equipped primary health centre clinics/ maternal and child care – family planning facilities for further diagnosis and treatment; routine screening of pregnant women for certain RTIs; and periodic screening of all 'high-risk' cases – female sex workers and their clients. These options are further elaborated in the following sections.

Management of symptomatic cases at the primary health care level

The problems inherent in relying solely on self reported symptoms and/or on a clinical examination, have been clearly demonstrated by the results of the community-based studies undertaken in India, and by a number of other studies undertaken elsewhere. The reports of studies evaluating the syndromic approach in women have not been very encouraging. Those dealing with the new risk-score approach have been mixed. However, according to the community-based studies, and reports of women seeking assistance from lay workers and maternal and child health/family planning clinics, a common presenting symptom is vaginal discharge with, or without vulval irritation, most often caused by candidiasis or bacterial vaginosis (BV), or concurrently with other STIs – trichomoniasis, gonorrhoea and chlamydia. For low risk women, who will hopefully return for a reassessment if symptoms persist, non-specialists, may, in the absence of laboratory facilities, be able to provide empirical treatment for candidiasis alone. A presumptive diagnosis of BV can be made relatively easily, and inexpensively, by testing the vaginal secretion pH (the procedure involves using the pH dipstick, and a strip of paper which changes colour); and by a positive amine test (using potassium hydroxide for the detection of characteristic amine odour in vaginal secretions). Women testing positive on both these tests, should be referred for a definitive diagnosis. An accurate clinical and sexual history, using a score-driven approach that ought to be evaluated, may be taken to identify and refer all high risk cases to an appropriate facility.

Current laboratory techniques for the detection of gonorrhoea and chlamydia in women are complex and expensive, and not cost-effective, especially for chlamydia. The need for simple, reliable and low-cost tests to diagnose gonococcal and chlamydia infections among women, particularly asymptomatic women, remains a high priority. Health workers at primary health care clinics can however, be trained to perform two simple microscopic tests: the 'wet-mount' test for detecting trichomoniasis and candidiasis in women; and the Gram stain test for diagnosing bacterial vaginosis in women, and gonorrhea in men. Microscopy can also be useful in detecting syphilis in both sexes, though detecting the syphilis pathogen requires some expertise.

Primary health care centres can send cervical specimen to the more specialised STD clinics or district hospitals for diagnosing gonorrhoea and possibly chlamydia infection in women, or for confirming syphilis diagnosis. In fact, one of the priorities for the National AIDS Control Programme is to target STD clinics to improve the diagnosis and management of all STIs (Anonymous,1994). Noting that such clinics are often used by 'high-risk' cases, they should ideally, be equipped to provide more comprehensive services – microscopy, culture of neisseria gonorrhoea, antigen detection of chlamydia trachomatis at certain referral centres, non-specific and specific tests for syphilis and tests for screening HIV. Unfortunately, such referral services are often more costly, time-consuming and logistically difficult. Selecting the appropriate site for culture may be difficult. Further, for either culture or immunologic techniques to be effective, adequate and appropriate specimens must be collected, rapidly transported to the laboratory, cultivated on appropriate media, and evaluated by an experienced laboratory personnel (Larsen, 1985; van Dyck et al, 1996). Experience has also shown that women at times fail to return to a health facility, whether it is to get results of diagnostic tests, or to confirm symptom resolution.

Effective STD clinical treatment also requires tracing all sexual contacts of the index patient and treating them also, if necessary (Toomey, Latif and Steen, 1996). Partner notification is needed to stop the chain of transmission of STIs. It also serves as an opportunity to provide focused education – how STIs are spread, the effects of infection, and how to reduce the risk of exposure to STIs. In fact, if primary health care clinics can use partner notification to identify core groups, they may have a greater impact on STD control. Unfortunately, as evident from the NGO experience, women are usually not very successful in getting their spouses, or sexual partners, to seek appropriate care.

Addressing Men With STIs

For several reasons, it is important to target STI services at men, though this should never be at the expense of providing high quality, comprehensive reproductive health care for women. As discussed earlier, STIs in women are hard to manage, because of the inadequate health-seeking behaviour of the sufferers, poor diagnostic facilities to detect STIs in primary health centre facilities, and the asymptomatic nature of gonococcal or chlamydial infections in many women. In contrast, men suffering from STIs are more likely to be symptomatic, and thus seek treatment, albeit mainly from pharmacists or traditional healers. Men do not face the many cultural constraints women do, in seeking treatment for STIs. The diagnosis of STIs in men is much more manageable at the primary health centre level, using the standard Gram stain technique: At the community-level, the syndromic approach in men – for both urethral discharge and genital ulcers – seems to work well in detecting STIs, though its use needs to be validated in India. More important, it is possible that men will be more likely, and able, to bring in their partners for treatment than vice versa, and this may well lead to the identification of asymptomatic women. Finally, an increased awareness in men themselves, will perhaps also make it easier for women to seek treatment.

There is the fear that public sector facilities providing STI services at the primary level are predominantly maternal child health/ family planning based, targetted mainly at women, and may be unavailable to men at risk. However, a recent study undertaken in rural Bangladesh, a relatively conservative society, demonstrates the feasibility of establishing STI clinics for men, within the existing maternal and child health and family planning system (Hawkes, 1998). In fact, in response to client demand, the clinics moved beyond simple STI care, towards the provision of comprehensive sexual health services for men. Addressing STIs in men will have certain financial implications. For example, it will entail the training of community-based male health workers in the management of STIs in men, forging links with pharmacists, and the private sector, and referring patients for medical evaluation and further counselling, when appropriate, though the cost of setting up a provider referral system may be too high.

Training Health Care Providers in Appropriate STI Diagnosis and Treatment

The effective treatment of STIs, also depends on the administration of the right type, and dosage of a drug. However, programmes often cannot afford, or do not have access to the more sensitive recommended antibiotics for STIs. In such circumstances, it is important to monitor the efficacy of the less expensive drugs. According to Mishra and Singh (1989), resistance to the recommended antibiotics for gonococcal infections for example, is reported to be quite rare (in 1989, 52 cases were reported nationwide). This however, may be due to under reporting of STIs in general, and inadequate laboratories and equipment to culture gonococcal strains at most centres.

In general, health care providers ought to be trained in the appropriate diagnosis, and use of recommended, effective therapies against STIs. They often treat patients without laboratory confirmation, and at times provide therapies which are not effective against possible pathogens; there is also a tendency to switch antibiotics at the first possible sign of treatment failure (Mishra and Singh,1989). For example, the results of a study of physicians treating STI patients in Chennai, revealed that 48 percent of the physicians, used a treatment effective against neisseria gonorrhoea and chlamydia trachomatis in men with urethritis; the corresponding figures for chancroid and syphilis in men and women with genital ulcers were only 12 percent and 10.7 percent, respectively (Kantharaj et al, 1995). Results of the same study also stressed the need to encourage providers to use this opportunity to provide focused patient education. Thus, while 79 percent of the physicians claimed to counsel their STD patients to use condoms, only 30 percent were observed to be actually promoting condoms for STD or HIV/AIDS prevention; further, barely 6 percent of STD patients were informed on how to use condoms, and just one patient was actually provided with condoms.

It is also important to realise that men and women often resort to the traditional or informal health sector for treatment. In fact, reports of health seeking behaviour for complaints pertaining to RTIs in women, suggest that herbal treatments are often the first to be tried, even where adequate services are available. They are culturally more acceptable, and often cheaper, than allopathic medicines, and prescribed by accessible healers. Inadequate and irregular supplies of medicines, through the government distribution system, is a frequent problem in many of the remote areas. In the light of problems related to sustainability, and to the possibility of growing antibiotic resistance, should consideration be given to the promotion of herbal remedies on a wider basis, especially for endogenous infections? For many women, especially pregnant women, a local treatment restoring the normal acidity and vaginal flora, without systemic effect, may be preferable to any other treatment. Of concern is the probable ineffectiveness of herbal remedies in treating women (and their sexual contacts) with STIs. Nevertheless, herbal treatments may have an important role to play in the management of endogenous conditions, and an assessment of the efficacy of these remedies is an urgent priority.

In addition to the traditional health sector, men often resort to buying drugs over-the-counter for their STIs at pharmacies and in market places, and treat themselves. Such self-treatment may lead to partially treated infections and lead to serious complications, not to mention the associated increased risk of contracting or transmitting STIs from having sexual intercourse while still infected. One priority is to study treatment-seeking behaviour among men with symptoms indicative of possible STIs (urethral discharge, pain in passing urine and genital ulcers). The results may identify ways of liaising with their various sources of care, to ensure that correct treatment is prescribed and that their female partners are traced and treated.

An interesting example is that of a pilot programme undertaken by Population Services International, in collaboration with Family Health International's AIDSTECH Project in Cameroon (Henry, 1995). A standard prepackaged therapy for male urethritis was tested out, and reportedly worked quite well. The package consisted of a pouch, containing antibiotics to treat gonorrhea and chlamydia (the two most common causes of urethritis in Cameroon), an educational brochure, detailed instructions on how to take the medication, two cards for referring sexual partners for diagnosis and treatment, and eight condoms.

Liaising with the informal sector is necessary, though obviously a huge undertaking, and will require a substantial degree of coordination and training, not to mention an efficient record-keeping system. In order for such an approach to work, however, local health care workers need to know which STIs are present in the region, the availability of effective drugs, and how the STIs respond to various treatment regimens. Given the degree of uncertainty involved in a diagnosis made on the basis of symptoms and signs alone, by lay workers at the community level, and the possibility of concurrent asymptomatic STIs, it is important that all cases grasp the importance of refraining from further sexual activity, as long as symptoms persist. Most important, the establishment of a standardised symptoms checklist, with a risk score approach, to use in interviews with women and men, and standardised diagnostic criteria for RTIs that include both the physician's diagnosis and laboratory results, deserves immediate attention. To this end, it is important to have an understanding of the patients' perceptions of symptoms, and their health-seeking behaviours. This is especially important, in the context of the cultural definition of 'white discharge' – the most important and commonest complaint reported by many women, and a major indicator of RTIs. It is important to realise that all women have vaginal discharge, and this varies in quantity and type; some women may have a copious discharge, others none, or little. It is therefore crucial to learn what women regard as 'excessive' and what they regard as 'abnormal' discharge.

Finally, if the available services are to be utilised, there are a number of important factors that are common to all health services and that need to be considered. For example, the availability of a female medical officer, or trained health worker, to examine women, a male trained worker for men, a convenient location, convenient operating hours, privacy, comfortable waiting areas, short waiting periods, and most important, a sensitive staff.

Routine screening of pregnant women

As discussed earlier, maternal child health/family planning clinics can easily be equipped to handle candidiasis, bacterial vaginosis (BV) and trichomoniasis in symptomatic women. Such facilities do not usually provide for the routine screening of pregnant women, but a strong case can be made for the screening of all pregnant women for BV; and for syphilis, in areas where its prevalence is known to be high. If left untreated, women suffering from syphilis may experience a miscarriage, foetal death, premature birth, or congenital syphilis. The diagnosis of syphilis however, will depend on the availability of non-specific tests (VDRL and RPR) for routine screening, and of specific tests for the confirmation of positive cases. The qualitative rapid plasma reagin (RPR) test alone is said to be sufficient to routinely screen pregnant women; it is also reported to be extremely cheap and simple to perform (Temmerman, Hira and Laga, 1996). Its use by community-based workers needs to be evaluated in India.

Bacterial vaginosis during pregnancy, has been associated with increased rates of second trimester miscarriage, and preterm labour, although a causal effect is not proven. Studies are in progress to determine whether the treatment of pregnant women with BV will improve the outcome of their pregnancies (Hauth et al, 1995; McDonald et al, 1997; Priestley and Kinghorn, 1996). The results of a study of asymptomatic pregnant women reporting for antenatal care at a large urban tertiary hospital in Durban, South Africa, showed that BV was present in 52 percent of the women studied, and was the commonest infection diagnosed, whereas mixed vaginal infections of BV and trichomoniasis were diagnosed in 14 percent (Govender et al, 1996) of the cases.. The results of another study, undertaken among pregnant women in Indonesia, showed that pregnant women with BV had more than a two-fold increase in chlamydia and a six-fold increase in gonorrhoea (Joesoef et al, 1996). It has thus been suggested that because detection of BV by the Gram stain method is easy to perform, and economical, the potential of BV should be considered as a prescreening marker for chlamydia and gonorrhoea among asymptomatic women. Overall, the role of sexual transmission of microorganisms in BV is controversial, and further work is needed to evaluate the usefulness of BV as a prescreening marker for chlamydia and gonorrhoea. Nonetheless, given the possible risks involved in the infant, and that around half the women with this condition are asymptomatic, it has been suggested that where the microscopic examination of a Gram-stained smear of vaginal secretions is possible, all women presenting for antenatal care should be screened and treated accordingly, in particular pregnant women at a high risk for preterm labour, and premature rupture of membranes (McCoy et al, 1995).

As noted earlier, a presumptive diagnosis of BV can be easily made in the field, and subsequently confirmed at the clinic level. It has also been suggested that any treatment aimed at pregnant women should be given no later than the beginning of the second trimester of pregnancy (Hay et al, 1994). Pregnant women do not commonly develop BV after 16 weeks gestation, and if present, it remits spontaneously in roughly half of those who reach term. Attempts will obviously need to be made to liaise with traditional birth attendants, and try to reach out to all pregnant women in their first trimester. However, women themselves are often not aware of their pregnancy status till they are well into the second trimester, at times due to their irregular menstrual cycle, and often as a result of their poor nutritional status. Screening for BV has also been suggested for women due to undergo any invasive gynaecological procedure (Priestly and Kingston, 1996). It is noteworthy that the recommended treatment for BV, chlamydia and trichomoniasis, is the same – metronidazole. Thus treating for one infection will invariably result in the resolution of the other two.

Targeting high-risk populations

Female sex workers

Female sex workers are especially vulnerable to HIV and other STIs (Das et al, 1994; Gilada 1993; Kanbargi and Kanbargi, 1996; Singh, 1995; Pandhi, Khanna and Sekhri, 1995; Rodrigues et al, 1995). They are an important source of STIs for the majority of male patients seen at STD clinics – adolescents, truck drivers and migrant workers. The majority of truckers in India have sexual relations with 50-100 female sex workers in a year, thereby making themselves one of the most vulnerable high-risk groups for receiving and transmitting STIs and HIV infections (Rao et al, 1994). Most female sex workers know nothing about contraception and STIs; and seek curative assistance from unqualified medical practitioners in red-light areas. Thus, besides encouraging symptomatic FSWs and clients to seek early care from STD clinics, or other appropriately equipped facilities, priority should be given for the periodic screening of all FSWs. Providing education, tracing a possibly infected partner, and condom promotion to a population known to engage in high risk behaviour is crucial in limiting the spread of STIs.

Training of community-based workers

If the public sector health programme is to make any effort towards developing comprehensive, women-oriented strategies, a major advocacy drive will be required to foster the necessary policy changes, from a model which emphasises operational targets, to one that focuses on the delivery of gender-sensitive services. This shift will also require an examination, and a redefinition, of the roles and responsibilities of existing family welfare staff. They will need to be trained to provide appropriate information, education and counselling in matters related to sexuality and infection prevention, and to diagnose and treat RTIs. Tracing sexual contacts is an essential part of a control programme for the prevention of STI. Interviewing patients about their contacts requires tact, sensitivity, and special communication skills. Health care workers may well have different moral and sexual attitudes from their patients. They have to accept, and come to terms with this, and their own sexuality, before being able to cope with patients.

The role of female grassroot workers in the public health sector, auxiliary nurse and midwives and female health workers in particular, is critical in bringing about effective intervention programmes in women's health. These female grassroot workers are usually the first point of contact with the health care delivery system that community women have. Equally important will be the role of male grassroots workers in promoting safe and responsible sexual behaviour, in promoting the use of condoms, and in detecting and encouraging men to seek treatment for symptoms indicative of STIs.

Significant lessons can be drawn from the experience of at least one innovative approach in the public health sector, the Briham Municipal Corporation project (Khanna et al, 1997). Using participatory methods, auxiliary nurse midwives in this project, were taken through a training process that enabled them to communicate with women on their reproductive and sexual health problems, and to undertake focus group discussions with them to explore the cultural and social definitions and practices surrounding PID. The training was conducted over a period of about 30 months. It resulted in a radical transformation of the auxiliary nurse midwives perspective on women's health; it improved their ability to communicate with women on sexual issues, and their knowledge about STIs and PID, and the social and mental constraints faced by women. The BMC project has moved beyond PID and is now in the process of becoming a 'women-centred health care' project, as it extends to 18 health posts and a number of post-partum centres in two wards in Mumbai. Auxiliary nurse midwives from the PID project are being used as resource persons; they are playing a crucial role in training other auxiliary nurse midwives and multipurpose workers who in turn will train others; gradually all will be trained in an ongoing process. The project has also led to the formation of sexual education sessions for adolescent girls.

Lessons can also be drawn from the various training programmes developed by NGOs. Their experience has shown that, at least on a small scale, it is possible to train community members to provide health care at the village level, but this process is intensive and time-consuming. Training is an ongoing process with heavy emphasis on actual doing and learning, using relevant and simple techniques such as role playing, actual case studies and audio-visuals. To enable women to discuss and seek treatment for reproductive health problems they had previously hidden, the training has to lead the women very gently through practical and confidence building exercises to talk more openly. Health workers are encouraged to take initiatives, make decisions and initiate action. Most important, they are treated with the respect and dignity they deserve.

All these programmes have demonstrated that given appropriate training, supervision, and back-up support, community-based health workers are able to provide the necessary services.

Prevention

The ultimate goal is to control the disease within the community as well as to protect the health of individuals who are symptomless and unaware of their disease. Prevention is obviously better than cure, and better and cheaper than late intervention. For women with gonococcal and chlamydial infections, the prevention of a costly disability is of paramount importance.

PID is a major cause of short- and long-term morbidity in women (Brabin, Raleigh, and Dumella, 1992). PID is often thought to be the direct result of a STI – usually gonorrhoea and chlamydia, though accurate assessment of the aetiology of PID is prevented by the lack of epidemiological data on STIs in different parts of the country. The primary means to prevent PID, due to STIs, are promotion of safer sexual behaviour and condom usage. In addition to its contraceptive effect, condom use reduces the risk of gonorrhoea, herpes simplex virus infection, genital ulcers, PID, HIV, hepatitis B virus, and chlamydia trachomatis (Faundes, Elias and Coggins, 1994). It has also been suggested that female-controlled barrier methods may prevent more STIs than condoms, because of their more consistent use (Cates and Stone, 1990).

A number of studies have suggested that much of PID may be due to poor quality medical procedures, especially in relation to sterilisations and IUD procedures (Bang, et al, 1989; Bhatia and Cleland, 1995; Sundari Ravindran, undated). It is possible that if lower tract infections, such as bacterial vaginosis and certain STIs are present and remain untreated, women undertaking medically invasive procedures, such as tubal ligation, IUDs and medical termination of pregnancy may be at increased risk of reproductive morbidity (Cates and Stone, 1990). However, findings from the BMC study clearly demonstrate that women, who had undergone sterilisations were at a much higher risk of PID, and that STIs, were not a major factor contributing to PID in these women (Brabin et al,1998).

All in all, reproductive tract infections should be of central concern to family planning service providers, because they not only affect the safety and quality of services, but also influence the demand for contraceptives (Elias, 1994). For example, it is not clear whether existing family planning services in India can ensure the safe use of IUDs. Recent data suggest that current IUDs increase the risk of RTIs only about two-fold, and that too, only during the first month after insertion (Cates and Stone, 1990). Nonetheless, the inability to identify women at risk of exposure to STIs, poses a special concern for IUD providers. A number of short-term strategies have been suggested to optimise the safe use of IUD (Winikoff, Elias and Beattie, 1994), some of which may be considered to include developing a risk-scoring system to identify appropriate IUD candidates (risk-factors need to be validated within the community where it may be used); possible therapeutic interventions to minimise risk, such as iron supplement for IUD users and prophylactic administration of antibiotics during IUD insertion. In the long term, steps need to be taken towards improving the overall quality of care of services such as well-equipped clinic facilities, trained staff, and mechanisms of client follow-up.

Poor menstrual hygiene has also been linked with heightened risk of RTIs, such as candidiasis and bacterial vaginosis (Huq and Khan, 1991). Similar findings have also been reported from studies undertaken in Egypt (Younis et al, 1993) and Bangladesh (Wasserheit et al, 1989). but, the evidence is not conclusive.

The emergence of HIV has placed primary prevention as an absolute priority. There, needs to be a balance, however, between providing basic RTI services at the primary health care level, creating referral links with well-equipped facilities, targetting the "high-risk" population, promoting safer sexual behaviour at the individual and at the community-level, and attempts at improving the overall quality of care of gynaecological services for women. It is therefore important to implement appropriate educational campaigns towards not only minimising the risks of contacting RTIs, but also encouraging symptomatic cases to seek timely care. Such information should be made available not only to married adults, but also, importantly, to unmarried adolescents. NGOs can play a crucial role in assisting the government sector, towards designing and implementing successful mass media campaigns on a broader scale, and towards developing focused health education interventions aimed at specific target groups.

In Thailand for example, STIs have been a major public health problem since 1967 (Limpaphayom, 1995). Prevalence of STIs increased rapidly during the early 1980s, then declined dramatically by 1992 following a highly successful mass media campaign. The decrease in the incidence of STIs was due to a combination of case finding, case management activities, contact tracing, counselling, promotion of condom use, and surveillance of female sex workers. In India, the Sonagachi experience has also demonstrated that client compliance was enhanced through the availability of condoms and primary care for STIs, along with increased client awareness and education by peer educators. Similar observations have been made by the AIDS Intervention Project in Chennai which was initiated in early 1989 (Swaminathan, 1993). Health education interventions aimed at the clients of female sex wokers were carried out over a 10-month period; 120 peer educators were trained in proper condom use. The family welfare programme of Tamil Nadu trained 463 medical and paramedical staff in the treatment and prevention of STIs. Evaluation after February 1992, showed a decline in STIs in 212 men who were tested. This decline was a result of increased condom use, availability of services and the improved treatment seeking behaviour of the clients.

To conclude, the difficulties of controlling RTIs emphasise the need to grapple with the conflict between what is ideal, and what is possible. RTI programmes may have their own objectives, but these need to be seen within the context of the overall objectives of the primary health care programme. It is pointless to develop strategies for the control of RTIs, if appropriate backup systems and public financing system are not in place for the delivery and adoption of services and health education. The discussion of any specific health activity, such as RTIs, raises a number of general issues that apply to all components of health programmes: how to generate the political will to do what needs to be done; how to put policy into practice; how to define priorities; how to generate and sustain community participation; how to develop the necessary management and diagnostic skills at the community level and how to maintain the enthusiasm and commitment of the health workers.

The Government can learn much from the several NGO programmes that have successfully addressed many of the above issues. The role of the voluntary sector is that of an innovator, and a facilitator. It is important for the work they do to percolate into the larger health system. There is a potential for significant upscaling of certain aspects of their programmes, but this is only possible if NGOs continue to document their experience, devise communication channels with the government, and strengthen the existing capacity for learning from each other.

The benefits of RTI programmes are no longer in question although cost data are as yet inadequate. But it is clear that that educational efforts towards preventing the occurrence of RTIs in the first instance, together with the early management of RTI cases are less costly than the treatment of the consequences of RTIs.

What needs much further work, however, is more precise and detailed information on cause-specific gynaecological morbidity; and the constraints women face in accessing appropriate care, and how health services can best meet their needs (Koenig et al, 1998). Such information would clearly be helpful when difficult choices arise, regarding affordability, cost-effectiveness and feasibility of specific services. Given the financial constraints, RTI services cannot realistically be provided for free. On the other hand, the NGO experience has shown that attempts at cost recovery are often not very successful. Even when fees are fixed at a nominal level, people are often not willing to pay for services that have, till recently, been provided free. At times, they are unable to pay. Clearly, services cannot be priced in such a way that those most in need, are unable to afford it. Government services will obviously need to experiment with various schemes that may include a health insurance system on a sliding scale depending on the patient's ability to pay, etc. What is clear is that there are unlikely to be any simple, universal solutions to these problems that will be 'right' in all settings. But, a long-term perspective on RTI programmes is essential, because the continued provision of services will be essential for many years to come.

References

Adler, M.W. 1996. Sexually Transmitted Diseases Control in Developing Countries. *Genitourinary Medicine*, 72: 83-88.

Adler, M.W. 1995. ABC of Sexually Transmitted Diseases. Third Edition. London: British Medical Journal Publishing Group.

Amin, A., Fatula, E., and Grenon, M.C. 1996. Men's Perceptions of Illnesses of the Nether Area. Evidence from Qualitative Studies Conducted in the Santrampur Taluka of Panchmahals District, Gujarat. SARTHI. Working Paper No.3.

Amin, A.,Fatula, E., and Khanna, R. 1997. Attitudes and Behaviours of Men in Relation to Gender and Sexuality. Evidence from Qualitative Studies Conducted in the Santrapur Taluka of Panchmahals District, Gujarat. SARTHI. Working Paper No.4.

Anonymous. 1994. India Confronts the Epidemic. AIDS Report. Spring: 8-10.

ARCH. 1996. Intervention of Community Health Workers in Women's Reproductive Health. Unpublished Paper.

ARCH. Undated. Primary Health Care: ARCH's Experience. Unpublished Paper.

Bang, R., and Bang, A. 1996. A Community Study of Gynaecological Disease in Indian Villages: Some Experiences and Reflections. In: S. Zeidenstein, and K.Moore, (eds.). Learning about Sexuality, 223-237, New York: The Population Council.

Bang, R., and Bang, A. 1991. Why Women Hide Them : Rural Women's Viewpoint on Reproductive Tract Infections. *Manushi*, 69: 27-30.

Bang, R., and Bang, A. 1994. Women's Perceptions of White Vaginal Discharge: Ethnographic Data from Rural Maharashtra. In: J.Gittelsohn, M. E. Bentley, and P.J. Pelto, et al. (eds.). Listening to Women Talk About Their Health. Issues and Evidence from India. New Delhi: The Ford Foundation.

Bang, R., Bang, A., Baitule, M., Chaudhury,Y., Sarmukaddam, S., and Tale,O. 1989. High Prevalence of Gynaecological Diseases in Rural Indian Women. *Lancet*, 8629: 85-88.

BCC, CINI, SEWA-Rural and Streehitakarini. 1995. Prevalence of Clinically Detectable Gynaecological Morbidity in India: Results of Four Community Based Studies. Unpublished Report.

Bhatia, J.C., and Cleland, J. 1995. Self- Reported Symptoms of Gynaecological Morbidity and their Treatment in South India. *Studies in Family Planning,* 26(4): 203-216.

Bhatia, J.C., and Cleland, J., Bhagavan, L., and Rao, N.S.N. 1995. Prevalence of Gynaecological Morbidity among Women in South India. The Indian Institute of Management, Bangalore, India. Unpublished Paper.

Bhattacharya, S. 1994. Gynaecological Morbidities among Women in West Bengal. Child in Need Institute, Calcutta, India. Unpublished Paper.

Bourgeois, A., Henzel, D., and Dilbanga, G., et al. 1996. Development and Evaluation of Screening Algorithms for Sexually Transmitted diseases in Pregnant Women in Libreville, Gabon. *Sante*, 6(2): 115-21.

Brabin, L. 1993. Pelvic Inflammatory Disease, *Africa Health*, 15(3):15-17.

Brabin, L., Kemp, J., Obunge, O.K., Ikimalo, J., Dollimore, N., Odu, N.N., Hart, C.A., and Briggs, N.D. 1995. Reproductive Tract Infections and Abortion among Adolescent Girls in Rural Nigeria. *The Lancet*, 8945 : 300-304 .

Brabin, L.,Gogate, A.,Gogate, S., Karande, A., Khanna, R., Dollimore, N., de Koning, K., Nicholas, S., and Hart, C.A. 1998. Reproductive Tract Infections, Gynaecological Morbidity and HIV Seroprevalence among Women in Mumbai, India. *Bulletin of the World Health Organization,* 76(3): ((In press).

Brabin, L., Raleigh, V.S., and Dumella, S. 1992. Pelvic Inflammatory Disease: A Clinical Syndrome with Social Causes. *Annals of Tropical Medicine and Parasitology*, 86 Supplement 1:1-9.

Bulut, A., Filippi, V., Marshall, T., et al. 1997. Contraceptive Choice and Reproductive Morbidity in Istanbul. *Studies in Family Planning,* 28(1): 35-43.

Bulut, A., Yolsal, N., Filippi, V., and Graham, W. 1995. In Search of Truth : Comparing Alternative Sources of Information on Reproductive Tract Infections. *Reproductive Health Matters*, 6: 31-39.

Cates, W., and Stone, K.M. 1990. Reproductive Tract Infections and Contraceptive Use/ Safety. Unpublished Paper.

Daly, C.C., Maggwa, N., Mati, J.K., et al. 1994. Risk Factors for Gonorrhoea, Syphilis and Trichomonas Infections among Women Attending Family Planning Clinics in Nairobi, Kenya. *Genitourinary Medicine,* 70(3):155-61.

Das, A., Jana, S., Chakraborty, A.K., Khodakevich, L., Chakraborty, M.S., and Pal, N.K. 1994. Community Based Survey of STD/HIV Infection among Commercial Sex Workers in Calcutta, India. Part-III: Clinical Findings of Sexually Transmitted Diseases (STD). *Journal of Communicable Diseases,* 26(4): 192-6.

Dixon-Mueller, R., and Wasserheit, J. 1991. The Culture of Silence: Reproductive Tract Infection among Women in the Third World. International Women's Health Coalition, New York, USA.

Elias, C. 1996. Determinants of RTI: Types, Prevalence and Consequences. Paper presented at a Workshop on Reproductive Tract Infections, Baroda, 27-29 February, 1996. Organised by the Society for Operations Research and Training. Baroda, India.

Elias, C. 1994. A Puzzle of Will: Responding to Reproductive Tract Infections in the Context of Family Planning Programs. In: Population Council, (eds.). Reproductive Health Approach to Family Planning, 5-23. Presentations from a Panel held on Professional Development Day at the USAID Cooperating Agencies Meeting, Washington, D.C. and New York, February 25, 1994. New York: The Population Council.

Elias, C. 1991. Sexually Transmitted Diseases and the Reproductive Health of Women in Developing Countries. Working Paper No.5. The Population Council, New York, USA.

Faundes, A., Elias, C., and Coggins, C. 1994. Spermicides and Barrier Contraception. *Current Opinion in Obstetrics and Gynecology*, 6(6): 552-8.

Family Health International. 1994. Improving STD Treatment for Women. Family Health International, AIDS Control and Prevention Project, Arlington, Virginia, USA.

Filippi, V., Marshall, T., Bulut, A., et al. 1997. Asking Questions about Women's Reproductive Health: Validity and Reliability of Survey Findings from Istanbul. *Tropical Medicine and International Health,* 2(1): 47-56.

Finger, W.R. 1992. What Should You Know About STDS? *Network,* 12(4): 2-3.

Germain, A., Holmes, K.K., Piot, P., and Wasserheit, J.N. 1992. Reproductive Tract Infections: Global Impact and Priorities for Women's Reproductive Health, New York: Plenum Press.

Gilada, I.S. 1993. AIDS and Sex Work: An Indian Perspective. In: Berer and Ray (eds.). Women and HIV/AIDS: An International Resource Book. Information, Action and Resources on Women and HIV/AIDS, Reproductive Health and Sexual Relationship, 276-9. London: Pandora Press.

Gittelsohn, J., Bentley, M.E., Pelto, P.J., et al. 1994. Listening to Women Talk About Their Health. Issues and Evidence from India. New Delhi : Har-Anand Publications.

Govender, L., Hoosen, A.A., Moodley, J., et al. 1996. Bacterial Vaginosis and Associated Infections in Pregnancy. *International Journal of Gynaecology and Obstetrics,* 55(1): 23-28 .

Government of India. (not dated). Reproductive and Child Health Programme. New Delhi: Ministry of Health and Family Welfare. New Delhi, India.

Grenon, M. 1996. Women's Health: Gender Relations and Illness Management Behaviour. Evidence from Qualitative Studies Conducted in the Santrampur Taluka of Panchmahals District, Gujarat. SARTHI Working Paper No.2.

Grenon, M., and Mawji,T. 1996. Women's Perceptions of Sexually Transmitted Diseases. Evidence from Qualitative Studies Conducted in the Santrampur Taluka of Panchmahals District, Gujarat. SARTHI Working paper No.1.

Hauth, J.C., Goldenberg, R.I., Andrews, W.W., DuBard, M.B., and Copper, R.I. 1995. Reduced Incidence of Preterm Delivery with Metronidazole and Erythromycin in Women with Bacterial Vaginosis. *New England Journal of Medicine,* 333(26): 1732-36.

Hawkes, S. 1998. Why Include Men? Establishing Sexual Health Clinics for Men in Rural Bangladesh. *Health Policy and Planning.* (In press).

Hay, P.E., Morgan, D.J., Ison, C.A., et al. 1994. A Longitudinal Study of Bacterial Vaginosis during Pregnancy. *British Journal of Obstetrics and Gynaecology,* 101 (12): 1048-1053.

Henry, K. 1995. AIDSCAP Seeks a Private Sector Solution to the STD Self-Treatment Dilemma. *AIDSCAPTIONS,* :26-9.

Huq, N., and Khan, M.R. 1991. Menstruation : Belief and Practices of Adolescent Girls. Bangladesh Rural Advancement Committee, Dhaka, Bangladesh.

Jejeebhoy, S.J., and Rama Rao, S. 1996. Unsafe Motherhood: A Review of Reproductive Health. In: M. Das Gupta, L. Chen, and T.N.Krishnan (eds.). Women's Health in India. Risks and Vulnerability. 122-152. Oxford: Oxford University Press.

Jejeebhoy, S.J. 1995. Infertility in South Asia: Priorities for Social Science Research. In: Issues in Women's Reproductive Health. Baroda : The Population Council.

Joesoef, M.R., Wiknjosastro, G., Norojono, W., et al. 1996 Coinfection with Chlamydia and Gonorrhoea Among Pregnant Women and Bacterial Vaginosis. *International Journal of STD and AIDS,* 7(1) : 61-64.

Kanbargi, R., and Kanbargi, S. 1996. Sexually Transmitted Diseases in Bangalore City: Some Findings from an Exploratory Study. *Journal of Family Welfare,* 42(1):30-7.

Kantharaj, K., Mertens, T.E., Davey-Smith, G., et al. 1995. Sexually Transmitted Disease Services in Madras: Could Their role in AIDS Prevention be Strengthened? *Indian Journal of Public Health,* 39(3) : 93-9.

Khanna, R., Pongurlekar, S., de Koning, K. 1997. Training Manual for Auxiliary Nurse Midwives in Communication and Research into Women's Sexual Health Issues. The Briham Mumbai Municipal Corporation, Mumbai, India.

Khanna, R. 1996: Shodhini Project: Gynaecological Self -Help and Use of Herbs, 1987-90. In: WAH! Curriculum Revision and Development. Report of a Workshop held at Pune 6-10 February 1996, 54-55. CHETNA, Ahmedabad, India.

Khanna, R. 1992. Taking Charge: Women's Health as Empowerment – the SARTHI Experience. SAHAJ/SARTHI, Baroda, India.

Koenig, M., Jejeebhoy, S., Singh, S., and Sridhar, S. 1998: Investigating Women's Gynaecological Morbidity in India: Not just Another KAP Survey. In: *Reproductive Health Matters*, An abridged version of Koenig, et al. 1996. (In press).

Koenig, M., Jejeebhoy, S., Singh, S., and Sridhar, S. 1996. Undertaking Community-Based Research on the Prevalence of Gynaecological Morbidity: Lessons from India. Paper presented at the IUSSP Seminar on Innovative Approaches to the Assesment of Reproductive Health , Manila, Phillipines: September 24-27, 1996.

Laga, M., et al. 1993. Non- Ulcerative Sexually Transmitted Disease as Risk Factor for HIV-1 Transmission in Women: Results from a Cohort Study. *AIDS*, 7:95-102.

Lalvani, A., and Shastri, J.S. 1996. HIV Epidemic in India: Opportunity to Learn from the Past. *Lancet*, 347(9012): 1349-50.

Larsen, B. 1985. Problems in Specimen Collection for Sexually Transmitted Diseases. *Journal of Reproductive Medicine*, 30(3 Suppl): 290-4.

Latha, K., Kanani, S., Maitra, N., and Bhat, R.V. 1994. A Quantitative and Qualitative Assessment of Morbidity among Urban Disadvantaged Women in Baroda, India. Baroda Citizens Council, Baroda, India. Unpublished Paper.

Limpaphayom, K. 1996. Status of STD Screening, Diagnosis and Treatment in Thailand. In: H.Sanghvi, and D. Lewison (eds.). Issues in Management of STDs in Family Planning Settings, 58-63. Proceedings of a Workshop held at Baltimore, Maryland: 19-21 April 1995. JHPIEGO, Maryland, USA .

Luthra, U.K., Mehta, S., Bhargava, N.C., Ramachandran, P. , Murthy, N.S., and Saxena, B.N. 1992. Reproductive Tract Infections in India: The Need for Comprehensive Reproductive Health Policy and Programmes. In: A. Germain, K.K.Holmes, P. Piot. and J.N.Wasserheit. 1992. Reproductive Tract Infections: Global Impact and Priorities for Women's Reproductive Health, New York: Plenum Press.

Mann, J., Tarantolem, D.J.M., and Netter, W.(eds.). AIDS in the World. Cambridge, Massachussets: Harvard University Press.

Mavalankar, D., 1996. SEARCH, Reproductive Health Services in a Primary Health Care Context in Rural India. Paper presented at an International Seminar on Management of Quality Reproductive Health Programmes: After Cairo and Beyond, Addis Ababa, Ethiopia: December 2-6, 1996. International Council on Management of Population Programmes, Malaysia.

Mayaud, P., Grosskurth, H., Changalucha, J., et al. 995. Risk Assessment and Other Screening Options for Gonorrhoea and Chlamydial Infections in Women Attending Rural Tanzanian Antenatal Clinics. *Bulletin of the World Health Organization,* 73(5): 621-630.

Mayaud, P., Uledi, E., Cornelissen, J., et al. Risk Scores to Detect Cervical Infections in Urban Antenatal Clinic Attenders in Mwanza, Tanzania. (In Press).

Mayaud, P., ka-Gina, G., Cornelissen, J., et al. 1998. Validation of a WHO Algorithm with Risk Assessment for the Clinical Management of Vaginal Discharge in Mwanza, Tanzania. *Sexually Transmitted Infections,* 74; (Supplement 1). (In press).

McCoy, M.C., Katz, V.L., Kuller, J.A., et al. 1995. Bacterial Vaginosis in Pregnancy: An Approach for the 1990s. *Obstetrics and Gynaecology Survey,* 50(6): 482-488.

McDonald, H.M., O'Loughlin, J.A., Vigneswaran, R.,et al. 1997. Impact of Metronidazole Therapy on Preterm Birth in Women with Bacterial Vaginosis Flora (Gardenerella Vaginalis): A Randomised, Placebo Controlled Trial. *British Journal of Obstetrics and Gynaecology,* 104(12): 1391-7.

Measham, A.R., and Heaver, R.A., 1996. India's Family Welfare Programme: Moving to a Reproductive and Child Health Approach. The World Bank, Washington D.C., USA.

Mehendale, S.M., Rodrigues, J.J., Brookmeyer, R.S., et al. 1995. Incidence and Predictors of Human Immunodeficiency Virus type 1 Seroconversion in Patients Attending Sexually Transmitted Disease Clinics in India. *Journal of Infectious Diseases,* 172(6):1486-91.

Mishra, D., and Singh, G. 1989. Penicillinase-Producing Neisseria Gonorrhoea Infection in India. *Indian Journal of Sexually Transmitted Diseases,* 10(2):45-7.

Morales, W.J., Schorr, S., and Albritton, J. 1994. Effect of Metronidazole in Patients with Preterm Birth in Preceding Pregnancy and Bacterial Vaginosis: A Placebo-Controlled, Double-Blind Study. *American Journal of Obstetrics and Gynecology,* 171(2) : 345-47.

Morse, S.A., Moreland, A.A., and Holmes, K.K. 1996. Atlas of STD and AIDS. Second Edition. London: Mosby-Wolfe.

Nag, M. 1996. Sexual Behaviour and AIDS in India. New Delhi: Vikas Publishing House.

Pachauri, S. 1994. Relationship between AIDS and Family Planning Programmes: A Rationale for Developing Integrated Reproductive Health Services. *Health Transition Review,* 4 Suppl:321-47.

Pal, N.K., Chakraborty, M.S., Das, A., Khodakevich, L., Jana, S., and Chakraborty, A.K., 1994. Community Based Survey of STD/HIV Infection Among Commercial Sex Workers in Calcutta, India. Part-IV: Sexually Transmitted Diseases and Related Risk Factors. *Journal of Communicable Diseases,* 26(4) : 197-202.

Pandhi, R.K., Khanna, N., and Sekhri, R. 1995. Sexually Transmitted Diseases in Children. *Indian Pediatrics,* 32(1) : 27-30.

Parekh, A. 1996. Women's Health in India: An Assessment of SARTHI's Village Health Programme. The Johns Hopkins School of Hygiene and Public Health, Department of International Health,. Baltimore, U.S.A.

Parikh, I., Taskar, V., Dharap, N., and Mulgaonkar. 1996. Gynaecological Morbidity among Women in a Bombay Slum. Streehitakarini, Mumbai, India. Unpublished Paper.

Priestley, C.J., and Kinghorn, G.R. 1996. Bacterial Vaginosis. *British Journal of Clinical Pract,* 50(6): 331-334.

Ramasubban, R. 1996. Patriachy and the Risks of STD and HIV Transmision to Women. In M. Das Gupta, L.Chen, and T.N.Krishnan (eds.). Women's Health in India. Risks and Vulnerability, 213-241. Oxford: Oxford University Press.

Rao, A., Nag, M., Mishra, K., and Dey, A. 1994. Sexual Behaviour Pattern of Truck Drivers and Their Helpers in Relation to Female Sex Workers. *Indian Journal of Social Work,* 55(4): 603-15.

Richter, R. 1990. Cervical Cancer. In: Special Challenges in Third World Women's Health, 17-22. Presentations at the 1989 Annual Meeting of the American Public Health Association. International Women's Health Coalition, New York, USA.

Rodrigues, J.J., Mehendale, S.M., Shepherd, M.E., et al. 1995. Risk Factors for HIV Infections In People Attending Clinics for Sexually Transmitted Diseases in India. *British Medical Journal*, (Clinical Research Edition) 311(7000) : 283-6.

RUWSEC. 1996. Comprehensive Reproductive Health Programme for a Rural Population. Annual Report, 1995 -1996. RUWSEC, Tamil Nadu, India.

Sabla and Kranti. 1995. Na Shriram Nadhi. (My Body is Mine). Saptahila Mudran, Pune, India.

SARTHI. 1996. Report of SARTHI's Health Programme, 1995-1996.

Satia, J., Dohlie, M.B., Patel, D., Patel, A., and Kapadia, R. 1996. ARCH. Reproductive Health Services in a Primary Health Care Context in Rural India. Paper presented at an International Seminar on Management of Quality Reproductive Health Programmes: After Cairo and Beyond, Addis Ababa, Ethiopia: December 2-6, 1996. International Council on Management of Population Programmes, Malaysia.

de Schryver, A., and Meheus, A. 1990. Epidemiology of Sexually Transmitted Diseases: The Global Picture. *WHO Bulletin,* 68(5): 639-654.

Schulte, J. 1994. Gonorrhea and Chlamydia – Their Cost to the Health of Women. In: *MotherCare Matters,* 4(3/4): 2-5.

SEWA-Rural Research Team. 1994. Gynaecological Aspects of Women's Health: A Cross-Sectional Study. SEWA-Rural, Jhagadia, India. Unpublished Paper.

Shodhini. 1997. Touch-, Touch-Me-Not: Women, Healing and Herbs. New Delhi: Kali for Women.

Singh, S. 1995. Three Year Sting at Sonagachi. An Exposition. The STD/HIV Intervention Programme at Sonagachi, 1992-1995. All India Institute of Hygiene and Public Health, Calcutta, India.

Sivaram, S., Gowda, B., Sogunro, R., 1995. A Community Based Approach to Behaviour Change: STDs and HIV/AIDS Education Among Devadaasi Women and Their Communities: Experiences from Rural Karnataka. Unpublished Paper.

Solomon, S., Anuradha, S., Ganapathy, M., and Jagadeeswari. 1994. Sentinel Surveillance of HIV-1 Infection in Tamil Nadu, India. *International Journal of STD and AIDS,* 5(6) : 445-6.

Starrs, A., and Measham, D., 1990. Challenge for the Nineties: Safe Motherhood in South Asia. New York and Washington: World Bank and Family Care International.

Sundari Ravindran, T.K. 1996. Women's Health in a Rural Poor Population in Tamil Nadu. In: M.Das Gupta, L.Chen, and T.N.Krishnan, (eds.). Women's Health in India. Risks and Vulnerability, 175-211. Oxford: Oxford University Press.

Swaminathan, S. 1993. AIDS Prevention Among Individuals with High-Risk Behaviour: The Madras Experience. In: P. Senanayake, and R.L.Kleinman, (eds.). Family Planning. Meeting Challenges: Promoting Choices, 339-45. The Proceedings of the IPPF Family Planning Congress, New Delhi, October 1992. Carnforth, England: Parthenon Publishing Group.

Temmerman, M., Hira, S., and Laga, M. 1996. STDs and Pregnancy. In: G.A. Dallabetta, M. Laga, and P.R. Lamptey, (eds.). Control of Sexually Transmitted Diseases. A Handbook for the Design and Management of Programmes, 169-186. Arlington, Virginia: Family Health International AIDS Control and Prevention Project .

Thomas, T., Choudhri, S., Kariuki, C., and Moses, S. 1996. Identifying Cervical Infection Among Pregnant Women in Nairobi, Kenya: Limitations of Risk Assessment and Symptom-Based Approaches. *Genitourinary Medicine,* 72 : 334-338.

Toomey, K.E., Latif, A.S., and Steen, R.C. 1996. Partner Management. In: G.A. Dallabetta, M. Laga, and P.R.Lamptey, (eds.). Control of Sexually Transmitted Diseases. A Handbook for the Design and Management of Programmes, 211-24, Arlington, Virginia: Family Health International and AIDS Control and Prevention Project. New York : International Conference on Population and Development, United Nations.

van Dyck, E., Behets, F., Crabbe, F., and Berkley, S. 1996. The STD Laboratory. In: G.A. Dallabetta, M.Laga, and P.R.Lamptey, (eds.). Control of Sexually Transmitted Diseases. A Handbook for the Design and Management of Programmes. Arlington, Virginia: Family Health International and AIDS Control and Prevention Project.

Vuylsteke, B., Laga, M., Alary, M., et al. 1993. Clinical Algorithms for the Screening of Women for Gonococcal and Chlamydial Infection- An Evaluation of Pregnant Women and Prostitutes in Zaire. *Clinical Infectious Diseases,* 17: 82-8.

Wasserheit, J.N., and Holmes, K.K. 1992. Reproductive Tract Infections: Challenges for International Health Policy, Programmes and Research. In: A. Germain, K.K. Holmes, P.Piot, and J.N.Wasserheit, 1992. Reproductive Tract Infections: Global Impact and Priorities for Women's Reproductive Health, New York: Plenum Press.

Wasserheit, J.N., Harris, J.R., Chakraborty, J., Kan, B.A., and Mason, K. 1989. Reproductive Tract Infections in a Family Planning Population in Rural Bangladesh. *Studies in Family Planning,* 20(2): 69-80.

World Health Organization/GPA. 1993. The Evaluation of Algorithms for the Diagnosis and Treatment of Vaginal Discharge. Informal Technical Working Group Meeting on STD Activities in GPA. Agenda Item No.IV, Background Paper No.5. Geneva : World Health Organization.

World Health Organization. 1991. Management of Patients with Sexually Transmitted Diseases. Report of a WHO Steering Group. WHO Technical Report Series 810. Geneva: World Health Organization.

Winikoff, B., Elias, C., and Beattie, K. 1994. Special Issues of IUD Use in Resource-Poor Settings. In: C.Wayne Bardin, and D.R.Mishell, Jr. (eds.). Proceedings from the Fourth International Conference on IUDs, 230-8. Boston, Massachusetts : Butterworth-Heinemann.

Younis, N., Khattab, H., Zurayk, H., et al. 1993. A Community Study of Gynaecological and Related Morbidities in Rural Eqypt. *Studies in Family Planning,* 24(3) : 175-186.

Zurayk, H., Khattab, H., Younis, N., Kamal, O., and El Helw, M. 1995. Comparing Women's Reports with Medical Diagnoses of Reproductive Morbidity Conditions in Rural Eqypt. *Studies in Family Planning*, 26(1):14-21.

Appendix

COMMUNITY-BASED PROGRAMMES ADDRESSING WOMEN'S REPRODUCTIVE HEALTH NEEDS IN INDIA

This project started in December 1994. Its prime objective was to document community-based programmes addressing women's reproductive health needs in India. The project consisted of four phases.

Phase One: As a starting point, around 300 organisations (non-governmental, academic institutions, women's groups, donors) were contacted. The objective was to identify a diverse range of reproductive health care programmes being implemented throughout the country.

Phase Two: A screening questionnaire sent to each of the organisations (mainly non-governmental identified in phase one), provided the initial information on the specific reproductive health needs being addressed. The return rate was around 80 percent. Every attempt was made to follow up on those NGOs that failed to respond.

Phase Three: Based on information obtained during phase two, field visits were made to 70 NGOs. The selection criteria were as follows: the programme had been established for at least five years; and, it should be somewhat innovative in its approach (other than the conventional maternal child care and family planning programmes). Another objective was to get a spread of groups across most, if not all, of the states across the country. Information from these preliminary visits has been compiled and published as a monograph entitled 'Community-based Programmes addressing Women's Reproductive Health needs in India: A Documentation' (Mamdani M (ed.), 1998). These documentations provide a 'snap shot' of reproductive health interventions being implemented by some of the community-based organisations within India.

Phase Four: Repeat visits were made to 33 of the programmes screened in the third phase. The objective was to get specific information on one or more of the following reproductive health interventions being implemented: reproductive tract infections; family planning (including spacing methods, infertility, abortion); safe motherhood; adolescent reproductive health; and, male involvement. Some issues of interest were: how these interventions are being implemented at the community level; the operational factors involved; the major obstacles met; and, where possible, get a notion of the incremental costs involved in implementing the specific intervention(s) of interest. About 4-7 days were spent with each of these programmes.

Apart from trying to get a geographic spread of programmes, a number of factors dictated the choice of groups selected. One obvious criterion was that the programme's approach was perceived as having been quite 'successful.' Another was to get a mix of 'models' (i.e., addressing the needs of a poor urban versus rural population, and clinic-based versus community-based programmes). The final choice also depended on the possibility of conducting another follow-up visit to that programme. Often programmes had several important items on their agenda and thus failed to accommodate our visit. Or, for example, due to unexpectedly bad cyclones in Andhra Pradesh, we failed to follow up on a number of programmes.

Major limitations:

1. We were unsuccessful in obtaining quantitative data of good quality, mainly because of a poor information system; a problem inherent in most programmes. A few programmes do have a systematic data collection procedure, but much of this information remains unanalysed.

2. It was not possible to get any valid information on the incremental costs involved in implementing a specific intervention. These are difficult to estimate for they are components of broader or larger programmes with which they share facilities and resources.

Information obtained from phase three and four has been used towards writing the following three issue-based monographs:

1. Community-based Management of Reproductive Tract Infections in Women in India: Lessons from the Field.

2. A Decade of Safe Motherhood: Initiatives in India.

3. New Priorities: Adolescent Reproductive Health in India.

5

Abortion in India: Current Situation and Future Challenges

M. E. Khan, Sandhya Barge,
Nayan Kumar and Stina Almroth

Introduction

Induced abortion has been practiced to varying degrees in all cultures by women facing unwanted pregnancies. Abortion can be a safe procedure when performed properly by trained health personnel. However, as abortion is legally restricted in many countries, women resort to unsafe abortion. It is a major cause of maternal deaths, injuries and illnesses worldwide. In India, according to the Office of the Registrar General of India, abortion is an important cause of maternal death and contributes to about 12 percent of maternal deaths every year (Registrar General of India, 1990).

Abortion at the International Conference on Population and Development

At the International Conference on Population and Development (ICPD) held in Cairo, September 1994, abortion was perhaps the most contentious issue and was discussed and debated at length. In the end however, by consensus, unsafe abortion was recognised as a major public health problem and the right to abort an unwanted pregnancy was acknowledged as a woman's basic right. The much debated paragraph 8.25 of the Programme of Action states:

"In no case should abortion be promoted as a method of family planning. All governments and relevant intergovernmental and non-governmental organisations are urged to strengthen the commitment to women's health, to deal with the health impact of unsafe abortion as a major public health concern and to reduce the recourse to abortion through expanded and improved family planning services. Prevention of unwanted pregnancies must always be given the highest priority and every attempt should be made to eliminate the need for abortion. Women who have unwanted pregnancies should have ready access to reliable information and compassionate counselling. Any measures or changes related to abortion within the health system can only be determined at the national or local level according to the national legislation process. In circumstances where abortion is not against the law, such abortion should be safe. In all cases, women should have access to quality services for the management of complications arising from abortion. Post abortion counselling, education and family planning services should be offered promptly which will also help to avoid repeat abortions".

India is a signatory to the ICPD Plan of Action and recognises women's right to seek and avail abortion services. The Ministry of Health and Family Welfare, under its recently launched reproductive and child health programme, has reiterated its commitment to strengthening abortion services to ensure that all women desiring abortion of unwanted pregnancies should have easy access to safe and hygienic abortion services.

Legal status of abortion in India: The Medical Termination of Pregnancy Act, 1971

In India, the need for liberalising abortion was debated as early as in the sixties. The Shantilal Shah Committee, which was formed at that time, deliberated for more than two years before submitting its report to the government in 1966. Seven years later, following further review and debate, the Medical Termination of Pregnancy (MTP) Act was placed before Parliament in 1971 and unanimously adopted by all political parties. Beginning in April 1972, the Act was implemented all over the country except in Jammu and Kashmir.

The MTP Act permits termination of pregnancy in the following cases:

(a) where the continuance of the pregnancy would involve a risk to the life of the pregnant woman or grave injury to her physical or mental health; or

(b) where substantial risk exists of the child being born with serious physical or mental abnormality.

The Act furthermore elaborates that pregnancy due to failure of contraceptive methods could also be aborted as the 'anguish caused by such unwanted pregnancy may be presumed to contribute a grave injury to the medical health of the pregnant woman' (MTP Act, 1971).

When the MTP Act was passed in India, only three other countries in the world had such liberal abortion policies. The initiative taken by the Government of India to liberalise abortion was pathbreaking in that it recognised that an unwanted pregnancy could cause serious mental anguish to a woman and, therefore, she should have the right to abortion.

The MTP Act, however, included several restrictions, which have proved counterproductive in making abortion services widely and easily accessible to women. Abortion procedures can only be performed by doctors who have received training in MTP. For the abortion of pregnancies up to 12 weeks, the certification of one qualified doctor is sufficient. For pregnancies between 12 and 20 weeks, two doctors must give their approval. In addition, abortion cannot be performed in any place other than a clinic or a hospital established, or maintained by the government or an institution approved by the government for this purpose. These restrictions have become major obstacles to making MTP services freely available.

After the introduction of the MTP Act in 1971, the number of approved institutions providing MTP services increased from 1,877 in 1976 to 8,511 in 1994-95. Similarly, as shown in Figure 1, the number of MTP cases rose from a mere 25 reported in 1972-73 to over 600,000 in 1994-95.

FIGURE 1: Trend of Reported MTP in India

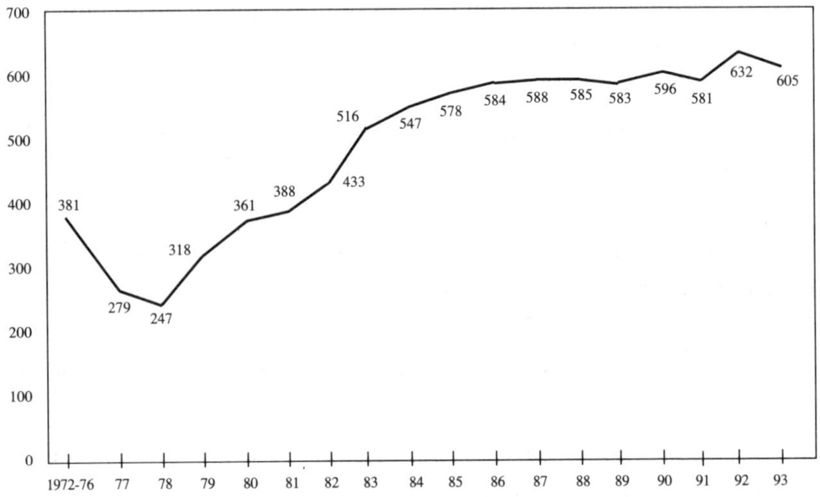

Source: Year Book, Government of India, 1993

Figure 1 also shows that since 1985, the number of reported abortions has remained stationary at around 600,000. However, this is only a fraction of the actual number of abortions performed in India. It is estimated that, every year, an additional five to six million abortions are carried out at unrecognised facilities by practitioners who are not qualified. As these abortions by definition are illegal, they are not reported in any statistics. Most of these unsafe abortions are conducted by unqualified health providers, traditional birth attendants and pharmacists in rural areas and result in 15,000 to 20,000 abortion-related deaths every year.

Twenty-seven years after the legalisation of abortion in India, it is of concern that, abortion services are very limited, especially in rural areas. After the ICPD, some efforts have been made to increase the number of MTP facilities both in rural and urban areas, so that women can have access to safe and hygienic abortion care.

This chapter presents a situational analysis of abortion in India, focusing on the demand for abortion services, the extent to which this demand is being met at current facilities and some of the obstacles. An attempt has also been made to examine the quality of services provided. We have compiled information from various sources including available government statistics, published articles and a rich data base on abortion services in the states of Gujarat, Maharashtra, Tamil Nadu, and Uttar Pradesh, maintained at the Centre for Operations Research and Training (CORT, 1995; 1996; 1997a; and 1997b). In particular, we are drawing on a large scale survey of MTP facilities in the four states.

Estimated Demand for Abortion Services

As explained above, government statistics on induced abortions pertain only to those carried out at recognised facilities. However, there are several unofficial estimates, based on different assumptions and calculated at different times, and hence varying considerably (Khan et al, 1996). In 1966, the Shah Committee assumed that for every 73 live births, there were 2 still births and 25 abortions (10 spontaneous and 15 induced), corresponding to a total number of 3.9 million induced abortions annually. Based on similar assumptions, Chhabra and Nuna estimated in 1994, that there were 6.7 million induced abortions. Assuming an abortion ratio of 200 per 1,000 known pregnancies and an abortion rate of 55 per 1,000 women aged 15-44 years, in 1970, the International Planned Parenthood Federation (IPPF), calculated that 6.5 million abortions were conducted in India every year. Karkal (1991) estimated the ratio of legal to illegal abortions and concluded that for every legal abortion, there were three illegal abortions in rural and four to five in urban areas. Gupte (1997) provided an estimate of eight illegal abortions for every legal abortion.

While it is difficult to arrive at any conclusive figure, the overall picture is clear. The total number of abortions conducted in India every year is about ten times higher than the officially reported service statistics. Even if it is assumed that of the illegal abortions, 10-20 percent are performed under safe and hygienic conditions at private clinics and nursing homes, it still means that up to 80 percent of all abortions are conducted by untrained providers at questionable facilities. Consequently, large numbers of women are exposed to the risk of post-abortion complications and death, essentially as a result of an unmet need for safe abortion services.

Availability of Abortion Services

Unequal distribution of abortion services

The number of clinics and hospitals, which have been approved by the government to conduct abortions, increased from 3,908 in 1981-82 to 9,467 in 1997. In view of the estimated incidence of abortions in the country, this pace of increase in the number of approved facilities is inadequate. Furthermore, the limited number of facilities is unequally distributed. There are more approved abortion facilities in urban than in rural areas. Table 1 shows, there are more approved facilities in the more developed states, which have smaller populations. For instance, in 1995, a more developed state like Maharashtra, with about ten percent of India's population, had 1,808 abortion facilities, constituting 21 percent of the total number of such registered facilities in the country. In contrast, less developed Bihar, also with about 10 percent of India's population, had one percent of the total number of facilities. Bihar, Madhya Pradesh, Rajasthan and Uttar Pradesh, the four least developed states, that account for about 40 percent of the country's population, had less than 17 percent of the number of approved abortion facilities.

Table 1: Geographical Distribution of Approved Abortion Centres Based on Service Delivery Statistics for 1995

State	No. of approved MTP centres (1995)	% of India's population	% registered MTP centres in India	No. of MTP centres per million population	No. of couples per MTP
Gujarat	557	4.9	10.0	21	8,400
Maharashtra	1808	9.4	21.2	23	7,650
Tamil Nadu	645	6.7	7.6	11	1,600
Uttar Pradesh	576	16.6	6.8	4	44,000
Bihar	116	10.3	1.2	1	1,76,000
Madhya Pradesh	297	7.9	3.5	5	35,200
Rajasthan	432	5.2	5.1	10	17,600
India	8511	100.0	100.0	10	17,600

Figure 2: Current availability of MTP services at Government Clinics

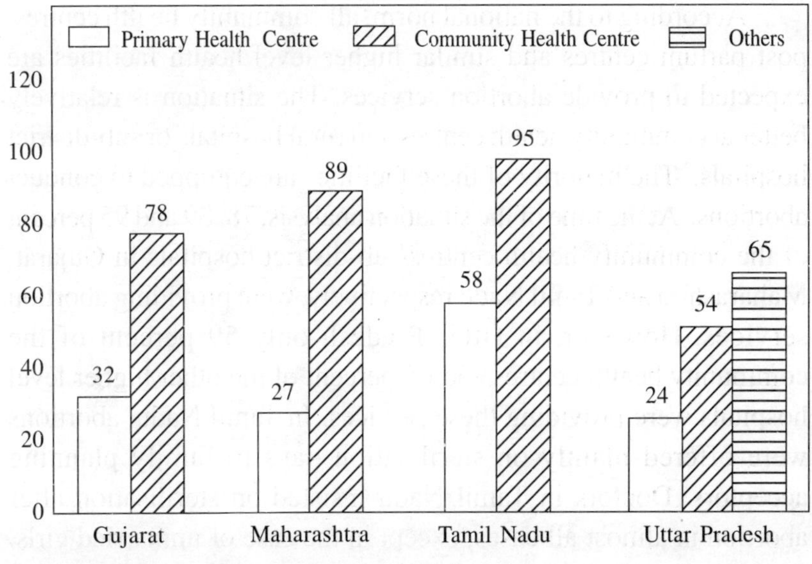

How functional are the facilities?

Available records of abortion facilities at the state and even district level do not provide an adequate answer to this question. We have therefore based our assessment on a situational analysis undertaken by the Centre for Operations Research in Gujarat, Maharashtra, Uttar Pradesh and Tamil Nadu. This analysis covered a total of 61 districts, 510 institutions approved for providing MTP services and 241 private health practitioners. Of the 510 clinics surveyed, 217 were primary health centres, 116 community health centres or rural hospitals, 50 post-partum centres/sub-district hospitals while the remaining 130 were private clinics.

The study showed that only about one-fourth of the primary health centres in Maharashtra (27 percent) and Uttar Pradesh (24 percent), one-third in Gujarat (32 percent) and more than one-half (58 percent) in Tamil Nadu were currently providing officially approved services (Figure 2). According to our analysis only 14 to 18 percent of all the primary health centres and community health centres in the states provided abortion services. This is indeed far short of the government's intention spelt out in the Seventh Five Year Plan (1985-90) to equip all primary health centres to conduct abortion services.

According to the national norm, all community health centres, post partum centres and similar higher level health facilities are expected to provide abortion services. The situation is relatively better at community health centres and rural hospitals or sub-district hospitals. The majority of these facilities are equipped to conduct abortions. At the time of the situation analysis, 78, 89 and 95 percent of the community health centres/sub-district hospitals in Gujarat, Maharashtra and Tamil Nadu respectively, were providing abortion services. However, in Uttar Pradesh only 59 percent of the community health centres and 65 percent of the other higher level hospitals were providing these services. In Tamil Nadu, abortions were offered mainly on sterilisation days to family planning acceptors. Doctors in Tamil Nadu insisted on sterilisation after abortion in almost all cases, except in the case of unmarried girls.

Such pressure for sterilisation was less in Maharashtra, Gujarat and even Uttar Pradesh.

A substantial proportion of the approved primary health centres (24 to 40 percent) had been providing MTP services in the past, but were not doing so currently, and 16-52 percent of these centres, after having been approved as MTP clinics, never offered the services. (Khan et al, 1998).

Given the relatively poor availability of MTP facilities, it is not so surprising that a majority of women seeking abortion services resort to private clinics, go to untrained practitioners or employ various traditional methods themselves.

Reasons for Not Providing Abortion Services

In all four states, 70 to 92 percent of approved clinics were not providing abortion services because they had no trained doctor. Another common reason for not providing abortions was lack of equipment. A substantial number of the clinics lacked both a trained doctor and equipment.

Since the lack of trained doctors and the non-availability of equipment were identified as the two main reasons for not providing abortion services at government approved clinics, we examined these problems in more detail. Our examination showed that, contrary to expectation, after the liberalisation of abortion, there had been no systematic effort by the government to train doctors to provide abortion services. According to available statistics, 162 institutions have been designated for training doctors in MTP. Each of these training centres can train up to 20 doctors a year. However, our study showed that, in most of the designated training institutions, only 6-10 doctors were trained in a year. The reasons for this included: government procedural delays in participants getting duty leave for training; lack of state health funds; lack of accommodation facilities at the training institutions, and inadequate case loads to provide sufficient practical training, (CORT, 1994;1997; Khan et al, 1998).

Furthermore, while 230 post-partum centres having an adequate case load of abortions should have been designated as MTP training centres, only 162 actually were. Thus, a number of factors led to an inadequate number of doctors being trained to perform abortion. Chhabra et al (1994) estimated that in 1992 only about 3,000 trained doctors were available compared to the approximately 21,000 required to serve all primary health centres, in rural areas.

A similar probing regarding the lack of equipment at approved clinics, revealed an apathetic attitude of the government to expand MTP facilities (Khan et al, 1996). Until recently, increasing access to MTP services was not an important issue for the Ministry of Health and Family Welfare. Since 1991-92, approximately US$ 350,000 has been allocated for the MTP programme annually. In 1995-96, influenced by ICPD recommendations, a serious effort was made to strengthen the services and increase the number of MTP centres and an amount of about US $ 2.3 million was requested. However, referring to financial constraints, the Ministry again allocated only about US$ 350,000 for this programme.

Ironically, even the small funds which were finally allocated to state government for the purchase of new equipment, remained partially unspent except in the case of Karnataka and Maharashtra. An enquiry revealed that the government required all equipment to be certified by the Indian Standards Institute (ISI) to ensure quality standards. As there is only one company in the country which provides MTP equipment and has the quality certification, the demand for the country cannot be met. For other manufacturers who cater mainly to the larger private sector, the small market offered by the public sector is not attractive enough to take the trouble of ensuring an ISI mark on their products.

Quality of Abortion Services

Research on the quality of services provided by public clinics has remained a neglected area in India. The quality of MTP services has received even less attention by researchers. Our study provides data that are analysed in this section.

Readiness of the clinics to provide abortion services

The study revealed a general inadequacy of equipment in most of the primary health centres providing abortion services. For example, out of 187 functional primary health centres, only 55 percent had all five sizes of dilators; 85 percent had at least four sizes of dilators. It is difficult to understand how the remaining 15 percent were performing abortions without having the minimum number of common size dilators. Similarly, only 21 percent of the functional primary health centres had a complete set of the nine different sizes of cannulas. About half (56 percent) of the centres had at least a set of the six most frequently used sizes of cannula. Surprisingly, 7 percent of the functional primary health centres did not even have a speculum.

We found that other support facilities at the clinics were also inadequate as shown in Table 2. Only one-third of the clinics had toilet facilities with adequate water supply. The operation theatres in general suffered from a lack of cleanliness and inadequate lighting. Auditory and visual privacy was unsatisfactory, particularly in Tamil Nadu where it was almost non-existent. While antibiotics and analgesics were generally available, sedatives and anti-haemorrhage drugs were often in short supply. Over all, our analysis indicated that there was considerable scope for improvement of logistics and management to improve the quality of services.

Percent clinics having each type of facility

TABLE 2: Availability of Support Facilities at Primary Health Centres

Other support facilities	Gujarat N*=54	Maha-rashtra N=60	Tamil Nadu N=38	Uttar Pradesh N=62
Physical facility				
Toilet facility with adequate water supply	37	52	34	29
Operation theatre				
Clean room	50	88	58	40
Operation table with clean rubber sheet	43	77	32	45
Washbasin	39	15	84	76
Adequate source of light	48	88	50	77
Privacy				
Auditory	61	68	11	42
Visual	54	60	13	40
Medicines				
Antibiotics	70	95	95	90
Analgesics	67	95	92	89
Sedatives	63	82	66	74
Anti haemorrhage drugs	33	38	40	76

* n = number of clinics

Competence of the doctors

We found that, of the 205 doctors providing MTP services, 31 (15 percent) did not have any training in conducting abortion. Thirty two doctors (around 15 percent) did not perform any abortions in spite of being trained. Eight of these 32 doctors expressed lack of confidence as the reason for not performing the procedure. As one of the doctors explained:

> *"Although after 4 weeks of training I was given a certificate, as the trainer was confident that I could do the MTP performance, but still I do not feel confident about my capability to perform MTP. I need to do several more MTPs under strict supervision of my senior before I could conduct MTP independently".*

Another doctor said:

> *"We could not do a single case in the whole of the training period. From where do I get the confidence?".*

Our analysis showed that doctors did not receive adequate practical training. In Maharashtra, the average duration of training was only eight days as compared to the prescribed norm of 30 days (now modified to 15 working days) and trainees had conducted only 13 abortions instead of at least 25 as prescribed by the government. Doctors in Tamil Nadu had performed only six abortions.

Attitude of providers

Abortion is a sensitive issue and many providers do not approve of it. Providers' negative attitudes can make a major difference to the quality of counselling, the provision of services and the quality of client-provider interaction.

Our analysis showed that the majority of the doctors as well as other health staff approved of abortion only conditionally. In all four states, less than 20 percent of the doctors and other staff approved of abortion unconditionally. Between 4 to 24 percent of the doctors and 23 to 52 percent of the workers were totally opposed to abortion (Table 3).

Our observations showed that the doctors' interactions with women seeking abortion were not generally sympathetic. They often insisted that the woman should agree to be sterilised. Such pressure was strongest in Tamil Nadu where it was an almost an unwritten

TABLE 3: Attitude of Providers to MTP

	Percent approving abortion							
	Gujarat		Maharashtra		Tamil Nadu		Uttar Pradesh	
Service Providers	UC	C	UC	C	UC	C	UC	C
Doctors	25	51	13	83	17	58	14	65
Other health staff	13	53	3	45	14	50	19	59

UC = Unconditional, C = Conditional

rule that an abortion must be followed by a sterilisation. A woman in Uttar Pradesh said (Khan et al, 1998):

> *"When I conceived unwantedly (3rd pregnancy), I wanted to get it aborted. When I contacted the lady doctor at the PHC, she discouraged me and persuaded me to continue with the pregnancy. She suggested that after delivery I could get sterilised. When I again requested her, she agreed and said, OK I will do it but you have to undergo sterilisation also".*

Some of the doctors and other providers confessed that they did not like conducting abortions. They therefore tried to discourage women from undergoing abortion. However, when a woman insisted on an abortion, the provider performed the procedure out of a sense of duty. As one of the lady doctors said:

> *"As a human being, I will also say that it is not good, but I am doing it because it is my profession".*

Interestingly, despite their dislike of abortion, some of the doctors and health workers supported it because abortions help them to get more sterilisation cases to meet their targets. As one of the health worker put it:

> *"Nobody will be in favour of abortion within. We are doing it because it is our duty. We have to bring cases for sterilisation, so if a women is ready to accept sterilisation after abortion, we cannot leave the case".*

Quality of counselling

Our analysis clearly showed that there is scope for substantial improvement of counselling services, particularly in terms of the quality of information provided to the women about the procedure, such as safety, the risk involved and the possibility of infection. While in about 70 percent of the cases, women were informed about the procedure and its safety, only 49 percent were told about the possibility of infection. Similarly, about half of the women were instructed to come back for a check-up, and even fewer were told what to do in the case of any complication. Eighty percent of the women reported that the humane aspect of the services, such as protection of modesty and efforts to make the women comfortable was satisfactory. In most states, more than 90 percent of the women were satisfied with the services they received.

Concluding Comments

Our analysis shows that there is a large gap between the demand for abortion services and the facilities available. Women who do not have access to safe abortion services, resort to unsafe abortion methods, thus risking their lives. However, studies also show that available facilities are not fully utilised. A time series analysis of service statistics showed that each approved institution performed only one abortion every four working days. This is an extremely low case load in view of the large number of abortions that take place every year. It indicates that merely increasing the number of approved abortion facilities may not be sufficient to ensure physical and social accessibility of abortion services for women who need them.

In a cultural context where sexuality, sexual health and reproduction are sensitive issues that are not discussed, abortion is especially sensitive because many feel that abortion is a sin. Even today, few women are aware that abortion is legally approved by the government. According to a study by the Indian Council of Medical Research (1989), 31 percent of women in Tamil Nadu and 75 percent in Uttar Pradesh and Haryana believe that abortion is illegal. In Bihar, only 28 percent of the people are aware of abortion being legal (CORT, 1996).

Therefore, to increase the accessibility to abortion services and to make the services socially appropriate, it is critical to understand the dynamics of decision making related to unwanted pregnancy and abortion, within the framework of partner relations. To enhance the utility of available services, it is equally important to understand women's perspectives in seeking abortion services; what they expect from these facilities; and how they want these services to be delivered.

Government Initiatives and Future Challenges

At a national consultation on safe abortion services organised by the Ministry of Health and Family Welfare in March 1998, the problem to prevent the growing number of illegal abortions was reviewed. Suggestions were made on how to bridge the gap between the demand for services and the availability of safe facilities. In addition to senior programme managers and state health officials, several NGOs and researchers were invited to this consultation. It was proposed that under the reproductive and child health programme, primary health centres that do not offer abortion services due to the lack of qualified government doctors should, on fixed days, obtain the service of doctors from the private sector on a contract basis. MTP equipment must be provided to well run and competent non-government medical clinics.

Recommendations of the National Consultation on Safe Abortion Services, Ministry of Health and Family Welfare, March 1998

- Functioning of the MTP programme should be reviewed every year at the national level.
- Establish MTP cells in every state.
- List of all recognised MTP clinics should be updated annually.
- Low performing MTP clinics should be reviewed.
- Existing MTP training programmes should be reviewed to improve the quality of training.
- The duration of the training should be at least of one month.
- Each trainee must assist in 10 MTP cases, perform 10 cases under supervision and 5 independently.
- Pre- and post-MTP counselling should be a part of the training.
- To encourage private institutions, income tax rebate should be provided for MTP and sterilisation.
- All recognised institutions should be reviewed every three years for recertification.
- Procedures for recognising institutions should be simplified and expedited.
- Focussed information, education and communication campaigns should be organised to inform all the sections of community about the legal status of abortion and available services.

These initiatives by the Ministry of Health and Family Welfare are certainly in the right direction and will be helpful in improving abortion care. However, the results of our analysis indicate that larger financial investments are needed to make abortion services available and accessible. On the medical front, the situation seems quite difficult and complex. Given the number of training institutions and the number of doctors who are trained every year, it would take more than a decade to train the required number of doctors unless a serious effort is made to provide adequate resources and train doctors. Yet, there is no assurance that even after they are trained, they will be available to serve in remote rural areas.

One way to address this problem could be to train paramedical staff like lady health visitors and public health nurses to conduct menstrual regulation and early first trimester abortions. In countries such as Bangladesh and Vietnam, paramedical staff are employed to provide these services. Such a move could enhance the availability of services and also reduce the social distance between providers and women, thereby, making these services more socially acceptable. However, the present MTP Act does not allow for such a possibility. The MTP Act of 1971 has a strong medical basis and unless it is modified and demedicalised, it will not be possible to involve paramedical staff to provide abortion services in India. We believe that it is time for a wider discussion and debate on the need for modifying the MTP Act and for redrafting its clauses from women's perspectives. It is highly likely that the medical lobby would oppose such a move. Therefore, a challenge for the Ministry of Health and Family Welfare would be to facilitate these changes without making abortion a controversial issue.

At the societal level, community members, both men and women must be informed that abortion is legal. They should know from where safe abortion services are available and should be made aware of the dangers of abortions performed by untrained providers. Local institutions such as *panchayats*, school teachers, *mahila mandals* (women's groups), NGOs and others could be effectively used for such educational campaigns.

The poor status of women and gender inequality within conjugal relations is a major cause of unwanted pregnancy and women's inability to access abortion services. Therefore, any serious effort to make contraception and abortion services easily accessible should be strategically planned within a gender framework, an aspect that has been ignored in the past and continues to be neglected. Strategic planning and sustained efforts are needed at all levels to operationalise these concepts.

References

Barge, S., Khan, M.E., Rajagopal. S., Kumar, N., and Kumber, S. 1998. Availability and Quality of MTP services in Gujarat, Maharashtra, Tamil Nadu and Uttar Pradesh – An Indepth Study. Paper presented at the International Workshop on Abortion Facilities and Post Abortion Care in the Context of RCH Programme, March 23-24, 1998. Centre for Operations Research and Training. New Delhi, India.

Centre for Operations Research and Training. 1995. Situational Analysis of Medical Termination of Pregnancy (MTP) Services in Gujarat. Monograph. Baroda, India.

Centre for Operations Research and Training. 1996. Situational Analysis of Medical Termination of Pregnancy (MTP) Services in Maharashtra. Monograph. Baroda, India.

Centre for Operations Research and Training. 1996. Situational Analysis of Medical Termination of Pregnancy (MTP) Services in Bihar, Family Welfare Programme in Bihar – A Baseline Survey. Monograph. Baroda, India.

Centre for Operations Research and Training. 1997a. Situational Analysis of Medical Termination of Pregnancy (MTP) Services in Tamil Nadu. Monograph. Baroda, India.

Centre for Operations Research and Training. 1997b. Situational Analysis of Medical Termination of Pregnancy (MTP) Services in Uttar Pradesh. Monograph. Baroda, India.

Chhabra, R., and Nuna, S.C. Undated. Abortion in India – An Overview. Delhi, India.

Government of India. 1998. Report of the National Consultation on Safe Abortion Services, Ministry of Health and Family Welfare. New Delhi, India.

Gupte, M., Bandewar, S., and Pisal, H. 1997. Abortion Needs of Women in India : A Case Study of Rural Maharashtra. *Reproductive Health Matters*, 9: 77-86.

Indian Council of Medical Research. 1989. Illegal Abortion in Rural Areas: A Task Force Study. Monograph. Delhi, India.

Jalnawala, S.F. 1975. Medical Termination of Pregnancy Act: A Preliminary Report of the First Twenty Month of Implementation. *Journal of Obstetrics and Gynaecology of India*, October 25(5).

Karkal, M. 1991. Abortion Laws and the Abortion Situation in India. *Issues in Reproductive and Genetic Engineering,* Vol. 4 No. 3.

Khan, M.E., Patel, B.C., and Chandrasekhar, R. 1993. Abortion Acceptors in India : Observation in India : Observations from a Prospective Study. Vol.3. Proceedings of IUSSP International Population Conference, Montreal, Canada.

Khan, M.E., Rajagopal, S., Barge, S., and Kumar, N. 1998. Situational Analysis of Medical Termination of Pregnancy Services in Gujarat, Maharashtra, Tamil Nadu and Uttar Pradesh. Paper presented at a Global Meeting on Post Abortion Care and Operations Research, Population Council, New York: January 19-21, 1998. Also published as Working Paper 13, CORT, Baroda, India.

Khan, M.E., Barge, S., and Philip, G. 1996. Abortion in India – An Overview. *Social Change*, Vol. 26 No. 3 and 4.

Khan, M.E., Sinha, R., Patel, B.C., Lakhanpal, S., and Khanna, P. 1998. Decision Making in Acceptance and Seeking Abortion of Unwanted Pregnancies. Paper presented at the International Workshop on Abortion Facilities and Post Abortion Care in the Context of RCH Program, March 23-24, 1998. Centre for Operations Research and Training, New Delhi, India.

Mathai, S.T. 1997. Making Abortion Safer. *Journal of Family Welfare,* 43: 71-80.

Mukhopadhyay, P., and Das. A. 1975. Termination of Pregnancy by Vacuum Aspiration With and Without Sterilisation. *Journal of Obstetrics and Gynaecology of India,* 25(5).

Registrar General of India. 1990. Survey of Census of Death, (Rural) Annual Report, 1990. Office of the Registrar General, New Delhi, India.

6

Promoting Safe Motherhood: Issues and Challenges

Dileep V. Mavalankar

Background

The maternal and child health programme was started in India in the early 1960s. Maternal health, however, remained a neglected problem. In 1987, the Safe Motherhood Conference organised by the World Health Organization (WHO) and other donors in Nairobi focussed attention on the high levels of maternal mortality in developing countries. Following this conference, the World Health Organization initiated the safe motherhood programme to lower maternal mortality in several developing countries, including India. More recently, the International Conference on Population and Development (ICPD) emphasised safe motherhood as a priority in its Programme of Action (United Nations, 1995).

In this chapter, the development of maternal health services in India are examined to critically analyse the achievements and problems in operationalizing the safe motherhood programme. Lessons are drawn from past experience and are related to plans for promoting safe motherhood within the new reproductive and child health programme.

Preventing Maternal Mortality

In the 1960s and 70s, maternal health services within the maternal and child health (MCH) programme focused on antenatal care and the high risk approach. It was believed that good antenatal care and using the high risk approach would reduce maternal mortality. Another effort of past programmes was training traditional birth attendants to improve their delivery practices. It was believed that training traditional birth attendants would also lead to a reduction in maternal mortality. However, the level of maternal mortality remained high in developing countries including India until the mid-1980s. Therefore, the causes of maternal death and the socio-medical factors contributing to maternal death were re-examined.

Research showed that, for mothers who develop complications during delivery, emergency obstetric care was needed to reduce maternal mortality. Since it is not possible to predict which mother will develop complications, the high risk approach could not really prevent maternal deaths. In fact, the high risk approach resulted in many women being referred, several of whom eventually had normal deliveries. This discredited the referral process. On the other hand, maternal death can occur within hours to days of developing complications and so it is important to promptly transport women to institutions equipped to manage complications. If obstetric complications are handled effectively, mortality can be substantially reduced. However, once major obstetric complications develop, a trained traditional birth attendant or a nurse can do little at home because surgical intervention is often necessary. Given these arguments it was proposed that first referral units where emergency obstetric care can be provided should be established. Such first referral units were believed to be the most cost-effective way of reducing maternal mortality (Maine, 1991).

The World Health Organization also changed its view from promoting the high risk approach to providing emergency obstetric care by establishing referral systems. As there was a consensus among several donors, emergency obstetric care became the main strategy for preventing maternal mortality.

The Child Survival and Safe Motherhood Programme

In the mid-1970s, following the success with small pox eradication and the expanded programme of immunisation, UNICEF helped to launch the universal immunisation programme with the objective of reaching 100 percent of children under 5 years of age and pregnant women with basic immunisations. By 1990, reported service statistics showed near 100 percent coverage of these groups. This was seen as a major achievement. The Government of India was encouraged to expand its focus from immunisation to a broader and more comprehensive programme which would include interventions for child survival and safe motherhood.

UNICEF and other donors played a key role in the development of the new child survival and safe motherhood programme. The programme was funded by the World Bank and UNICEF provided technical support. The budget was about $ 330 million for five years. About half of this amount was earmarked for safe motherhood activities (World Bank, 1991).

Programme design

The programme had two major objectives: (1) to reduce infant and child mortality; and (2) to reduce maternal mortality. It, therefore, included interventions for child survival as well as for safe motherhood. These interventions are listed in Table 1 (Government of India, 1994).

The goal of the safe motherhood component of the programme was to reduce maternal mortality from 4 per 1,000 births to 2 per 1,000 births by the year 2000. The key strategy for reducing maternal mortality included establishment of first referral units for providing emergency obstetric care. These first referral units were to be established within existing community health centres to provide emergency obstetric services including caesarean section. Another strategy was to improve maternal care at the village level. The

TABLE 1: Key Interventions Included in the Child Survival and Safe Motherhood Programme

Child survival interventions	Safe motherhood interventions
Essential new born care	Immunisation for pregnant women
Immunisation	Prevention and treatment of anaemia
Management of diarrhoea	Antenatal care and early identification of maternal complications
Management of acute respiratory infections	Delivery by trained personnel
Vitamin A prophylaxis	Promotion of institutional delivery
	Management of obstetric emergencies
	Birth spacing

mother was expected to receive antenatal care and high risk cases would be identified and referred. Training of traditional birth attendants would continue. They would be provided with disposable delivery kits to perform hygienic deliveries. Sub-centres would be provided with equipment and drugs. Auxiliary nurse midwives would provide maternal care at the sub-centre level. A monitoring system would be developed to assess programme output and impact. In addition, information, education and communication activities would be undertaken to make people aware of this new programme and staff would be trained to orient them to the new initiative and to upgrade their skills (World Bank, 1991; Government of India, 1994).

Implementation issues and problems

For various reasons, only some of the activities planned for the programme were in fact implemented. Among the child survival interventions, immunisation was reasonably well implemented as it was a continuation and consolidation of the earlier universal immunisation programme which had received high priority during 1985-90 with active support of UNICEF. Other child survival interventions such as treatment of diarrhoea and acute respiratory infections, received relatively less attention. These activities depended on the regularity of visits by health workers which could not be ensured.

Training problems

All key staff were expected to receive orientation as well as training to upgrade their skills. A short orientation-cum-skills development training programme of five to six days duration was implemented. It covered all components of the programme including modules on planning and monitoring. Instead of relying on existing training institutions, special teams of trainers were employed.

Our analysis of the training programme, however showed that the training was too brief to upgrade skills and that training on safe motherhood interventions was particularly inadequate (Government of India, 1992). There were very few practical sessions. Many of the newer concepts were presented in a confusing and unclear manner. The importance of emergency obstetric care was not conveyed clearly and forcefully. The training programme did not cover life saving skills that auxiliary nurse midwives and medical officers could employ to deal with obstetric emergencies. The quality of training was inconsistent and was not linked to supplies of medicines and equipment or to the monitoring. Supplies and equipment reached the facilities long after the training programme and so the skills which staff learned could not be used (Mother Care, 1996; Christensson et al, 1997).

Skills development for maternal health was neglected. Skills development was especially important because most staff, including the doctors, did not have the skills for providing emergency obstetric care. It also became clear that it would not be possible to staff facilities with qualified obstetricians and, therefore, it was important to train general doctors and lower level staff (Mother Care, 1996).

Equipment, supplies and logistics

High quality, imported and potentially very useful equipment was purchased and supplied to the first referral units, primary health centres and sub-centres. The procurement of quality equipment and supply on such a large scale, however, became a major logistic exercise as India has more than 1,700 first referral units, 20,000 primary health centres and 130,000 sub-centres. There were substantial delays in procurement and supply of equipment and this hindered the implementation of the programme. On the other hand, equipment was not always put to use. Some of the equipment could not be used because trained staff were not in place and because of the lack of reliable electricity (Mother Care, 1996).

Staffing issues

The most critical problem was staffing. Estimates indicate that not even half of the 1,748 first referral units were fully functional (Government of India, 1998). Many did not have key staff such as an obstetrician, a paediatrician and an anaesthetist (Government of India, 1997). Data from one of the advanced states highlighted the problem. Of the 88 first referral units in the state, only 19 had an obstetrician, 18 had a paediatrician and 7 an anaesthetist. In another such state, only 14 out of 123 first referral units had all four specialists. The problem is not lack of specialists but their reluctance to be located in rural areas and small towns.

Emergency obstetric care can be provided by doctors with an MBBS degree, provided they can be trained and their skills upgraded. However, these doctors are reluctant to provide such services for fear of being sued since the Consumer Protection Act now covers health services, too. The auxiliary nurse midwife, too, can provide obstetric first aid with some skills training. However, such training was not organised.

Information, education and communication, and community participation

Information, education and communication activities were limited in scope and implementation. The educational materials produced and communication efforts made for safe motherhood received low priority, further limiting the effectiveness of maternal health interventions. The design of the programme had a limited component of community participation.

Service delivery problems

Many of the safe motherhood interventions were not implemented. The content of antenatal care remained weak and was in most places limited to tetanus toxoid vaccination and distribution of iron and folic acid tablets. A study in 24 districts in 13 states by the Indian Council of Medical Research (ICMR) showed the limited range of maternal services provided. There was poor identification of high risk mothers and complications during delivery were not handled systematically. Emergency obstetric care was not really operational in most places (ICMR, 1997).

Access to blood

No systematic efforts were made to improve the blood supply at the first referral units. On the contrary, during this period access to blood became more problematic because the Supreme Court passed an order to ensure blood safety. The order decreed that only those blood banks which complied with the government's guidelines should be allowed to function. As the government's guidelines were very idealistic, many of the government and private blood banks had to be closed down.

Supervision and monitoring

Supervision and monitoring of the programme focussed mainly on interventions for child survival such as immunisation and a few safe motherhood interventions including immunisation and the provision of iron and folic acid tablets. The functioning of the first referral units was not monitored. It was, therefore, difficult to get data on basic parameters such as how many facilities were fully functional and how many emergency obstetric care procedures, including caesareans were conducted at these centres. Although detailed guidelines were developed to monitor the functioning of the first referral units, these were not operationalised. It seems that even at the national, state and district levels monitoring efforts were focussed primarily on the family planning and immunisation programmes.

The World Bank had intended that maternal mortality review committees be established at national and regional levels to monitor, evaluate and assist the Ministry of Health and Family Welfare in the development of a future strategy and for reporting maternal mortality and morbidity (World Bank, 1991). However, these committees were never established. Therefore, basic data on the number of maternal deaths and their causes were not available in most states.

A key reason for the lack of supervision and monitoring was the low priority given to the safe motherhood component. UNICEF, the technical agency supporting the programme, also did not focus its efforts on safe motherhood and did not have adequate technical staff to monitor the programme.

Impact of the Programme

Assessment of the impact of a major national programme requires a good data collection system. In India, vital registration is incomplete and important outcome data for programme monitoring are not available. In this case, no systematic efforts were made to develop a management information system to provide information on maternal health interventions. A review of the programme in 1996 showed that less than 10 percent of maternal deaths were reported in the required format (Mother Care, 1996). Recent information from one of the more advanced states showed that only about 20 percent of maternal deaths were reported. Data were reported on antenatal registration rather than on antenatal examination. Data from three districts in an advanced state showed that on an average about 22 caesarean sections were conducted per first referral unit in one year while the estimated need for caesarean sections was about 600 per first referral unit per year; thereby, underscoring the low level of performance of the first referral units.

There has not been any national survey or any systematic study to assess the impact of the programme. Only a small number of quick reviews provide some information on programme implementation and outcomes (Mother Care, 1996; Christensson, 1997; Mavalankar, 1996). The second round of the National Family Health Survey (equivalent of Demographic and Health Surveys) will include some indicators to examine the impact of the safe motherhood programme but these data will become available only in late 1999. Multi-indicator cluster surveys supported by UNICEF provide district level data on maternal and child health indicators. The selection of districts in these surveys, however, does not ensure that they are representative of the country in any one round, and comparison of data between rounds is problematic. These surveys provide some information on the coverage of services but national compilations of these data are not readily available.

As there are no systems to measure maternal mortality or morbidity, it is not possible to study change. Surrogate indicators such as the proportion of deliveries attended by trained staff and the proportion of institutional deliveries can provide an idea of coverage of maternal health services. The infant mortality rate, an outcome indicator, is affected by child survival as well as maternal and perinatal interventions. Data compiled from various secondary sources are provided in Table 3 . It shows that there has not been any substantial improvement in these indicators except for tetanus toxoid immunisation and iron and folic acid tables distribution.

TABLE 3: Infant Mortality Rate, Coverage of Tetanus Toxoid Immunisation, and Distribution of Iron and Folic Acid Tables, Institutional Deliveries, and Attendants at Delivery

Programme/Year	1981	1983	1990	1991	1992	1993	1994	1995	1996	1997
Infant mortality rate	110	105	80	80	79	74	74	74	72	72
Tetanus toxoid (%) Immunisation					55*			66**		
Iron and folic acid coverage		51*				69**				
% Births in institutions@		19	23	24	24	25	22	25		
% births (at home) attended by trained professionals@		18	21	22	23	24	28	28		

@ data from Sample Registration System,
* data from National Family Health Survey (International Institute of Population Sciences, 1995),
** data from management information system.
Note: The programme started in 1992.

Lessons Learned

The planning and implementation of safe motherhood interventions in the child survival and safe motherhood programme provides several key lessons for future programming:

1. Lack of co-ordination

There was no co-ordination between programme inputs, process and outputs. There was a mismatch between these three key elements. For example, one objective was to establish first referral units to treat emergency obstetric problems. Equipment was supplied but training was neglected. Performance was not monitored in terms of treating emergency obstetric cases. Therefore, data on how many first referral units were functional and how many procedures were performed were not available. The lesson is that inputs should be well co-ordinated and outputs should be measured to ensure effectiveness.

2. Need for micro-level planning and monitoring
Safe motherhood interventions were not worked out in detail at various levels along with the indicators to monitor their implementation and effectiveness. For example, there were no guidelines to measure the prevention and treatment of nutritional anaemia. There was no way to assess compliance with iron and folic acid tablets that were given to the mothers. There was also no effort to assess whether anaemic women were getting adequate amount of drugs for an adequate duration. There was no monitoring of haemoglobin levels in anaemic mothers. All this lead to a situation where high coverage of iron folic acid distribution was reported but with no data to show that it made any difference to the status of anaemia in pregnant women.

3. Complexity of programme interventions and management capacity
In a country of the size and diversity of India, complex programmes with many different interventions are difficult to operationalise. Programmes take time to actually get implemented on the ground due to administrative delays within the bureaucracy at the central, state and district levels. For example, the immunisation programme took almost 15 years to reach a coverage of 70-80 percent even though it received high priority by the government and donors. The child survival and safe motherhood programme included many more interventions and was much more complex. It therefore needed a higher level of managerial capacity, administrative commitment and resources to have a reasonable chance of success.

4. Need for around-the-clock services

Emergency obstetric care and delivery care must be provided for 24 hours and throughout the year. More staff and resources are therefore needed. Most states have found it difficult to staff first referral units with specialists, especially obstetricians and anaesthetists, partly because of the shortage of specialists and partly because of the unwillingness of these specialists to work in sub-district hospitals and community health centres. The alternative is to train medical officers so that they can provide emergency obstetric care.

5. Skewed programme priorities

The major priority of the programme was child survival and more specifically immunisation. The safe motherhood component received lower priority and therefore substantially less attention.

The Reproductive and Child Health Programme

Post-ICPD, the Government of India is in the process of reorienting the family planning and maternal and child health programmes to a reproductive and child health programme (Government of India, undated a). The budget of the programme ($ 1.2 billion) is almost four times that of the child survival and safe motherhood programme. The objective of the new programme is to improve reproductive health, including maternal and child health. The key elements of this programme are: immunisation, essential obstetric care, emergency obstetric care, 24-hour deliveries at primary health centres and community health centres, referral and transport for disadvantaged families, blood supply at first referral units, essential new born care, medical termination of pregnancy, treatment of reproductive tract infections and of sexually transmitted infections. Thus, safe motherhood is a part of the essential package of reproductive and child health services.

Independent district surveys are underway to assess the availability and utilisation of services. However, only four maternal health indicators are included: (1) percentage of institutional deliveries; (2) number of cases referred to primary health centres, first referral units and postpartum centres for the management of complicated deliveries; (3) number of patients treated for reproductive tract infections; and, (4) the proportion of women completing three antenatal visits. These indicators do not provide information on other aspects of maternal health. It is not clear why this programme has not adopted the indicators suggested by the WHO for maternal health and reproductive health (WHO, 1994; 1997).

The reproductive and child health programme will not make a substantial difference until the basic barriers in provision of maternal health services and problems in the utilisation of these services are systematically addressed (Mavalankar, 1998). Lessons learned from past experience should be used to inform the programme.

Recommendations

To ensure that the safe motherhood agenda does not get neglected yet again, we offer the following recommendations based on the analysis of past experiences:

1. Need for high priority, clear objectives, and well worked out strategy for safe motherhood

The objectives to promote safe motherhood should be articulated clearly and should be measurable in the terms of a reduction in maternal mortality, an increase in institutional deliveries, the number of deliveries conducted by trained staff, and universal access to emergency obstetric care. The objectives should be followed by a well thought out strategy to achieve them.

2. Conceptual clarity and detailed implementation guidelines

For any programme to be implemented effectively, a very clear conceptual framework is needed. In addition, there is a need to develop implementation guidelines for various levels of service delivery. The concept of maternal care should be specified in terms of normal maternity care and emergency obstetric care. The roles of staff at the centre, state and district levels must be clearly delineated. A detailed plan for supervision with some flexibility is needed to enable the programme to be adapted to local realities. Contingency arrangements should be built into the plan, and local managers should have the power and the resources to purchase and repair equipment and contract staff so that there is no interruption in the provision of services.

3. Co-ordination and consistency between objectives, inputs, process, supervision, and monitoring

It is necessary to ensure that all inputs such as staff, training, equipment and supplies are provided in a co-ordinated way. Supervision and monitoring are important. For example, if emergency obstetric care is to be strengthened, monitoring indicators are needed to measure how many first referral units are functional and what proportion of the expected need for such care is being served by these facilities.

4. Ensuring accountability

The supervision and monitoring system should ensure accountability of staff at various levels. It should ensure that staff are present at the place of work; are providing high quality care in a gender sensitive way; and, are accountable for the outputs of the services they provide. Accountability should include reporting, investigating and monitoring all maternal deaths and major complications in the area and taking steps to prevent deaths. A national maternal mortality study must be carried out every 10 years to ensure that there are reliable data to indicate progress towards the ultimate goal of safe motherhood.

5. Decentralising management and problem solving

Programme planning should be decentralised so that local managers make adaptations to local conditions. The focus should be on solving problems so that the services are available. Supportive supervision is especially important as staff have to deal with emergency situations.

6. Providing good quality technical support

As safe motherhood interventions include substantial technical components, high quality technical support is needed at various levels from public health and management professionals, and obstetricians.

7. Training and human resource development

This is an important input that is generally neglected. Skill development is required for staff at all levels. Lower level staff should be trained to provide basic emergency obstetric services even in the absence of an obstetrician.

8. Information, education, and communication, and community participation

Information, education and communication to make the community aware of the availability of services and the community's participation and mobilisation arc needed to ensure that there is early recognition of complications and timely transportation of women for emergency care.

Concluding Comments

This review of safe motherhood efforts in India shows a mixed picture. The challenge now is to make motherhood safe through the reproductive and child health programme. The government must give it high priority and the society, including NGOs, donors, professional organisations, media and academic institutions must support the programme. Long-term planning with consistent, concerted and sincere efforts is needed to ensure that the programme is implemented in the spirit in which it had been conceptualised.

References

Christensson, I., David, L., Hutter. I., Johansson, E., and Roy, T. 1997. Evaluation of UNICEF- Child Survival and Safe Motherhood Programme in India. Draft Report.

Government of India. 1992. National Child Survival and Safe Motherhood Programme: Module for Health Workers. Department of Family Welfare, Ministry of Health and Family Wefare, New Delhi, India.

Government of India. 1994. National Child Survival and Safe Motherhood Programme. Maternal and Child Health Division, Department of Family Welfare, Ministry of Health and Family Wefare, New Delhi, India.

Government of India. (Undated, a). Reproductive and Child Health Programme. Department of Family Welfare, Ministry of Health and Family Welfare, New Delhi, India.

Government of India. (Undated, b). A Manual on Target Free Approach to Family Welfare. Department of Family Welfare, Ministry of Health and Family Welfare, New Delhi, India.

Government of India. 1997. Reproductive and Child Health Programme: Schemes for Implementation. Department of Family Welfare, Ministry of Health and Family Welfare, New Delhi, India.

Government of India. 1998. Reproductive and Child Health Programme: Implementation Issues. Department of Family Welfare, Ministry of Health and Family Welfare, New Delhi, India.

Indian Council of Medical Research. 1997. A Baseline Survey of Reproductive Health Care Services in 23 Districts (14 States) in India. New Delhi, India.

International Institute of Population Sciences. 1995. National Family Health Survey, India, (1992-93), 239. Mumbai, India.

Maine, D. 1991. Safe Motherhood Programs: Options and Issues. Centre for Population and Family Health, Columbia University, New York, USA.

Mavalankar, D.V. 1996. Can PHC System in India Deliver Emergency Obstetric Care? A Management Perspective on Safe Motherhood Programme. Working Paper No. 1198. Indian Institute of Management, Ahmedabad, India.

Mavalankar, D.V. 1998. Management Constraints on Operationalisation of Reproductive Health Program Interventions in PHC System in India. Indian Institute of Management, Ahmedabad, India. (Unpublished)

Mother Care. 1996. Child Survival and Safe Motherhood Programme Review and Assessment: Lessons Learned and Recommendations – An Evaluation Report Prepared for the Ministry of Health and Family Welfare of India. Mother Care, John Snow Inc., Arlington, USA.

Pachauri, S. 1995. Defining a Reproductive Health Package For India: A Proposed Framework. South and East Asia Regional Working Paper No. 4. Population Council, New Delhi, India.

United Nations. 1995. Summary of the Programme of Action of the International Conference on Population and Development, 1994, 13. United Nations, New York.

World Bank. 1991. Staff Appraisal Report: India Child Survival and Safe Motherhood Project. World Bank Report No. 9849-IN. Washington D.C., USA.

World Bank. 1995. India's Family Welfare Program: Toward a Reproductive and Child Health Approach. World Bank Report No. 14644-IN. Washington D.C., USA.

World Bank. 1997. Project Appraisal Document (India): Reproductive and Child Health Project. World Bank Report No. 16393-IN. Washington D.C., USA.

World Health Organization. 1994. Indicators for Monitoring Maternal Health Goals. WHO/FHE/MSM/94.1 Geneva: World Health Organization.

World Health Organization. 1997. Draft Report of the Interagency Technical Meeting on Reproductive Health Indicators for Global Monitoring, April 1997. Geneva: World Health Organization.

7

Sexuality and Sexual Behaviour: The Current Discourse

Pertti J. Pelto

Introduction

This paper reviews the current state of knowledge concerning sexuality and sexual behaviour in India and the development of new programmes aimed at safer, healthier, better-informed sexual practices. Research interest in sexuality and sexual behaviours has developed rapidly during the decade of the 1990s, mainly as a response to the mounting alarm about the HIV/AIDS epidemic. Although most of this research is connected with the need to develop interventions to prevent HIV/AIDS, there are other good reasons why more knowledge about sexual behaviours is needed. Practically all aspects of reproductive health relate directly or indirectly to sexual behaviours. Issues concerning abortion practices and abortion-seeking arise directly or indirectly from sexual behaviours; programmes focussed on contraceptive practices require knowledge about the sexual negotiations and practices of married couples; and various gynaecological problems also have their direct links to sexual practices.

Beyond the direct concerns about reproductive health problems, recent research attention has turned to the importance of sexual relations as major factors in domestic violence and other aspects of gender relations. Coercive sexual relations are a major element in violence instigated by men toward their wives. In addition, conflicts regarding sexual relations provoke other forms of domestic violence. Very few studies have explored these sexual behaviours but some research is now emerging that deals with this sensitive area.

Programmatic Guidelines from the International Conference on Population and Development (ICPD)

The programme of action adopted at the ICPD called for a dramatic shift away from a narrow family planning orientation to policies that encompass a wide definition of reproductive and sexual health. Concerning the topical area of 'sexuality and sexual behaviours', the main elements of the ICPD guidelines are listed below (Pachauri, 1996):

1. Women and men should be enabled to make informed choices about their own sexuality, reproductive fulfillment, and reproductive health. Achieving these ends requires services for screening, education and counselling in addition to clinical health services.

2. Programmes directed to general reproductive health should involve men in a variety of direct ways, in order to bring about more effective, well-informed, actions on behalf of both women and men.

3. Reproductive health programmes aimed at both women and men will need to recognise, understand, and promote changes in the prevailing norms of gender relations. For men to become more responsible partners in all aspects of reproductive decision-making, programmes will need to foster much greater levels of communication between male and female partners. Also, steps must be taken to lessen the power differentials – in levels of information, access to resources, decision-making practices, and other sectors of control – within families and between sexual partners. Thus, reproductive and sexual health programmes must develop, and make use of, systematic knowledge of the varieties of social constructions of gender relations and sexuality.

4. Community participation should be built everywhere into reproductive and sexual health programmes. Wherever feasible, reproductive and sexual health programmes should seek to decentralise and to devolve power to regional and local community levels. Such community participation is particularly vital for programmes for sexually transmitted infections (STIs), HIV/AIDS, and related sexual health problems.

5. To accomplish these goals, a great deal of research would be required on current practices and knowledge of people (women and men) in the areas of sexuality, sexual behaviour, and the social contructions of power relationships around sexual and reproductive issues.

State of the Art at the Time of the ICPD

At the time of the ICPD, various governmental and non-governmental bodies in India had begun awareness campaigns and other interventions in the face of the HIV/AIDS epidemic, but these activities had been developed with very little systematic information about sexuality and sexual behaviours. Some authoritative sources argued that there is no problem in India because of the prevailing morality favouring strict adherence to standards of monogamous marital sex. Others argued quite the opposite, pointing to the relatively large numbers of sex workers and alleging that large numbers of married and unmarried Indian men were engaged in non-marital sexual activities. Few data were available to support either position. Also, there were very few data concerning sexual behaviours in the daily lives of married couples. That kind of information is needed for dealing with a variety of reproductive health issues in the new agenda mandated by the ICPD.

In 1994, the year of the ICPD, *The Indian Journal of Social Work (IJSW)* published a special issue entitled 'Sexual

Behaviour and AIDS in India.' The papers in that volume had originated in a workshop at the Tata Institute of Social Sciences, sponsored by the Ford Foundation in 1993. These papers provide a useful picture of the 'state of the art' at the time of the ICPD. The lead paper by Moni Nag pointed to "the limited amount of studies done on sexual behaviour in contemporary India..." (Nag, 1994). Nonetheless, he cited several surveys, particularly some carried out among students, as well as a questionnaire survey carried out by the magazine, *Debonair*. The *Debonair* survey was among the first widely publicised studies of reported sexual behaviours of the 1990s (Savara and Sridhar, 1992). Other surveys provided evidence of the changing standards concerning premarital sex, particularly among young people (mainly students). The studies indicated that a considerable minority of them (more males than females) felt that sexual intercourse before marriage is permissible, particularly if the partners are 'in love,' or are engaged to be married. In one of the attitude surveys cited by Nag, 35 percent of male students answered yes to the item, 'A couple in love may have premarital sex.' Thirteen percent of females also replied positively to that statement. However it is important to note that about one-third of the respondents 'didn't know' or did not respond. Nag compared the data of the 1990s with studies from the 1960s and 1970s, and found that "...the perceived limits within which sexual freedom should be allowed to unmarried boys and girls have widened..." (Nag, 1994).

In the early stages of the HIV/AIDS epidemic, news media and health programme people focussed most attention on female sex workers, especially in the larger cities. Research and interventions in Calcutta's brothel areas developed mainly in 1992-93, although there had been a major survey in 1987. Interventions coordinated by the All India Institute of Hygiene and Public Health began to have impressive effects on increasing the use of condoms among female sex workers in the Sonagachi brothel area. A survey carried out in November-December 1993, found that condom use had increased to nearly 50 percent from a reported 1 percent in 1992 and the prevalence of STIs had declined from previous levels (Jana et al, 1994).

The second focus of attention was on truck drivers and their assistants. Studies in other countries, particularly in Africa, had shown that major truck routes were major conduits for the spread of sexually transmitted infections. In 1992 and 1993, some unpublished studies on truckers began to appear in conferences and workshops. In June 1993, a workshop was organised on 'Developing An Action Plan for control of AIDS Among Truck Drivers in India', in Jaipur (Rao et al, 1994).

A study based on in-depth interviews with 100 truck drivers at a halt point 55 kilometers outside Calcutta was conducted in a context that included clinical services, which undoubtedly led to a sampling bias toward more sexually active individuals. The researchers reported very high rates of sexual contacts with female sex workers. Ninety-seven of their 100 informants reported visiting sex workers; most of them said they had such contacts several times per week. The researchers also reported that one-third to almost half of the truckers had experienced oral and/or anal sex with other men. In some of these male-to-male sexual contacts, young helpers (*khalasis*) were forced to submit to the sexual demands of the drivers. (Rao et al, 1994).

Data on male-to-male sex among 813 Indian men living in 'the West' (UK), and 387 men living in India obtained from letters, telephone conversations, and direct conversations emphasised the strong social stigmatisation of male-to-male sex in Indian society (Khan, 1994). Hence, such behaviours are very secretive and even males who have strong preferences for same-sex intercourse are forced to accept conventional marriages. Most of Khan's sample were engaged or married. Only a very small percentage indicated that they would be able to resist marriage. "Marriage is a duty, a necessity, and not very often a matter of personal choice.....[avoiding marriage would bring] shame and dishonour to their families..." (Khan, 1994). The most common first initiation to sexual behaviour, was that of masturbation (489 men), followed by femoral sex (between the thighs) (225), anal sex (190), 'frottage' (178), and oral sex (118). Approximately this same rank ordering of sexual practices was found in the men's current practices and preferences

(Khan, 1994). These data seemed to indicate that male-to-male sex acts are often 'safe' from the standpoint of infections. Both masturbation and femoral sexual contact are unlikely to result in transmission of serious infections, least of all, HIV infection. On the other hand, anal sex has a very high probability of infection transmission.

This study and the other (meagre) sources of data about sex among males showed that up to 1994 at least, men had little awareness of HIV/AIDS and condom use was rare. Even the men of Indian origin in the United Kingdom reported low rates of condom use (Khan, 1994). The same applied to the truck drivers. In 1994, studies and interventions on truckers had only just started in various parts of India. Apparently the truckers in these studies were somewhat aware of the use of condoms for prevention of sexually transmitted infections (STIs) but had much less exposure to information about HIV infections.

These studies conducted during the first half of this decade are only a small sample from the inventory of research in sexual behaviours. They do, however, give a fairly clear picture of the state of affairs around the time of the Cairo conference. The overall situation existing in 1994-1995 could be summarised as follows:

1. Pre-marital and extra-marital sexual encounters were found to be more frequent in the Indian populations than had earlier been assumed but there was practically no data concerning the behavioural contexts of these sexual activities.

2. General surveys on the attitudes and behaviour of young people suggested that moral attitudes about pre-marital sex were changing rather rapidly.

3. By 1994, there was an increasing number of reports in newspapers and magazines about the threat of AIDS. However, the dominant beliefs among the general population seemed to be that AIDS was only found among female sex workers and truck drivers. These popular beliefs were from the news media and some AIDS activists who were focussing attention primarily on the HIV prevalence among sex workers in Mumbai and Chennai. For example, "The Indian Health Organisation's report on the rapid

rate [of increase] of HIV infection from 1 percent in 1986 to over 30 percent in 1992 based on a sample of (female sex workers) in Bombay is often cited by the news media...." (Nag, 1994).

4. Interventions had been initiated to raise awareness of AIDS and STIs, and to bring about behavioural changes (especially greater condom use) in redlight areas and among truck drivers. Some sectors of the news media as well as some government health officials were still taking the view that the HIV/AIDS epidemic would not affect India severely, since pre-marital and extra-marital sexual activities, they felt, are rare. Solid research on sexuality and sexual behaviours in 'ordinary' populations was extremely scanty.

5. Most people, even in 'targetted populations' such as truck drivers, had rather scant knowledge of the use of condoms for protection against sexually transmitted infections.

6. Information about male-to-male and female-to-female sexual behaviours was even rarer than data on heterosexual behaviours. "Very little is known about the current practice of male or female homosexuality in India." (Nag, 1994). The *Debonair* study showed that about ten percent of the male respondents reported that their first sexual experience was with another male.

7. Researchers were becoming disillusioned with broad-based surveys and were turning to small-scale qualitative methods as a means of getting more systematic and detailed information about actual sexual practices among the various segments of the population. Some methodological studies have demonstrated, for example, that broad-based surveys resulted in considerable under-reporting of sexual behaviour. A study in Uganda made systematic comparisons between quantitative survey results and in-depth interviews and demonstrated that there was significant under-reporting among both males and females with regard to extra-marital sex partners. In the in-depth interviews among males, the estimated frequency rose from 35 percent to 45.5 percent. Among women, the under-reporting was more dramatic: the survey data showed 14 percent having 'at least one non-regular partner,' but in-depth interviews indicated that 32 percent (more than double) had multiple partner sex in the past year (Konings et al, 1995). When we consider

that sex outside marriage is more highly stigmatised in India than in east Africa, it would appear that all survey data must be assumed to include systematic under-reporting of sexual behaviour. The extent of under-reporting is likely to be much greater among female respondents. Although we have no studies in India comparable to the Konings study in Uganda, it may not be misleading to regard the extent of women's non-marital sexual behaviours to be at least double the frequencies reported in specific surveys.

The '65 Cities Study' of the National AIDS Control Organisation

In 1994-95, the National AIDS Control Organisation (NACO) embarked on an ambitious project to develop inventories of sexual activities among designated high risk subpopulations in the major cities of India. The research methodology was largely qualitative, with a considerable emphasis on mapping of locations of high risk sexual activities. The individual research groups were expected to find knowledgeable key informants (NGO workers, community health workers, health providers, and others) who could direct them to specific locations of: sex worker activities, homosexual contacts, drug-user areas, sexual activity areas of students, and trucker locations near the city. In addition to mapping locations of sexual activities, the researchers were expected to get in-depth interviews with persons in the various 'high risk situations,' in order to collect detailed information of the actual context, constraints to practising safer sex (including availability of condoms), and related information concerning actual sexual practices (Sethi et al, 1995).

The project was seriously under-funded during its actual operations, but researchers went about the research in a dedicated, often innovative manner. Reports from the individual city studies varied considerably in depth and quality. However, the results indicated widespread prevalence of 'risky sexual practices,' and also showed that qualitative, free-form data gathering methods could produce useful information about sexual practices for intervention programmes.

Some informal comparisons among the different cities showed large differences in local situations affecting the pattern of risky sexual behaviours. It was found that in some cities, there was strict surveillance of female sex workers, where there were no regular, established brothels (for example, Chennai), and sex workers were contacted through a more complex system of brokers, in dispersed locations. Reports suggest considerable differences in the degree of police control of commercial sex workers, the extent and locations of casual sexual encounters, and other relevant features.

For a variety of reasons, neither the individual reports from the '65 Cities Study', nor an overall summary of the findings were distributed to wider audiences in India. Nonetheless, the experience of qualitative research in a large number of study areas contributed to a growing realisation among researchers and programme planners that combinations of in-depth interviewing, mapping, and other qualitative techniques could generate extremely useful descriptive data for intervention projects.

Research on Sexuality and Sexual Behaviour: The 'Sexual Behaviour Research Network'

The Workshop on Sexual Behaviour and AIDS in India (1993) occurred on the eve of rather ambitious new research in sexual behaviour. The Ford Foundation, ODA (later DFID), USAID and a number of funding agencies developed a series of research-cum-intervention projects that led to a rapid increase in information about sexuality and sexual behaviours. Some individual researchers have also contributed to the accumulation of knowledge during the past four to five years. Not all of these research projects are described here, but I will review some examples from different parts of India, in order to delineate common features as well as possible regional variations. Regional variations are especially important for developing locally appropriate intervention programmes. 'Locally appropriate' means not only the use of appropriate local terminology in interviews and other interactions with local people, but also points to the fact that the obstacles to 'safe sex behaviours' and other objectives are different in different areas. In some areas, the array of local practitioners of health may be quite different from other areas, thus suggesting different approaches.

Starting in 1995, the Ford Foundation research network developed gradually. As individual research groups (NGOs and others) were funded by the Ford Foundation, it became evident that communications among these groups would enhance the understanding and productivity of all the participants. Meanwhile, the International Center for Research on Women (ICRW) also developed research projects in four sites to study adolescents' sexuality and behaviours. These researchers were invited to join in the network. During 1997-98, the network expanded to include other researchers.

Many of the studies presented below are from the network, but I will include some other data wherever needed to complete the picture of current knowledge of sexuality and sexual behaviours in India.

The Picture at the End of the Century

Data from increasing numbers of studies in different parts of India show that there are pre-marital and extra-marital sexual behaviours in both urban and rural communities. Individuals involved in non-marital activities are certainly only a minority in these communities. Nowhere in the newer data is there indication that 'everybody' is involved in these sexual activities. No research methodology available to us can provide actual, precise percentages. Therefore, estimates are provided. There are serious problems of possible under-reporting because of the social sensitivity of information about sexual behaviours.

However, the actual numbers or percentages are not really the most important feature. More important, by far, is information about the pattern of sexual relationships and the sexual habits of partners, including the obstacles and facilitating features that affect the possibilities for people to practice safer sex (lessening the likelihood of pregnancy and STIs including HIV), and to engage in relationships that would be healthier and more satisfying to both partners.

Studies of Sexual Behaviour in Rural and Urban Communities

Almost all the data I am reporting in this section are unpublished, though extensive reports have been written for the funding agencies. Several studies have presented in-depth data on sexual behaviours in rural communities. The data presented here will deal mainly with rural communities in Gujarat (Deepak Charitable Trust [DCT], 1997), Haryana (SWACH, 1998), and Orissa (AIMS, 1997). In each of the studies, the researchers have carried out in-depth interviews with men and women to learn about their sexual histories and recent sexual bchaviours. Key informant interviews and group discussions were also used to gather data on sexual activities and related information.

In each of the study areas, individual interviews and group discussions are in strong agreement that both pre-marital and extra-marital sexual activities are very common in the communities.

Sexual histories of men in rural communities around Baroda reported contacts with female sex workers, relatives (married women) and unmarried girls. In the study carried out in Gujarat, there was frequent mention of the nearby national highway, and sex workers at various locations along this major thoroughfare. Young men reported many sexual contacts with female sex workers, but in practically all cases, there were also sexual relations with women in the villages. On the other hand, in the study by Joshi and colleagues in an area farther from the national highway (in south Gujarat), the researchers found much less contact with sex workers. Of the total 124 males interviewed, only 25 reported contacts with female sex workers. Most of the men in that study reported that they had no desire or need to utilise the services of sex workers, as there is ready availability of unmarried girls for sex. In one of the group discussions the men said: "Why should we go 'outside' [visit female sex workers] when we get girls in our village?" Married men who reported extra-marital relations said that their liaisons were mainly with women within their community (Joshi and Dhapola, 1998).

Research in rural Haryana, near the Uttar Pradesh border, also produced evidence of high rates of non-marital sexual activities. However, these data suggested considerable contact with female sex workers and other local women who were sexually available in exchange for money or materials (particularly grass for their animals). Very few men reported going to sex workers in the urban centres (SWACH, 1998).

In rural Orissa, the Asian Institute of Marketing Studies carried out a wide range of research activities, culminating in a carefully constructed quantitative survey. Group interviews, in-depth interviews with individuals, and other qualitative data-gathering methods were also used. There appeared to be important variations in the patterns of sexual activities, partly reflecting different kinds of exposures to outside influences. In areas with higher rates of foreign and Indian tourism, there was more evidence of sexual activities. Recent survey data from Orissa are undoubtedly the best quantitative estimates of the prevalence of pre-marital sex in a rural region. A total 2,096 men were interviewed, divided between rural and urban areas. Approximately one-quarter of the married men in the rural portion of the sample reported that they had engaged in pre-marital sex. However, in the higher tourism area – Puri district – half of the married rural men (49.3 percent) reported having engaged in pre-marital sex, compared with men in a more isolated area (Ganjam) with only 15 percent. On the other hand, men from

Ganjam reported much higher rates of first sex with female sex workers, 15 percent as compared with 7 percent in Puri (Collumbien, personal communication).

A survey of sexual behaviours in a rural region of south Gujarat (Khan et al, 1997) found that 27 percent of married men said they had had non-marital sexual experiences. Pre-marital sexual experiences (only) were 18 percent; 6 percent said they had been engaged in extra-marital sex, and 3 percent reported both pre-marital and extra-marital activities. Most of the reported non-marital sexual contacts were with 'friends' and 'relatives.' Apparently, contacts with sex workers were quite few. These data suggest rates of non-marital sex somewhat lower than the situation in Orissa. Overall, the data from these quantitative studies, and others like them, point to the importance of regional variations in both the prevalence of non-marital sexual activities as well as the types of behaviours involved.

Multi-Partner Women in Rural Areas

Researchers have found that almost every village has one or more women who are known to be available for sexual contacts, though not all should be classified as 'sex workers'. The data are particularly interesting in Haryana's rural areas, where SWACH researchers have categorised 'available women' into five different categories. These categories, with slight modifications, would seem to apply very widely to the villages of rural India:

1. Village women who are engaged in sex-for-money in their own village.

2. Village women who 'commute' to sex work locations in urban or semi-urban brothels or lodges. [Such 'commuter sex workers' are particularly noteworthy in reports from Calcutta.] (Bhattacharya and Senapati, 1994).

3. Village women who go to the nearest major highway to serve the trucker population. (Also reported in the DCT study in Gujarat.)

4. Village women who exchange sex for fodder, firewood, and other necessities, mainly with the landowners from whose lands they obtain those necessities.

5. Village women who engage in some multi-partner sex, at least occasionally, but without expectations of regular payments. These might be labelled as 'miscellaneous others.' (Also reported in the DCT study.)

In the Haryana interviews, it appeared that categories 4 and 5 in particular should not be labelled as 'sex workers.' In the Gujarat studies also, it became clear that many of the women identified as 'sexually available' should not be considered commercial sex workers in the usual sense. Category 4 above, is particularly clear, and some of the male informants in Haryana pointed out that they did not refer to these women with the same labelling (local term = *taxi*) as the other women. Some of the 'available women' were quite frank about the need to 'do something' to get money if the husband does not earn, or if the husband does not give his wife enough money for the children and her own needs. Here is an excerpt from one such interview:

> *"After a while she added...'we are poor, if we indulge in such activity, there is always a reason..but what about those women who belong to upper castes and have big homes..even they are involved in...(earning out of sin)....sometimes one has to do it for funding themselves...'*
>
> (SWACH, 1998)

Many of the sex workers in Gujarat and Haryana narrated sad tales about how they entered the sex trade. In some cases dire poverty came about because of the death of the husband, but the more usual pattern appeared to be abuse and neglect by husbands, often accompanied by serious alcohol abuse. Another variation was the marriage of a young woman to a much older man. Informants said that such age discrepancy can sometimes be the explanation for why women in relatively wealthier families turn to multi-partner sexual activities. In some cases in Haryana, the husband forced his wife into selling sex for money:

> *"She looked at me with a little sadness and narrated the story [being thrown out of the house by her husband's aunt, who had sexual relations with her husband]. One day her husband (who was a drunkard) took her to the [urban centre] to his friend's house. He gave alcohol to his friend and took money from him. Then he locked me in the room with the friend. After that he got into that practice [selling her sexual services]. After that, a male friend introduced her to a small brothel, where she began earning quite well for herself."*
>
> (SWACH fieldnotes, 1998)

The extent to which men's non-marital sexual activities are directed to female sex workers seems to vary considerably from community to community, and region to region. A large number of sexual episodes described by Haryana men involved sex workers. Many of those episodes involved 'group sex,' in which two, three or four men hired a sex worker (sometimes two sex workers) and brought her to some secluded location.

The following are some examples from in-depth interviews in Haryana:

> *"One day, we were having liquor outside the village at the house of [friend]. Then we planned to bring [He named a particular sex worker from another village.]. No matter if it will cost how much." DR [informant] further added "My friend and myself brought that girl from [that other village] in the evening after deciding the amount of Rs 500. We kept her at [the friend's] house for whole of the night.*

BS (interviewer) asked DR: " How many of you were there?
DR: 'We were four boys.
BS: 'How did you decide who would go first?'
DR: "Sabse pehle mein hi gaya. Hamne usko dere par sari raat rakha aur sharab bhi pite rahe."(I was the first one. We kept her there for whole of the night and continued drinking alcohol also)."

Another young informant described a chance encounter in which three young men had sex with a customer who came to a provision shop:

"B [informant] said that he forget to tell us that again [about one and a half years ago] a Muslim woman from [names her village] was hooked up by Kabir [shop owner]
... She was a taxi (sex worker) and used to came to his shop for buying groceries. She was a chalu woman and we fixed up (set kar liya). We used the backside of the shop by guarding one another."
DS [interviewer]: "How do you decide who will go first?"
Informant: " I went first."
DS: "Did you pay her anything?"
B: (Laughs) "Where was the need to pay her any money. We used her free... or she must have taken some things from Kabir's shop."

The interviewer asked one informant about whether such group sex activities are difficult for the women:

DS [interviewer]: "How does a woman cope up with 6-7 men at one time when there is a group sex kind of activity?"
HS [Informant]: "I also asked the same question from a taxi' [local term for sex worker]. She said that men who go for sex outside are scared of being found out so they are in a hurry. Some men are 'babujees', some are drunk, so the sex act takes half a minute or one minute. The woman does not have much of a problem.

If a man has sex in a house, or a single man does the act, he takes about 20-30 minutes. In a group it happens quickly.

The narratives concerning group sex activities were more numerous in interviews from Haryana than in Gujarat or Orissa. That may be accidental. On the other hand, there is a possibility that there are social and economic factors involved that bring about real differences between the study areas. Many of the narratives about group sex mentioned alcohol. In at least one such group sex event in Orissa, the informant mentioned that one of their group went to get condoms.

First Sexual Experience

The first sexual experience for many of the men in various study sites was masturbation. In some cases, masturbation was taught by some older boy; sometimes it occurred among a small group of boys. Here are excerpts from interviews:

RS (informant): " When I was in 8th class and used to go to (big village). There were 3-4 boys from [a village] who were senior to me. They only taught me masturbation. Before that I did not even know what masturbation was. They (senior friends) used to say (Marlan Mathole, Rukke Na Role). (You should masturbate, it neither creates hue and cry, nor anyone objects to it.)
DR (informant): "There was one boy from Gujjan. (Backward caste) a village. He got us involved in these bad habits."
BS (interviewer): "For how long did you masturbate?"
DR: " For three years."
BS: "Why did you stop this?"
DR: "Phir maine (big village) ki Kumharon ki chokri pata li thi. Sara din usko raja ke bag ki bar mein lekar para rehta tha.(Then one girl of Kumhar from (big village),I got her involved with me and used to lie down with her for the whole

day in the lodges of Raja's garden.)
BS: "Then how did your studies go on?"
DR: "What to talk of studies! I got involved in this business and passed my 7th class after 4 years.

Probably many young men in rural communities have experienced the following sexual phase in their adolescence: *"Our friends taught us about masturbation during school time only. They only taught us that there is no other thing better than this. There is no need of going anywhere or to catch hold of any girl."*

For many, masturbation ended when they were able to find sex partners, as we see in the following comment:

RD (informant): "Then a girl from the village got hooked with me and I stopped masturbating."

Sex With Relatives

In some situations reported by men, their first sexual experience beyond masturbation was initiated by a relative, in some cases a slightly older married woman. In the quite ambivalent 'lore' about sex in Indian culture, the *bhabhi* (brother's or cousin's wife) is often singled out as a likely sex partner for young unmarried men. Thus, while one version of Indian culture maintains that married persons, especially women, do not engage in extra-marital affairs, the other side of the ambivalence frequently refers to the sister-in-law as a likely sexual partner, particularly for unmarried members of extended families. Beyond the extended family, the concept of *bhabhi* is often extended to a wide range of 'sisters-in-law' in more distantly related households. A study among college students found that 'one half of all the first sexual partners of 72 college students in Hyderabad were married women, older than themselves, and a large majority of the partners were relatives.' (Goparaju, 1994).

One of the informants in south Gujarat told a particularly poignant story of his ignorance of sex, and how his *bhabhi* introduced him to heterosexual intercourse. This narrative also illustrates the fact that rural informants (both male and female) are often quite eloquent in describing their sexual experiences, provided that the interviewer is open, sympathetic, and non-judgemental:

"Once we got a T.V. in our village. Everybody went there to watch 'Chitrahaar'. There was a lot of rush because everybody wanted to watch 'Chitrahaar'. We boys were more in number. That day, my friend's wife (my sister-in-law) agreed. She had also come and there was a nice song on the T.V. So my bhabhi looked at me and while watching 'Chitrahaar,' she whispered in my ear, 'come to my house'. I was wondering about what work she could have. She got up, and went first, and I went after her. She asked me to come to her house at 10:00 o'clock. 'Your brother is going for second shift and night shift and I really get scared when I'm alone. So come and sleep here.' So I told her that I'll inform my people at home and then come. She said: 'Come and have your dinner with me. I've prepared it. There is none to eat it so you come and have it.' I said yes and I went home and told my mother that I would be sleeping at my bhabhi's house.

Interviewer: "Your mother let you go to sleep there?"

Informant: "Of course, she would let me go. It was my friend's house, and bhabhi got along well with my family, so she let me go. Me and bhabhi ate together and then she said 'I'll put a cot outside and you can sleep on that'.... and my bhabhi finished her housework and slept.... After everybody slept she woke me up and took me near her. I was scared about what she would do. And my bhabhi straight away opened my chain and so I was even more scared. I thought that bhabhi must've come to know that I masturbated. After opening my chain she took me in her arms and took me on top of her and took off her blouse and skirt – everything. Then she caught hold of my penis and I liked it a little. It had become stiff so I did not say anything."

(Deepak Charitable Trust. Fieldnotes. 1997)

For other young men, (a small minority in the study areas), the first initiation to sex beyond masturbation was with sex workers. Often the 'expedition' to the sex worker was arranged as a group activity. The following narrative came in response to the interviewer's request that the informant describe his first heterosexual experience:

DS (Interviewer): "Can you tell us in details who did the fixing up for you?"
Informant: "A boy from [another village] had come to tractor repair shop and I was also sitting there in that shop as the mechanic was our friend and mechanic said to him: 'Yaar nothing is getting fixed up for us' (Kahi judar hi fit nahi hota). That boy from [the other village] said 'you came over to our village; I will do the fixing up for all of you. But all of you must pay at least Rs 50 each.' All of us agreed and went to [village] at about 6 p.m. It was winter time and we all went to an animal shed in the fields and this woman came at about 8 p.m., after a long wait. We were three men and Anand went first then me and last the mechanic went and after we finished that the woman went back.
DS: 'How many times did you do it?'
B: 'Just once or twice.'
DS: " Did you pay the money to her?'
B: 'We paid the money to that boy who had done the fixing up.'
DS: 'Did that boy also have her or not?'
B: 'I don't know , may be. He is an agent may be once in a while he also does it.'
DS: 'Did you use condom?'
B: 'No, we did not use it.'

Understanding About the First Sexual Experience

The first sexual experience among young men appears to be an unplanned, often unanticipated experience. The age range during which heterosexual experience occurs is apparently rather large. Small numbers of precocious individuals have their first sexual experiences in the early teens, some as young as 12 or 13 years. But the average age at first sexual contacts is much more. For most men in India, according to the available studies, the first sexual experience (like those of their wives) occurs at marriage. The very large spread in age at first sexual intercourse is important to keep in mind when people develop intervention projects. In almost any group of unmarried men (for example in reproductive health camps) the majority of the participants will not have experienced sexual intercourse!

In the Orissa survey, mentioned earlier, only about one quarter (27 percent) of the men reported sexual experience before marriage. This statistical picture seems in startling contrast to the prevalent narratives about sexual experiences in the informants' interviews. With the average age at marriage somewhere around 23 years, the majority of men in the Orissa study area, and other parts of India, experience their first sexual encounters with women after the age of 20. Clearly, there is a great need for research programmes to carefully identify that minority of young boys and men who become heterosexually active well before marriage. Despite their being a minority in the population, they represent very large numbers in India. Those are the people who immediately are most in need of better information concerning reproductive processes, prevention of pregnancy, and how to avoid risks of infection (including HIV) in sexual encounters.

The Sexually Active Minority of Unmarried Men

All the data from quantitative surveys, in various different rural areas of India, present a picture in which only a minority of men have sexual experience before marriage. The usual percentages in the surveys range from around 20 percent to 35 percent of men having pre-marital sexual activity. The highest rates thus far in sufficiently large random sample surveys, are from the Puri district of Orissa, where half (49 percent) of the rural sample reported pre-marital sexual contacts (Collumbien, personal communication). The usual survey data, however, give no indications of the situations of sexual activities, other than figures on numbers of contacts with sex workers and other sex partners. The current challenge in research is to uncover much more descriptive information about the contexts, the situations, and sequences of sexual behaviours.

A study by Joshi and associates from the Operations Research Group (ORG) provides much needed descriptive details about the sexual behaviours of the more sexually active persons of the local population in rural south Gujarat (Joshi and Dhapola, 1998). The research team interviewed 124 men (78 married men; 46 unmarried) in repeated in-depth contacts. The men were contacted through a sequential referral process, in which the first informants referred the researchers to their friends and other people who 'would be willing to talk with the interviewers.' The informants were from 8 different villages, and from different neighbourhood clusters in those villages. No attempt was made to find sexually active individuals, but it is clear, in retrospect, that the sample is biased toward persons who had non-marital sexual experiences. (Thus, 97 of the 124 men reported pre-marital experiences.) Each informant was contacted at least 2 or 3 times, and the more sensitive topics about sexual behaviours were brought out in the later interviews.

All the key informants in the villages and the group discussions, revealed that non-marital sexual activities are extremely common in the area.

Only 25 informants reported contacts with sex workers, and the usual partners in sexual activities were unmarried girls in the villages (Joshi and Dhapola, 1998). Several informants reported that there was no need to go to sex workers, as sex was easily available with the village girls. The men reported 116 contacts with unmarried girls and only 26 contacts with married women. The overwhelming proportion of sexual partners were reported to be in the age range of 15 to 19 years.

The major additional feature provided in this study is the fact that a large number of the sexual relationships were relatively long-term 'affairs' involving emotional attachments. The men made frequent references to 'love' (using the English word) and *prem* (the corresponding Hindi/Gujarati word). Of the 97 men reporting pre-marital activities, 58 spoke of 'love' in their descriptions of sexual activity. Considerable numbers of these encounters continued as long-term relationships. One result of these continuing sexual relationships was the numbers of unmarried girls who became pregnant, due to the general lack of contraceptive measures, including very infrequent use of condoms. Thirty of the men reported involvement in seeking abortion services for their girlfriends. (These data emerged unexpectedly in the in-depth interviews, as they were not anticipated by the research team.) The men's involvements in seeking abortion services for the girls registers yet another unexpected feature that provides leads for practical interventions. It is quite evident from these data that men are an important part of the process of seeking abortion services for unmarried girls and that they need to have much more detailed information about safe abortion services, prevention of conception, and other reproductive health topics.

Another finding in this study was that longer term emotional attachements in pre-marital sexual relationships not infrequently continue after marriage. Although the girlfriend married, the relationship continued (in 10 cases among these interviews). Such a continuation of a pre-marital relationship is practically unthinkable in Western cultures, where marriages are mostly contracted as 'love marriages.' However, in the case of arranged marriages, in which the girl has no established emotional tie to her new husband, it is much more understandable that she might continue a relationship with her pre-marital lover. Practically no research is available on this subject.

The discussion here has focussed entirely on men and their pre-marital sexual experiences. The numbers of women involved in pre-marital sex are much smaller than the men, though they are much more numerous than survey results indicate. There is every reason to believe that all surveys of sexual behaviours among Indian women result in serious under-reporting.

Sexual Experiences of Married Women

Until recently, there has been very little information available concerning the sexual experiences of married women, in either rural or urban areas. Most studies have examined pre-marital and extra-marital sexuality and sexual behaviours and have focussed on men. A recent study presents quite interesting information on the experiences of rural women in the Vadodara district of south Gujarat (Joshi et al, 1998). The qualitative research consisted of in-depth, sequential interviews with 69 women in 8 villages. On average, the researchers conducted five interviews with each woman, in order to get extensive data on reproductive health problems, treatment seeking, sexual experience, and related information.

Most of the women were married at quite a young age; 48 of them became pregnant at, or before the age of 18. More than one-third (29) were married before they attained puberty. It is therefore not surprising that almost all of these women knew practically nothing about sex and married life until the moment they entered conjugal relations. As the authors report, "Most of the women (43 out of 69) stated that they were totally unaware of sex prior to marriage...only 10 women reported that they knew about the nature of the sexual relationships between a man and a woman." (Joshi et al, 1998).

Because these women were so poorly informed about physical sexual relations, the majority reported that their first sexual experience was negative, often traumatic. Only 19 of the women reported that the first sex was pleasant (though painful). The following quote is typical of the more negative recollections:

> "...*When it happened for the first time....I felt as though something had hurt me...while urinating, it used to burn a lot. Yet my husband insisted on doing 'it' every day. I did not enjoy it at all. I used to pray that the night should not come...After this I developed a fear of sex.*" (Joshi, p. 15)

Contrary to research and impressions from other areas, these researchers found that the majority of the women in their sample developed positive attitudes toward sex with their husbands (Joshi et al, 1998). Over a third of the women (29) spoke of sex with the husband as pleasurable, using words such as *anand mate* (happiness), *maja mate* (enjoyment), and *shaukh mate* (interest); others were more neutral in talking of sex with their husbands. On the other hand, 16 of the 69 women were quite negative about their current sex lives, saying things like, "I never liked it from the beginning...." Somehow, despite the decidedly negative first experiences, a majority of the marriages had developed in a positive direction. The evidence concerning women's positive attitudes toward sex is supported by the fact that over half of the women spoke about how they communicate sexual desire to their husbands. In 28 cases women communicated through direct physical contact with the men; 15 women reported various forms of verbal communication, including direct statements such as:

> *"I have the desire."*
> *"I want to do it." (mane karwanu che).*
> *"Come we will do intercourse." (chal havei kam karia).*
> *"I am in the mood." (Mane bahuj mood thai che).*

These reports of rural women communicating their sexual desire to husbands contradict many reports from other areas according to which women are not supposed to acknowledge or communicate any desire or anything else positive about sex. Joshi and her colleagues felt that their repeated in-depth interviews, usually with at least 5 sessions with each woman, resulted in a more accurate, valid portrayal of women's sexual lives. They also suggested that the rural Gujarati women are more 'empowered' and more assertive than women in other parts of India.

Some studies in rural regions of Uttar Pradesh and elsewhere present a more negative picture of women's marital experiences. A study in two villages of central Uttar Pradesh about experiences of marital sex found that, of 98 women respondents, "...67 reported sexual coercion – 21 percent reported physical violence, 14 percent reported anger [whose anger?] ....However, about one-third of the women did not report any coercion by their husband." (Khan et al, 1996). These data resulted from multiple in-depth interviews with the women, similar to the research methods followed by Joshi and her research team. The overall picture of sex life in marriage in the Uttar Pradesh study is dramatically different from the data for south Gujarat. The hypothesis of strong differences in women's situations in Gujarat as compared with rural women in Uttar Pradesh is supported by data from the same rural region (Gujarat); a survey of 342 males randomly selected from 28 villages. In the interviews, 69 men (20 percent) reported that they encountered occasional refusals of sex from their wives. Of the men reporting such refusals, 61 percent said they kept quiet and did not do anything. Fourteen of these (sexually rejected) men said they 'persuaded their wives,' while 18 men admitted to violence, forced sex, and verbal abuse (Khan et al, 1997). These data indicate considerable violence in a rather small minority of men, but the scale of sexual coercion directed to wives in this study seems strikingly less than the report from Uttar Pradesh, even allowing for the likelihood of under-reporting. Unfortunately, there are no available studies comparing husbands' and wives' reports of sexual coercion and violence, so we have no guidelines for estimating the likely degree of under-reporting by males.

A study in the Kheda district, north of the Vadodara area, presents another perspective on a Gujarat rural population. This research was conducted in a village "adjacent to the national highway...frequented by truckers 'for the purpose of obtaining wine and women." (Sharma et al, 1998). It is clear from several indicators that this village is quite unusual in terms of contact with both extra-marital sexual activities and alcohol consumption (in a 'dry' state). Almost 27 percent of the 109 women in the sample reported addiction to either tobacco or alcohol and 62 percent (68) said their men were addicted. Almost 24 percent of the women admitted that they had had extra-marital sexual contacts. The authors point out that "the population studied by us may not be considered as representative of the rural population of the district." That is certainly the case, as there are no other studies of rural populations in India in which one quarter of the women acknowledged extra-marital sexual activity. In the Vadodara study, 4 of the 69 women (6 percent) admitted to having extra-marital sexual activity.

The data of most interest to us in the study in Vadodara, Gujarat, are those concerning the husbands' reactions to denial of sex by their wives. According to these women, in 48 cases (44 percent) the man does nothing (except perhaps sulk); 25 women reported coercive sex; 23 said he 'tended to go' to other women; 7 reported physical violence against her or the children; and 6 women reported abusive language (Sharma et al, 1998).

Although this rural Gujarat population is heavily influenced by its dealings with the truck drivers of the national highway, and there is reportedly heavy use of alcohol among the men, the rates of physical violence and coercive sex toward their wives are much lower than the figures reported in Uttar Pradesh where the large majority of women reported coercive sex or physical violence.

Sexual Patterns of Married Couples in Urban Slums

Several studies in the period from 1994 to 1998 have produced data on sexual behaviours in urban settings, some of them focussed on married men and women. In 1993-94, an innovative groundbreaking study was carried out with a small group of women in a low-income slum area of Mumbai. The researchers continued to meet with the same group of women in a number of sessions over several weeks and also had individual sessions with the women in their sample (George and Jaswal, 1995). Subsequent research provides further important data on sexual interactions of married couples in the slums of Mumbai (George, 1997).

The results of these studies present one of the more graphic and compelling portraits of the situations of low-income urban women, and the extent to which intrafamily power relationships result in sexual exploitation and other abuses. Urban slum populations are one of the most rapidly growing sectors in Indian society. All the larger cities of India are experiencing a rapid influx of people from rural areas, coming to seek jobs and better incomes, often pushed out from rural communities because of crop failures, reduced prices of agricultural products, and other economic factors.

Although the people crowding to cities are very often family groups, they come without their extended family networks, usually settling in the city as nuclear families. As a result, the wives are very often cut off from the support of their natal families. Conflicts in the family, from economic hardships and other factors frequently result in exacerbated tensions between husband and wife. Many other special conditions in the urban setting contribute to family breakdowns. There seems to be no doubt that conditions in urban slum populations put greater stress on husband-wife relations than those encountered in rural areas. A major manifestation of these increased domestic tensions appears to be in sexual abuse and conflicts about sexual behaviours.

Another study of the Mumbai slum population consisted of in-depth, multi-session interviews with 65 married women (ages 20 to 38 years); and 23 men (ages 26 to 45). The respondents were approximately equally divided among Hindus, Muslims and Buddhists. Approximately half of the women (32) reported being beaten by their husbands. Excessive use of alcohol appeared to be an important contributor to domestic violence. The husband's inability or unwillingness to provide adequate financial support of the household was also a factor.

Concerning women's approach to, or expression of interest in sex, the women in this study felt that:

> *"...it was not appropriate for a woman to admit that she had sexual feelings; it was more acceptable to deny these feelings or to deny interest in sex. Most women felt that expressing their sexual desire and initating sex, even with their husbands, would decrease their honour. They expected men to be the sexual initiators." (George, 1997)*

As one of the respondents expressed it:

> *"You see, many women must be feeling that (sexual feelings) but they feel shy to tell their husbands. Even if the woman feels like (sex), still she feels shy. Earlier even if I had the desire, I would get sharam. I would feel that my husband may think that this woman is bad or she must be of bad character, that's why she wants (so much sex)." (George, 1997).*

Another woman said:

> *"Those who read the Times (Times of India newspaper), who are doctors know that a woman wants to have sex just like a man does. But due to some reasons, only men come forward. We (women) cannot say it ourselves because we don't think it proper to even talk about it." (George, 1997).*

On the other hand, the author found some women who could express their sexual desires to their husbands.

> *"Sangeeta and her husband discuss many aspects of their sexual life together. For instance, they use signals to each other to indicate when they both want to have sexual relations." (George, 1997).*

Physical violence was a common occurrence, according to the women, including physical violence in conflict over whether to engage in sexual activity. In addition to physical violence, the men in this study used other means to coerce wives to engage in sex. Some men argued about sexual activity in front of other family members, particularly the children. Those husbands *"count on the woman's feeling of embarrassment in making a public issue of a private affair...."* Others, if the woman refused sex, regularly expressed doubts about her fidelity. *"There must be someone else for you...."* Or, in another case, *"...you may be loving someone, that's why you say no to me."* Another technique was to a cast a slur on the woman's family honour. The most common verbal technique for forcing the woman to have sex was, the threat to break up the marriage. Either he would threaten to send her back to her family; or else he threatened to take another wife or mistress. Marriages in the urban slums are more unstable than unions in the villages, so the threat of desertion or taking a second woman carries force. Those threats, of course, are more convincing under circumstances where the woman has only marginal support from her own natal family.

The author found that despite the threats of physical beatings and various forms of verbal violence and abuse, a number of women regularly denied sexual access to their husbands under certain circumstances. The most usual situations for denying sexual access to husbands were: 1) if he was drinking heavily, and 2) if he was not bringing in money to support the family. The male is supposed to support the family, in return for which the wife takes care of his household and also serves him sexually. 'No money, no sex,' according to some of the informants.

One other important feature of urban life deserves mention here. Compared with situations in rural villages, urban slums provide little privacy, for sex or for other sensitive, private matters. Some of the women in this study use the lack of privacy as an excuse to avoid sex. In other households, its the other way around, as the man used the lack of privacy as his weapon to make the wife comply.

There were few interviews with men in this study (23 men) but they raised important points for more comprehensive research:

1. The men too expressed their frustrations at the lack of privacy in the tiny, one-room houses in the slums. The issue of privacy must certainly have important effects on sexual behaviours.

2. Contrary to the ideas of 'shyness' and 'honour' expressed by the women, several men spoke of their irritation that the women never took the initiative in sexual relations. As one man put it, apparently negatively, "I don't remember a single time when she told me on her own that she wants (sex)."

3. Some of the men admitted that they forced their wives to have sex whenever they themselves wanted it. The men gave explanations, mostly based on the simple assumption that access to sex was bestowed on the man through the marriage (Khanna's research team reported that a number of women in their study appeared to accept that male dominant attitude: *"we cannot say anything because it is our duty..."*).

4. The concept of 'control' was mentioned by several men, in the sense of controlling themselves (sexually) and not going to sex workers. Also, too much sex could set a bad example for one's children. 'Control' was also seen as necessary to avoid sexual health problems (STIs and others). This concept of 'control' among urban low-income males, which appears to hark back to a Vedic concept, suggests a need for much more detailed research. The data could be useful for designing messages to enhance awareness of HIV/AIDS and STIs and designing other interventions.

The contrast between rural data (Joshi, 1995) and from Mumbai slums is stark. Despite the fact that both samples were small, the contextual information, and the richness of the individual sets of interviews (in each case more than one interview with each woman) point to strong differences in marital life in the urban slum setting as compared with rural Gujarat. It is tempting to suggest that the situations of women in rural Gujarat are more 'typical of the Indian culture', whereas life in the slums of Mumbai displays, in many ways, a breakdown of social norms and values, with higher levels of frustrations, aggression, and consequent sexual exploitation of women. The contrast between the Uttar Pradesh and Gujarat is also striking. People who are familiar with both of the areas are likely to conclude that the differences are really there – that the Gujarati woman really are more empowered in many ways, less coerced by their husbands in sexual matters, than their sisters in Uttar Pradesh and the women in the slums of Mumbai.

Sexual Behaviours and Reproductive Health Knowledge Among Adolescents

Recent research among adolescents in a low-income area of Delhi focussed on patterns of sexual behaviour in relation to developing programmes aimed toward improving reproductive health knowledge. Qualitative in-depth interviews provide an unusually multifaceted picture of teenage romantic encounters, exploration of relationships, and pathways to risky sexual encounters. The interviews were carried out by youth from the community, in order to maximize the social communication between researchers and their informants. In-depth interviews of boys and girls (71), case studies, group discussions, and key informant interviews provide rich, complex scenarios of sexual behaviours. The study community seems to have high levels of sexual activity and consequent high levels of vulnerability to unwanted pregnancies, STIs, HIV infection, and other problems (Sodhi et al, 1998).

The study results suggest that young girls are supposed to be tightly controlled by their families with regard to contacts with boys. As a result, girls are confused about possible 'friendships' (*dosti*) with boys. Many of them say they want to avoid *dosti*, yet their statements reveal emotional conflict, partly at least brought on by romantic impressions made by contemporary Indian movies, which are an important source of entertainment and information for young people. Romantic encounters are often modelled from movie songs and movie heroines/heroes. In a culture where boys and girls have few opportunities to practice heterosexual conversations, the currently popular movies provide some of the scripts.

One 18-year old girl became friendly with a boy because they liked the same film stars. She described how the relationship developed. The boy approached her by saying, *"I find you very good. Just like Karishma Kapoor (a famous Indian movie star)."* According to her story, *"He liked Karishma Kapoor and I also like her. Once he asked me which hero do I like. So I said I like Amir Khan. Our views seemed to be alike so we got friendly."* (Sodhi et al, 1998).

Unfortunately, the romantic intentions and expectations of the girls in this urban community were rather naive, and ill-suited for the advances of boys whose definitions of *dosti* relations are much more explicitly sexual. Encounters described by the girls (and corroborated by some of the boys' narratives) showed that the girls were drawn into situations where they were forced to engage in sex against their will. Some informants described situations where a girl would be forced to have sex with more than one boy:

> *"Situations like these put the girls particularly at risk. The vulnerable girl can be coerced into multiple partner relationships where her boyfriend introduces her to another friend of his and she is forced to have sex with him because of threats of defamation. A 19 year old student remarked, '...friends also help in establishing physical relations with his girlfriend and the process goes on. And if the girl says no then boys defame her in her gali (lane) and colony. Because there is no effect on boy's character." (Sodhi et al, 1998a).*

> *"One 14 year old student related an incident where a boy lured a girl into a deserted building with a temptation of Rs 100. The witness related, 'Once he showed Rs 100 to a girl and took her to the – and don't know what he did with her....that girl had tied two ribbons in her plait and when she came back her clothes were torn. Marks were made on her face and on her hands also her marks were made and she came out crying. When she came back I asked her what happened to you. So*

she started telling me that one boy gave me temptation of Rs 100 and he took me inside. So I said, '...and you went inside?' So she said that 'How would I know that he would do this to me?'..... She was saying that he took off her salwar and [began to force her]. Those who were working there [near the building] saved her." (Sodhi et al, 1998a).

Many of the interviews with both boys and girls reported instances of coercion, including outright rape. It is often evident from the stories that the victimised girl did not know what would happen. It seems that the strong attempts (by the families) to minimise contacts between boys and girls have resulted in increased vulnerability. *"All this inhibits the development of a girl's skills to negotiate terms of intimacy and/or decision-making capabilities. This results in her physical and emotional exploitation."* (Sodhi et al, 1998b).

This study is important because it gives a detailed picture of the situations and sequences by which initial contacts develop into 'friendships' (*dosti*), leading to unplanned sexual intimacies. These scenarios, or 'scripts for developing relationships' provide insights into the kinds of specific information needed by adolescents and crucial points of intervention for planning action programmes.

In the latter part of this decade, after the ICPD, there has been a considerable increase in attention to the sexual behaviours, and information levels, among adolescents in different parts of India. Beginning in 1995, the International Centre for Research on Women (ICRW) sponsored a four site study of adolescents in Maharashtra (Mumbai and two rural sites) and Tamil Nadu. These studies reported evidence of increased sexual activity among adolescents and the distressing lack of basic information concerning reproductive processes and related reproductive health topics.

It was evident in all of these studies that girls have few sources of information. They are ill-prepared for their first experience of menstruation, and are still worse prepared for marriage and family life. Those who remain unmarried into their late teens, or later, are at risk of unwanted pregnancy if they engage in sexual activity, as they have little or no knowledge about conception, or how to negotiate relationships with males. One of the ICRW studies in rural Maharashtra (Pune District), reported that less than one percent of girls knew anything about STIs, and 8 and 16 percent of the boys had some knowledge of these infections. About 30 percent of the married men in this study reported multiple partner relations (pre-marital and extra-marital) (Apte, 1997). A recent review of the general state of knowledge of adolescent sexuality and fertility shows that there is still a serious dearth of information concerning this particularly vulnerable age category (Jejeebhoy, 1996).

Sexual Health Problems: The Male Perspective

A recent study, also in Mumbai, provides excellent data on the sexual health problems experienced by men in an urban slum, as well as the treatment-seeking behaviours and local resources utilised (Verma et al, 1998). The interviewers asked the men to "tell us all the different illnesses and symptoms of sexual health problems (*gupt rog*)". This freelisting technique produced an extensive listing of locally recognised sexual problems. The same freelisting technique was also used to gather lists of *gupt rog* from the local health practitioners (most of whom were not qualified in allopathic medicine). Analysis of the *gupt rog* lists and further in-depth interviews brought forth the following:

The most frequently mentioned *gupt rog* were not sexually transmitted infections (STIs). They were 'illnesses' associated with semen loss, or 'semen deterioration.' These conditions included *swapnadosh* (nocturnal emissions), masturbation, *dhat girna* (white discharge) and *dhat patla hona* (semen becomes thin). The leading *gupt rog* mentioned by the community men (35 of the 56 respondents) was *kamjori*, which can be translated as 'sexual weakness.' Anxieties about sexual performance, including lack of erection and 'lack of desire,' were also common complaints. Among the most frequently mentioned sexual problems, symptoms of STIs appeared further down the listings. Illnesses such as gonorrhoea and syphilis were only infrequently mentioned, as most people do not know these medical terms. AIDS was mentioned by 16 percent of the community men and the same percentage of providers. It appears that HIV/AIDS as a sexual health problem is not salient among the slum dwelling men – at least they do not perceive it as a serious threat to themselves.

Similar freelisting of sexual health problems was carried out in Orissa, with much the same results. Concerns about *dhatu padiba* (semen discharge) topped the lists along with *jadu* (itching) and *swapnadosh* (nocturnal emissions). Men in the more urbanised sector, around Bhubaneshwar, mentioned AIDS relatively frequently (50 percent of respondents) (AIMS, 1997; Pelto et al, 1997). The freelisting question was included in the large-scale survey, mentioned above. The data showed large variations in awareness of AIDS, ranging from quite high frequencies of mention among unmarried urban men, to relatively low awareness among rural married men. The same generalisations apply to mention of gonorrhoea and syphilis. Similar to the Mumbai results, most of the different sectors of this survey showed frequent mention of the 'non-contact' sexual health problems and somewhat less awareness or concern about the symptoms related to STIs. Interviews with informants in the various communities indicate, however, that men are quite aware of the sexual transmission of infections.

Similar data concerning mens' perceptions of sexual health problems have been collected in Gujarat, Haryana, and other locations. The following generalisations have emerged from these studies:

1. Males throughout India have anxieties and concerns about 'semen loss' and 'weakening of semen,' reflecting cultural theories about the importance of semen, derived from ancient vedic texts (Nag, 1996). Concerns about loss of sexual vigour are common, and result in the frequent mention of *kamjori* as a sexual health problem (notably in the Mumbai study).

2. Thus, the various sexual health problems (*gupt rog*) known and mentioned by males can be broadly grouped into:

a. 'non-contact' complaints (including nocturnal emission, masturbation, 'bent penis,' and many others;

b. infectious conditions such as sores and boils, swelling, itching, and other symptoms, often arising from sexual contacts.

3. Various medical practitioners, both qualified and non-qualified, (allopathic, ayurvedic, unani, homeopathic and others) provide treatment for men who complain of 'semen loss,' *kamjori,* and other conditions, many of which well-trained medical people would regard as non-pathological.

4. Males in both rural and urban areas are well aware of the sexual transmission of infections, but they also believe that these conditions can be caused by diet, excessive heat, and other causes.

5. Awareness of AIDS is reflected to varying degrees as a 'sexual illness' in various communities. In Orissa, AIDS awareness as evident in freelistings, is highest among urban, more educated, unmarried men.

6. In practically all areas studied thus far, men are not very aware of the use of condoms to prevent sexually transmitted infections. That awareness does seem to be higher among men in Orissa where there has been more extensive marketing of condoms.

7. Throughout India and nearby areas, there is a widespread concept of *garmi* (heat) as a cause of various sexual health problems which is sometimes used to refer to a sexually transmitted illness. For example, truckers use "the term *garmi* for some illnesses which included *ghav* (ulcer), whitish urethral discharge, *peep* (pus), and *sujak* (genital swelling)" (Rao et al, 1994). Some of the truck drivers in this sample reported that long distance driving <u>causes</u> heat in the body (evidently excess *garmi*). Thus, the concept of *garmi* appears to be closely related to STIs, both as a cause and as a label for the actual disease condition.

One immediate conclusion of these studies of men's sexual health problems is that sexual health clinics for men should be prepared to deal with a variety of 'non-contact sexual problems' in addition to treating STIs. This implies that there is a need to develop counselling training for medical practitioners, including training about various local 'vocabularies of sexual health problems' and the belief systems surrounding men's concepts of *gupt rog* and *garmi*.

Progressing from Research to Action

Most of the research projects described in this paper were carried out in the study areas of intervention projects. Some NGOs were already involved in interventions related to sexual behavioural issues contemporaneously with the research. At the time of this writing there are a number of interventions underway in these study areas.

The research projects in Orissa conducted by the AIMS group, are all linked to interventions sponsored by the British Department for International Development (DFID). The interventions that are on-going in Orissa are in the sectors of social marketing of condoms, mass media awareness of HIV/AIDS, and development of sexual health clinic facilities for men. The research carried out in Delhi is connected with on-going contacts with adolescents, including developing awareness of sexually transmitted infections, HIV/AIDS, and counselling young people. The research findings suggest that there is a need to change the social environment within which adolescents are coping with their sexuality. That is, in the long run there should be more information access and more open exploration of boy-girl communications, because "the controlling family structures and values while seeking to protect adolescents may paradoxically increase their vulnerability" (Sodhi et al, 1998b).

The terminologies concerning men's sexual health problems are all given here in more or less Hindi versions. Similar terms are found widely in languages related to Hindi. We have much less data about the concepts and terminology used in south India, among Dravidian language speakers. That remains an area in need of study.

In Haryana, the staff of the NGO are involving health practitioners to develop ways to deal with men's sexual health problems. They are also encouraging them to play more active roles in raising awareness about STIs and HIV/AIDS in the district.

In Gujarat, HIV/AIDS control programmes are now linked to a support system labelled Programme Support Unit (PSU), funded by the DFID and the AIDS Cell of the Gujarat state government. The PSU has organised training workshops to develop research skills among the interested NGOs and researchers in academic institutions. They are also actively developing guidelines for designing interventions. A similar network, established in Kerala, is also supported by the DFID. In all these networking activities, there is an effort to explore the best ways to develop specific intervention relevant to the local area.

The Deepak Charitable Trust (DCT) programme, cited above, has held feedback sessions in the study communities, and has hired local, in-community 'coordinators' to develop community participation and to supply condoms. Contacts are being developed with local health providers, both qualified and less qualified, to expand effective treatment of STIs, and to develop counselling in relation to non-pathological sexual concerns of the local men.

In collaboration with the ICRW, the Sexual Behaviour Research Network sponsored by the Ford Foundation will develop specific guidelines for feedback of information to local communities and for generating participation in policy development. The guidelines will be especially directed towards influencing policy makers and opinion leaders at the local, regional and state levels.

Directions and Goals for the Next Five Years

The various research programmes outlined above point to major challenges ahead to develop an effective understanding of the complexities of sexuality and sexual behaviours. Some of the main areas in which more research is needed are:

1. Sexual and reproductive health communications and negotiations between husbands and wives constitute an area where research has just begun. A few pioneering studies provide a glimpse of the complex issues where sexual behaviours and communications are linked to family structures, gender roles, and economic and political issues. Follow-up research should probe more deeply into these issues. Similar information is needed from other cities and rural regions.

2. Much more specific information is needed about the patterns of domestic violence as it relates to sexual relations and reproductive health. Serious research on the patterns and processes of domestic violence has only just begun. Key issues of methodology, ethics, and other issues are yet to be dealt with.

3. Much more research is needed on male-to-male sexual behaviours in order to develop effective programmes aimed at safer sexual practices as well as for counselling and other support for this very much hidden category of 'people at risk.'

4. A major challenge during the next five years will be to develop the methodological and conceptual tools for identifying the 'exposure factors,' contributing to non-marital, multi-partner sexual activities. Current data show that only a minority of males in rural and urban populations are actively involved in extra-marital and pre-marital sexual relations. Programmes of information and counselling are needed for all sections of the Indian population, but special interventions are needed to reach those 20 to 30 percent of men (for example), to reduce the risks of unwanted pregnancy, STIs, and other undesirable consequences.

5. Aggravated sexual coercion and violence in families appears to be a special problem in many households. The special characteristics of those family situations 'most at risk of sexual violence' must be identified, in order that governmental and non-governmental outreach workers can effectively focus attention and interventions on those 'at risk' cases.

6. Collaborative programmes with both governmental and private health providers have begun in some locations, but these explorations are in very early stages. More careful studies are needed to identify best practices for enlisting participation of health providers in treatment of sexual health problems (both contact and non-contact illness), counselling of sexually active people with regard to healthier sexual practices, and other aspects of the sexuality-reproductive health domain.

7. Careful, innovative, evaluation research is needed to study intervention programmes. Which parts of awareness campaigns are successfully reaching the hard-to-reach segments of the population? What are the best techniques for getting grassroots participation in rural and urban communities? What methods of contact with policy makers can succeed in getting structural changes? Which levers of women's empowerment work best for bringing about non-reversable changes in gender relations – in households, workplaces, and other situations?

During the next phase, research programmes should continue to be closely linked with the interventions, and there should be well-planned, thoughtful feedback between research and action. Vitally useful new information will emerge from the action programmes themselves, but those experiences can only add to our body of knowledge if there is careful documentation and analysis, through well-planned evaluation procedures.

Concluding Comments

Research on sexuality and sexual behaviours now requires much more sophisticated conceptual models. Instead of merely singling out instances of sex acts, researchers must now follow the lead of those who see sexuality as a complex web of relationships and processes. The relationships are within families (married couples and their many relatives) and outside marriage, among couples from different households – with different backgrounds. These relationships develop through fairly structured processes and communication mechanisms. These processes seem to be quite similar in different regions of the country but the patterns are quite different between urban and rural environments. Even the relationships between sex workers and their clients are complex involving 'agents,' 'fixers,' and other intermediaries.

Researchers need to become more sophisticated about the intra-community variations. The examples from the research in urban and rural areas point to the need to understand more about the complicated reasons why some women report much more amicable, loving relationships than others – in the same communities. Poverty is a factor, yet economic status and education seem to have rather small effects on the large differences in sexual interactions.

Violent episodes in households, like sexual relationships, have their developmental histories. In many households, it appears that violence builds up over time. There are ebbs and flows of violence, only part of which seems related to peoples' economic cycles. Women in households, as well as women in sexual relationships have wide differences in their coping abilities and coping strategies. Some women, in rather difficult urban conditions, are successfully able to defend themselves against physical aggression. The levels of knowledge and modes of acquiring information differ significantly. These variations in processes and relationships require much more carefully constructed 'theories of Indian sexuality and gender relations.' Some of the new knowledge will come from the practical experiences of intervention programmes. It is extremely important that their successes and failures are systematically documented.

References

AIMS RESEARCH. 1997 Attitudes Towards and Use of Condoms Among Men in Orissa. Report sumitted to the British Council Divison and Department for International Development.

Apte, H. 1997. Adolescent Sexuality and Fertility: A Study in Rural Western Maharashtra. Workshop on Research Related to Male Involvement in Reproductive Health and Contraceptive Use. Population Council, Baroda, India.

Bhattacharya, S., and Senapati, S. K. 1994. Sexual Practices of the Sex Workers in a Red Light Area of Calcutta. *The Indian Journal of Social Work,* (Special Issue: Sexual Behaviour and AIDS in India) LV (4): 547-556.

Bhende, A. A. 1994. A Study of Sexuality of Adolescent Girls and Boys in Underprivileged Groups in Bombay. *The Indian Journal of Social Work,* (Special Issue: Sexual Behaviour and AIDS in India) LV (4): 557-572.

Collumbien, M. (Data analyst from London School of Hygiene and Tropical Medicine). Personal communication.

Goparaju, L. 1994. Discourse and Practice: Rural-Urban Differences in Male Students' Sexual Behaviour in India. Paper prepared for the International Union for the Scientific Study of Population Seminar on Sexual Subcultures, Migration and AIDS, Thailand: February-March, 1994.

Jejeebhoy, S.J. 1996. Adolescent Sexual and Reproductive Behaviour: A Review of the Evidence from India. Working Paper No. 3. International Center for Research on Women. Washington D. C., USA.

Jejeebhoy, S. J. 1997. Implications of Domestic Violence for Women's Reproductive Health: What We Know and What We Need to Know. Biennial Report 1996-97. World Health Organization, Geneva, Switzerland.

Joshi, A., Dhapola, M., Kurian, E., and Pelto, P.J. 1998. Rural Women's Experiences and Perceptions of Marital Sexual Relationships. Ford Foundation Working Papers Series, The Ford Foundation, New Delhi, India.

Joshi, A, and Dhapola, M. 1998. Male Involvement in Seeking Abortion Services in Rural Gujarat. Paper presented at a Workshop of South Asian Reproductive Health Initiative. Colombo, Sri Lanka, December, 1998.

Khan, M.E., Townsend, J.W., Sinha, R., and Lakhanpal, S. 1996. Sexual Violence Within Marriage. *Seminar*, 447: 32-35.

Khan, M. E., Khan, I., and Mukerjee, N. 1997. Males' Attitude Towards Sexuality and Their Sexual Behaviour: Observations from Rural Gujarat. Workshop on Research Related to Male Involvement in Reproductive Health and Contraceptive Use. The Population Council, Baroda, India.

Khan, S. 1994. Cultural Contexts of Sexual Behaviours and Identities and Their Impact Upon HIV Prevention Models: An Overview of South Asian Men Who have Sex with Men. *The Indian Journal of Social Work,* (Special Issue: Sexual Behaviour and AIDS in India) LV (4):633-646.

Khanna, R., de Koning, K., Pongurlekar, S., Ubale, U., and Manjiri, S. 1998. Sexual Coercion and PID in Slum Women of Mumbai: The Role of the Health Care Provider. Paper presented at an International Conference on Preventing Violence, Caring for Survivors, and Role of Health Services in Violence, November, 1998. Centre for Enquiry into Health and Allied Themes, Mumbai, India.

Konings, E., Bantebya, G., Carael, M., Bagenda, D., and Mertens.T. 1995. Validating Population Surveys for the Measurement of HIV/STD Prevention Indicators. *AIDS.*

Kulkarni, V. 1998. Networks, Language and Sexual Behaviours of Men Who Have Sex With Men. Report to The Ford Foundation, New Delhi, India.

Lakhani, A., Ganju, S., and Pelto, P.J. 1997. Use of Qualitative Research Methodologies for Situation Assessment of the Sexual Behaviours in the Nandnagar Area in Vadodara District, Gujarat. Unpublished Report to the Department for International Development, New Delhi, India.

Maitra, S. 1999. Sexual Negotiations Among Muslim Married Couples in a Mumbai Slum. Report submitted to The Ford Foundation, New Delhi, India.

Nag, M. 1994. Sexual Behaviour and AIDS in India: State-of-the-Art. *The Indian Journal of Social Work,* (Special Issue: Sexual Behaviour and AIDS in India) LV (4): 503-546.

Nag, M. 1996. Sexual Behaviour and AIDS in India. New Delhi: Vikas Publishing House.

Pachauri, S. 1996. The Problem (Introduction to a Symposium on Reproductive Health). *Seminar*, 447: 12-15.

Pelto, P. J. 1994. Focused Ethnographic Studies on Sexual Behaviour and AIDS/STDs. *The Indian Journal of Social Work,* (Special Issue: Sexual Behaviour and AIDS in India) LV (4): 589-602.

Pelto, P. J. 1996. Qualitative Data-Gathering for Reproductive Health Research. *Social Change*, (September-December): 161-189.

Pelto, P. J., Das, B., Das, R. N., and Bohidar, N. 1997. Men's Sexual Health Concerns: A Freelisting Approach. AIMS. Unpublished Paper.

Rao, A., Nag, M., Mishra, K., and Dey, A. 1994. Sexual Behaviour Pattern of Truck Drivers and Their Helpers in Relation to Female Sex Workers. *The Indian Journal of Social Work,* (Special Issue: Sexual Behaviour and AIDS in India) LV (4): 603-617.

Savara, M., and Sridhar, C.R. 1992. Sexual Behaviour of Urban, Educated Indian Men: Results of a Survey. *Journal of Family Welfare,* 38 (1): 30-43.

Savara, M., and Sridhar, C.R. 1994. Sexual Behaviour Amongst Different Occupational Groups In Maharashtra, India and the Implications for AIDS Education. *The Indian Journal of Social Work,* (Special Issue: Sexual Behaviour and AIDS in India) LV (4) 617-632.

Sethi, G., Deshmukh, M., and Dorrell, P. 1995. High Risk Behaviour Study. Paper presented at the Indo-US Workshop on Behavioural Priorities: Developing Effective Strategies for the Prevention of HIV in India. Tata Institute of Social Sciences, Mumbai, India.

Sharma, V., Sujay, R., and Sharma, A. 1998. Can Married Women Say No to Sex? Repercussions of the Denial of the Sexual Act. *Journal of Social Welfare,* 44(1): 1-8.

Sodhi, G., Verma, M., and assistants. 1998a. Report of Research: Exploring Adolescent Sexual Behaviour. Report submitted to Rockefeller Foundation from Swaasthya. New Delhi, India.

Sodhi, G., and Verma, M. 1998b On the Threshold – Exploring Adolescent Sexual Behaviour. Information Bulletin. Swaasthya, New Delhi, India.

SWACH (Survival for Women and Children) Foundation. 1998. An In-depth Study to Understand Men's Reproductive Health Behaviour and Feasibility of Specific Intervention. Progress Report. The Ford Foundation, New Delhi, India.

Verma, R., Rangaiyan, G., Narkhede, S.L., Agrawal, M., and Pelto, P.J. 1998. Cultural Perceptions and Categorisation of Male Sexual Health Problems by Practitioners and Men in a Mumbai Slum Population. Paper presented at a Workshop on Reproductive Health. Indian Institute of Health and Family Welfare. Hyderabad, India.

Annexure

Notes on Research Methods and Strategies

Most of the data reported in this paper come from studies employing a variety of qualitative methods. The single most important research tool in the 'qualitative toolbox,' is the in-depth interview, used in almost all the studies reported above. 'In-depth' means that the interview style is relatively open, and the interviewer probes for additional explanations, examples, and other narrative from the informants. In many of the projects described here, individual informants were contacted more than once – sometimes five or more times.

Another important technique used in some of the studies is social mapping. This method, widely known in association with PRA (participatory rural appraisal), is often used nowadays in locating the specific sites where sexual activities and other behaviours occur. Often social mapping is used to motivate local people to participate in the research activities. Social mapping is usually carried out as a group-interviewing activity, though the mapping can be done in one-on-one interviews as well. In the group situation the mapping sessions often lead to identification of good key informants for later follow-up through one-on-one interviews.

Free listing, pile sorting, and rating are techniques referred to as 'structured qualitative interviewing.' Freelisting is particularly useful in many studies because extensive listings concerning a topic (e.g. 'sexual health problems,' 'health providers in this area,' 'types of sexual behaviours,' 'places men go for sexual contacts' etc.) can be obtained quite quickly from small numbers of informants. Such lists can then be used to develop systematic 'inventories' of places, persons, or other topics. The freelisting technique is also a quick way to accumulate vocabularies of local language used on topics related to sexuality and sexual behaviours. More detailed discussion about these and other qualitative research methods are presented in Pelto 1994; and Pelto, 1996.

An ideal research strategy, if there is time and money, is to have a phase of intensive qualitative research, followed by a carefully designed quantitative survey. The purpose of the quantitative survey is to provide estimates of the frequencies of specific behaviours within a defined population; and also to test hypotheses concerning statistical relationships of background variables, 'causal variables,' etc. to selected dependent variables that one is trying to explain. Well constructed quantitative survey questionnaires usually include local vocabulary and other features developed during the qualitative phase of the research.

During the past five years, since the ICPD, various NGOs and other researchers in India have taken steps toward computerising their data management and data analysis. Also, a considerable portion of communications among the various research groups, and with the funding agencies, is now carried out through E-mail. It is to be hoped that the continuing process of computerisation of research, even in small organisations, will add to the depth of applied studies in sexuality and sexual behaviours, and also contribute to the volume of exchanges among different organisations and individuals.

Abbreviations

AIIHPH	All India Institute of Hygiene and Public Health
AIDS	Acquired Immuno Deficiency Syndrome
AIMS	Asian Institute of Marketing Studies
ANE OR/TA	Asia Near-East Operation Research/Technical Assistance
ANM	Auxiliary Nurse Midwife
ARCH	Action Research in Community Health and Development
ASHA	AIDS/STD Health Action
BCC	Baroda Citizens Council
BMC	Brihan Mumbai Municipal Corporation
BV	Bacterial Vaginosis
CAM	Charutar Arogya Mandal
CASP-PLAN	Community Aid and Sponsorship Programme in Alliance with Foster Parents Plan International
CBR	Crude Birth Rate
CDR	Crude Death Rate
CHETNA	Centre for Health, Education, Training and Nutrition Awareness
CHW	Community Health Worker
CINI	Child-in-Need Institute
CNAA	Community Needs Assessment Approach
CORT	Centre for Operations Research and Training
CPR	Couple Protection Rate
CSSM	Child Survival and Safe Motherhood
CSO	Civil Society Organisation
DCT	Deepak Charitable Trust
DDS	Deccan Development Society
DFID	Department for International Development (British)
DWCRA	Development of Women and Children in Rural Areas
EOC	Emergency Obstetric Care
FHI	Family Health International
FPAI	Family Planning Association of India
FRCH	Foundation for Research in Community Health

FRHS	Foundation for Research in Health Systems
FRU	First Referral Unit
GDP	Gross Domestic Product
GOI	Government of India
GSCPT	Gujarat State Crime Prevention Trust
HIV	Human Immuno-deficiency Virus
HPV	Human Papiloma Virus
ICDS	Integrated Child Development Scheme
ICMR	Indian Council of Medical Research
ICPD	International Conference on Population Development
ICRW	International Center for Research on Women
IEC	Information, Education and Communication
IIHMR	Indian Institute of Health Management Research
IIPS	International Institute of Population Sciences
IJSW	Indian Journal of Social Work
IMR	Infant Mortality Rate
IRDP	Integrated Rural Development Programme
ISST	Institute of Social Studies Trust
IUD	Intra Uterine Device
IVDU	Intra-Venous Drug User
KEM	King Edward Memorial Hospital Research Centre
KNBMCT&HC	Krishan Nath Baba Memorial Charitable Trust and Health Centre
LBW	Low Birth Weight
LHV	Lady Health Visitor
MASUM	Mahila Sarvangeen Utkarsh Mandal
MCH	Maternal and Child Health
MCH-FP	Maternal and Child Health/Family Planning
MTP	Medical Termination of Pregnancy
MOH&FW	Ministry of Health & Family Welfare
NACO	National AIDS Control Organisation
NCAER	National Council of Applied Economic Research
NFHS	National Family Health Survey
NGO	Non-government Organisation

NRR	Net Reproduction Rate
OMRAH	Orissa Institute of Medical Research and Health Services
ORG	Operation Research Group
PALWHA	People Living with HIV/AIDS
PCO	Programme for Community Organisation
PCR	Polymerase Chain Reaction
PHC	Primary Health Centre
PID	Pelvic Inflammatory Disease
POA	Programme of Action
PRC	Population Research Centre
PSS	Parivar Sewa Sanstha
PSU	Programme Support Unit
RCH	Reproductive and Child Health
REAC	Rural Education and Animation Centre
RTI	Reproductive Tract Infection
RUWSEC	Rural Women's Social Education Centre
SAARC	South Asia Association of Regional Cooperation
SARTHI	Social Action for Rural and Tribal Inhabitant's of India
SEARCH	Society for Education, Action and Research in Community Health
SECRT	Sex Education, Counselling, Research and Training/Therapy Centre
SED	Social Education for Development Trust
SEWA	Self-Employed Women's Association
SEWA-Rural	Society for Education, Welfare and Action -Rural
SIDH	Society for Integrated Development of Himalayas
SDT	Social Development Trust
SIFPSA	State Innovation in Family Planning Service Agency
SMAM	Singulate Mean Age at Marriage
SRED	Society for Rural Education and Development
SRS	Sample Registration System
STD	Sexually Transmitted Disease
STI	Sexually Transmitted Infection

SUTRA	Society for Social Uplift Through Rural Action
SVDS	Sardar Valley Development Society
SWACH	Survival of Women and Children (Foundation)
TBA	Traditional Birth Attendant
TFR	Total Fertility Rate
TNSACS	Tamil Nadu State AIDS Control Society
TPHA	Treponema Pallidium Haem Agglutination
UIP	Universal Immunisation Programme
UNAIDS	United Nations Programme on HIV/AIDS
USAID	United States Agency for International Development
UNICEF	United Nations Children's Fund
VDRL	Venereal Disease Research Laboratory
VHAI	Voluntary Health Association of India
WHO	World Health Organization
WHOTRAC	Women's Health Training Research Advocacy Centre

Contributors

Anrudh Jain, Ph.D., a sociologist and demographer, is Senior Director, Policy and Regional Programs, International Programs Division, Population Council, New York, USA.

Anjali Nayyar, BA, a communication specialist, is Project Director, Population Council, New Delhi, India.

Asha A. Bhende, MPH, Ph.D., a sociologist, is an independent consultant based in Mumbai, India.

Dileep V. Mavalankar, MD, Dr.P.H., a public health physician and health management expert, is Chairman, Public Systems Group, Indian Institute of Management, Ahmedabad, India.

Faujdaar Ram, Ph.D., a demographer, is Professor and Head, Department of Fertility Studies, International Institute for Population Sciences, Mumbai, India.

Geeta Sethi, MA, a social scientist, is Senior Project Operations Officer, United Nations Development Programme Sub-Regional Project on HIV and Development for South and South-West Asia, New Delhi, India.

Jagdish C. Bhatia, MA, MPH, Ph.D., a social scientist, is Chairman, Foundation for Research and Education in Health Management, and Consultant in Health Systems Management, Bangalore, India.

John Cleland, MA, a demographer, is Professor of Medical Demography and Head, Centre for Population Studies, London School of Hygiene and Tropical Medicine, London, UK.

John W. Townsend, Ph.D., a social psychologist, is Director, FRONTIERS Project, Population Council, Washington D.C., USA.

Jyotsna Sivaramayya, MA, M.Phil., a sociologist, is Research Associate, Institute of Social Studies Trust, New Delhi, India.

K. B. Pathak, Ph.D., a demographer, is Director, International Institute for Population Sciences, Mumbai, India.

Leela Visaria, Ph.D., a sociologist and demographer, is an independent researcher, based in New Delhi, India.

Masuma Mamdani, MPH., a public health professional, is Research Fellow at the London School of Hygiene and Tropical Medicine. She is currently based in Tanzania.

M. E. Khan, Ph.D., a sociologist, is Senior Programme Associate, FRONTIERS Project, Population Council, Dhaka, Bangladesh.

Nayan Kumar, MA., a communication specialist, is Manager, Field Operations, Centre for Operations Research and Training, Baroda, India.

Nirmala Murthy, MA, MPH, DSc., a management specialist, is Chairperson, The Foundation for Research in Health Systems, Ahmedabad, India and Consultant to the World Bank, India.

Pravin Visaria, Ph.D., an economist and demographer, is Director, Institute of Economic Growth, New Delhi, India.

Pertti, J. Pelto, Ph.D., an anthropologist, is Consultant, John Hopkins University, Washington D.C., USA.

Purnima Mane, Ph.D., a social scientist, is Chief, Executive Director Office, UNAIDS, Geneva, Switzerland.

Radhika Ramasubban, Ph.D., a social scientist, is Director, Centre for Social and Technological Change, Mumbai, India.

Ravi K. Verma, Ph.D., a demographer, is Senior Faculty Member, Department of Extra Mural Studies, International Institute for Population Sciences, Mumbai, India.

Sagri Singh, M.Sc., a social scientist, is Project Director, Population Council, New Delhi, India.

Sandhya Barge, Ph.D., an anthropologist, is Associate Director, Centre for Operations Research and Training, Baroda, India.

Sangeeta Subramanian, MBA, is a health management consultant, New Delhi, India.

Saraswati Raju, Ph.D., a social geographer, is Associate Professor, Jawaharlal Nehru University and Consulting Associate, Population Council, New Delhi, India.

Saroj Pachauri, MD, Ph.D. DPH, a public health physician, is Regional Director, South and East Asia, Population Council, New Delhi, India.

Stina Almroth, Ph.D., a researcher, is a nutrition and reproductive health consultant, New Delhi, India.

Swapna Mukhopadhyay, M.S., Ph.D., an economist, is Director, Institute of Social Studies Trust, New Delhi, India.

ERRATA

Page xxiv; line 26: '..client's face in ..' to be read as '..clients' face in..'

Page 83; line 10: '..decentralised planning was recognised..' to be read as '...decentralised planning were recognised..'

Page 130; line 13: '..performance dropped from 10 to 50 percent' to be read as '..performance dropped by 10 to 50 percent'

Page 137; subhead: 'Effect of the target free approach to reproductive and child health' to be read as 'Effect of the target-free approach on reproductive and child health'

Page 137; line 27: 'It does not include delivery..' to be read as 'It does not include deliveries..'

Page 139; line 5: 'Reduced pressure of target' to be read as 'Reduced pressure of targets'

Page 150; line 5: '..the net reproductive rate..' to be read as '..the net reproduction rate..'

Page 192; line 22: '(International Institute of Population Studies, 1995)' to be read as '(International Institute of Population Sciences, 1995)'

Page 222; lines 5&6: '..parastic..' to be read as '..parasitic..'

Page 284; line 5: '..patriarchichal framework' to be read as '..patriarchal framework'

Page 367; line 19: '..practised by men who or may not...' to be read as '..practised by men who may or may not..'

Page 391; line 12: '..of the project, a procurement, and..' to be read as '..of the project, procurement, and..'

Page 391; line 21: '..as one pertaining foreigners..' to be read as '..as one pertaining to foreigners..'

Page 409; line 17: '..training resource groups..' to be read as '..technical resource groups..'

Page 410; line 3: '..the family wefare programme' to be read as '..the family welfare programme'

Page 438; line 20: '(Luthra et al, 1992; Nag, 1993..)' to be read as '(Luthra et al, 1992; Nag,1996..)'

Page 491; line 2: '..female sex wokers ..' to be read as '..female sex workers ..'

Page 543; line 17: 'All this lead to a situation...' to be read as 'All this led to a situation..'

Page 587; line 4: '..and 8 and 16 percent of the boys..' to be read as '.. And 8 to 16 percent of the boys..'